**William S. Hein Sr.
Memorial Biblical Library**

LOCATED AT THE TABERNACLE
3210 Southwestern Blvd
Orchard Park, New York 14127

716-675-3070 / 716-675-2888

THE WHOLE BOOK OF HEALTH

BY O. Quentin Hyder, M.D.

The Christian's Handbook of Psychiatry
The People You Live With
Shape Up
Don't Blame the Devil
The Whole Book of Health (Editor)

THE WHOLE BOOK OF HEALTH

O. QUENTIN HYDER M.D.
EDITOR

FLEMING H. REVELL COMPANY • PUBLISHERS
OLD TAPPAN, NEW JERSEY

Unless otherwise identified, Scripture quotations in this book are based on the King James Version of the Bible.

Scripture quotations taken from the HOLY BIBLE: NEW INTERNATIONAL VERSION. Copyright © 1978 by the International Bible Society. Used by permission of Zondervan Bible Publishers.

Scripture quotations identified AMPLIFIED are from the Amplified New Testament © The Lockman Foundation 1954–1958, and are used by permission.

Acknowledgment is made for the use of copyrighted material from the following:

Flab: The Answer Book by Jim Krafft, M.D., copyright © 1983 by Fleming H. Revell Company.
Fitness: The Answer Book by Cecil B. Murphey, copyright © 1983 by Fleming H. Revell Company.
Headaches: The Answer Book by Joan Miller, Ph.D., copyright © 1983 by Joan Miller, Ph.D.
Heart Attacks: The Answer Book by Daniel J. MacNeil, M.D., and Larry Losoncy, Ph.D., copyright © 1983 by Fleming H. Revell Company.
Junk Food: The Answer Book by Virginia and Norma Rohrer, copyright © 1983 by Fleming H. Revell Company.
Vitamins: The Answer Book by Virginia and Norman Rohrer, copyright © 1983 by Fleming H. Revell Company.
Don't Blame the Devil by O. Quentin Hyder, M.D., copyright © 1983 by O. Quentin Hyder.
Shape Up by O. Quentin Hyder, M.D., copyright © 1979, 1984 by O. Quentin Hyder.
None of These Diseases by S. I. McMillen, M.D., with David E. Stern, M.D., copyright © 1963, 1984 by Fleming H. Revell Company.

Library of Congress Cataloging in Publication Data
Main entry under title:

The Whole book of health.

Includes index.
1. Health—Addresses, essays, lectures.   2. Mental health—Addresses, essays, lectures.   3. Christian life—1980–   —Addresses, essays, lectures.
I. Hyder, O. Quentin, 1930– .
RA776.W566   1985   613   84-24987
ISBN 0-8007-1406-7

Copyright © 1985 Fleming H. Revell Company
All Rights Reserved
Printed in the United States of America

The material in this book is only for the reader's general information and should not take the place of consultation with a physician.

Contents

Preface	*O. Quentin Hyder, M.D.*	9
Introduction	*O. Quentin Hyder, M.D.*	11

PART I

Exercise and Nutrition

1.	Flab	*Jim Krafft, M.D.*	16
2.	Fitness	*Cecil B. Murphey*	62
3.	Junk Food	*Virginia and Norman Rohrer*	94
4.	Vitamins	*Virginia and Norman Rohrer*	111

PART II

Self-destructive Habits

5.	Marijuana	*O. Quentin Hyder, M.D.*	150
6.	Alcohol	*O. Quentin Hyder, M.D.*	156
7.	Smoking	*S. I. McMillen, M.D.* *with David E. Stern, M.D.* *O. Quentin Hyder, M.D.*	160

PART III

Common Medical Problems

8.	Stress	*Angharad Young, Ph.D.*	184
9.	Heart Attacks	*Daniel MacNeil, M.D.* *Larry Losoncy, Ph.D.*	211
10.	Pain	*David P. Armentrout, Ph.D.*	247
11.	Headaches	*Joan Miller, Ph.D.*	270

PART IV

Common Emotional Experiences

12.	Grief	Burrell Dinkins, S.T.D., and Larry Losoncy, Ph.D.	302
13.	Depression	O. Quentin Hyder, M.D.	330
14.	Anxiety	O. Quentin Hyder, M.D.	369
15.	Nervous Breakdown	O. Quentin Hyder, M.D.	377

PART V

Physiological Needs

16.	Relaxation and Sleep	O. Quentin Hyder, M.D.	384
17.	Sexuality	O. Quentin Hyder, M.D.	391

PART VI

The Spiritual Dimension

18.	The Spiritual Dimension	O. Quentin Hyder, M.D.	400

Index   407

Preface

The Whole Book of Health is a compendium of ten short monographs written originally for the Revell Wellness Series. All the original contributions are included in part in this book, deletions having been made mainly to avoid duplication, or to reduce anecdotal examples because of space limitations.

In addition, the section on Smoking is taken from an updated very popular best-seller *None of These Diseases,* by S. I. McMillen, M.D., with David E. Stern, M.D. Sections on Marijuana, Alcohol, Relaxation and Sleep, and Sexuality are extracted from a revised edition of my book on physical well-being for Christians, *Shape Up.* To supplement my own original contribution on Depression, I have added sections on Anxiety and Nervous Breakdown.

Since it is my belief that one cannot have "whole health" without being healthy in the Spiritual Dimension, the book concludes with a chapter on that subject.

The eighteen chapters in the book are divided into six major divisions containing related topics. They can be read in any order since every section is self-contained. My hope and that of the Fleming H. Revell Company is that this book will provide a useful reference for Christians on many topics that have to do with the protection and proper use of their physical minds and bodies, "the temple of the Holy Spirit" (*see* 1 Corinthians 3:16,17 and 6:19,20).

O. QUENTIN HYDER, M.D.

INTRODUCTION
Christianity and Well-Being

I was alone, very alone, piloting a tiny, single-engine airplane over London when I became trapped in some low clouds. Suddenly I could no longer see the ground and was unable to tell if I was flying straight and level or going out of control.

In front of me were the essential instruments: the turn-and-bank indicator, the artificial horizon, the climb-and-descent indicator, two others that showed my airspeed and altitude, and a directional compass. With uninterrupted, intense concentration on these, I was for a short while able to keep the plane on an even keel.

Within a few minutes, however, my concentration lapsed, and I began to rely on my own sense of attitude from the balance mechanisms in my inner ears, but these only work in conjunction with a firm basis of sight or touch, which I lacked. I could see only cloud all around me and could touch only the stick and rudder pedals, since I was tightly strapped in.

Suddenly I realized that the nose of the plane was pointing steeply up, my airspeed quickly dropped, and the plane stalled and started to go into a spin toward the ground.

"Lord, save me," I muttered, half-terrified of being killed, and half-mad at myself for my stupidity.

The spin quickly took me below the cloud base, and the instant I saw the ground I was immediately able to restore level flight. Mercifully I still had a few hundred feet to spare. I thanked God that there were no high hills in the area and that I was safe. I remembered His promise in Deuteronomy 33:27: "The eternal God is thy refuge, and underneath are the everlasting arms...."!

This incident has become an analogy, for me, of the Christian life, in which we need to keep our attention on the facts that form the foundation of our faith and the principles of physical well-being. As long as I relied objectively on the instruments, I could keep the airplane on course. Once I started relying on my own subjective feelings, I was headed for destruction.

I am a Christian, a physician, and a psychiatrist, and each day I see many people who have wandered off course with a wide range of problems. These vary from psychosis to marital communication breakdowns, from obsessive thoughts to obesity, from anxiety to guilt, and from self-destructive behavior to the need to keep physically fit.

Most of my patients have in common the need to keep themselves in better physical shape and to straighten out internal personal or external relationship problems that they have been unable to deal with themselves. They need to get their lives back on course.

The causes of a few of these problems are purely spiritual in nature, requiring of the believer a fresh understanding of the essentials of the Christian faith and a renewed willingness to make a rededication to a new commitment to Christ as Lord. Many such Christians are living like a pilot who is not relying on his instruments to guide him.

Some patients experience emotional or psychological problems that respond to counseling: They need to talk out their inner tensions and to make some life-changing decisions to improve their ability to cope with routine responsibilities. These people are like a pilot who wants to watch his instruments, but whose internal tensions prevent his concentration on them.

Others face physical, social, or marital problems and need to discover the basics of how to improve their interpersonal relationships, communications, priorities, and bodily fitness. These live like a pilot who disregards the fundamental information his instruments give.

A fourth group suffers from medical problems due to biochemical imbalances in the brain, causing upsets in mood, thought processes, or behavior. These are like a pilot who has lost the use of his instruments through an electrical failure in the plane.

However, nothing in life is black and white. Almost all those whom I see have several overlapping problems, which are frequently interrelated. For example a depression of medical origin can result in a believer fearing he has lost his salvation. Anxiety can lead to uncontrollable, repetitive, unwanted sexual or blasphemous flash thoughts. Neurotic feelings may cause physical aches and pains. Anger, resentment, bitterness, hostility, or jealousy can lead to ulcers, colitis, or high blood pressure. Being overweight and underexercised can lead to physical illness. Physical illness can lead to spiritual depression, with negative thinking leading to loss of faith in God's love and care.

Some well-meaning Christians believe that any mental illness is of demonic origin and teach that the cure is purely spiritual. While not denying the devil's activity in this world, I am convinced that Christian healing, in addition to prayer and biblical counseling, should include the medical resources that God has given us to use. This includes the principles of good nutrition and regular vigorous exercise.

In my practice, I see many persons who have psychological, personality, or relational difficulties which benefit from discussion or counseling. Others have neurotic experiences caused by chemical imbalances, and these respond to medical treatment. Almost all need spiritual help through increased fellowship, Bible study, and prayer.

Most sufferers need an integrated approach that involves the physical, psychological, and spiritual components. Total health is to be well in body, mind, and spirit. If any one part is sick, the whole person is incomplete. It is my goal to effect total healing.

God is the ultimate healer, "... for I am the Lord that healeth thee" (Exodus 15:26). Sir William Osler said, "I treat: God heals." I also do all I can to bring healing to my patients through sharing relevant Bible passages, counseling, listening, and when necessary, through the prescription of specific medications. I also use and rely on prayer. I pray for all my patients daily, and whenever they are willing, I pray with them as well, usually at the end of our sessions together.

God heals, but He usually chooses to use human means. All physicians need to be humble enough to recognize that God sometimes chooses to step in and produce miraculous cures they cannot account for. More often God seems to take time producing the healing by means of the spiritual, psychological, and medical treatments He has made available, and the preventive measures of sensible diet and exercise He has revealed to us. I pray that this book will help to bring total health and healing to you and your loved ones.

Part I

Exercise and Nutrition

The opening section of this book zeroes in immediately on the two most fundamentally important elements in sustaining a fit and healthy physical body. The reduction of unwanted fat and the maintaining of good cardiovascular fitness are thoroughly examined in the first two chapters, with detailed recommendations on how to get into great physical shape and then to keep that way.

The Rohrers' expertise on good nutritional habits is the flip side of the coin. What you put into your body is as important as the exercise you put out of it. The avoidance of sugar and animal fat is stressed, and a diet high in fresh fruits, vegetables, and whole grain cereals, with vitamin supplements as needed, is well-taught.

1
Flab
Jim Krafft, M.D.

THE FIRST WORD IS NOT *DIET*

How does one get rid of fat? Easy, you say. Just follow Dr. XYZ's super don't-eat-ever diet, and it will all come off rapidly and easily. Success is guaranteed within sixty days or sooner, right?

Wrong! True, you can lose weight on a crash diet. But losing *weight* is not what you who are overfat need to do. You need to get rid of *fat,* not *weight.*

With a crash diet you lose muscle and water and some fat, but confirmed studies show that 99-plus percent of those who lose weight by diet alone will regain it. Not only that, you regain the weight as 100 percent fat! *Crash dieting is one of the surest ways to gain fat, not lose it.* Weight loss by dieting only means you will lose muscle and fat but regain only the fat. Sooner or later you will have a net gain in fat!

It is important to realize that we are all bombarded daily by powerful advertising "hype" about diets and dieting. We have a rash of new miracle diets each year that draw millions of gullible takers. Where I come from we believe in miracles, but the miracle of losing fat comes slowly and steadily in every instance I have ever seen. Sudden hurry-up diets are almost always flagrant examples of bad diet advice.

In "miracle" diets that have been popularized in recent months and years, the dieter's calorie-and-protein intake is cut to starvation levels. True, you can shed pounds quickly with these diets, but while you are battling the bulges of flab, you are running the risk of losing valuable muscle mass that is so important to the entire body, especially the heart.

At least one study has shown that such diets have been associated with heart irregularities that resulted in the deaths of fifty-eight women. One popular diet drink provides a daily supply of under 400 calories (starvation level) and less than forty grams of protein (well below the recommended minimum of sixty grams). Persons on this kind of weight-loss plan may experience irregular heart rhythms within a week of starting the diet.

Such miracle diets claim to include vitamin-and-mineral supplements, but they do not alter the bad effects of inadequate dietary protein. Such diets also claim there will be no significant muscle loss, but as a medical doctor who has spent many years in nutritional and weight-control work, I say categorically this is pure hogwash.

The miracle-diet substances or plans preach nutritional nonsense and propagate inaccuracies that can result in life-threatening side effects. For example, one untruth is that undigested food accumulates and becomes fat, while digested food cannot cause weight gain. Precisely the opposite is true. Another myth states that enzymes cannot work together and often cancel each other out in the digestive tract. Again, the facts are exactly the opposite.

In short, *don't use miracle diets!* In the long run they do not work, and they can cause serious harm.

I know what your next question is going to be, and it's a very logical one: "If I can't count on dieting only and miracle diets are downright dangerous, what *can* I do?"

The answer is simple, but it may not thrill you. You don't get rid of fat by diet only. Dieting is important but it is secondary. When trying to lose fat, your primary weapon is aerobic exercise. Aerobic exercise is the kind anyone can do. Aerobic exercises are long, slow, easy, endurance-type activities. I repeat, you do not have to be an Olympic champion to engage in aerobic exercise that fits your abilities and life-style.

So, let's get the cart properly placed *behind* the horse. Exercise (the horse) is first. Diet (the cart) is second.

Please note that when I talk about aerobic exercise, I am not including calisthenics or stretching activities. The exercises you see on TV shows are usually calisthenics or stretching of some kind. These are excellent, but do almost nothing to help you lose fat. Also, spot-reducing aids such as hip-shaker belts at your local health spa do nothing whatsoever to burn fat either, not even in the spot where you are being jostled. When you want to lose fat, engage in aerobic exercise. These are the long, slow, endurance exercises such as walking, jogging, bicycling, and swimming.

As director of Student Health Services at Oral Roberts University for the last ten years, I have seen mild and easy aerobic exercise (note the *mild* and the *easy*) work with hundreds of men and women. Daily, my staff and I guide overfat people in losing weight *and fat,* while toning and building muscles through good nutrition, proper diet, sports activities, and aerobic exercises that are right for the individual. Yes, it's slower than the miracle crash diets, but it's safer and more effective over the long haul. The weight stays off. There is no regaining of pounds that are composed of more fat than previously.

One example of how our program works is a girl named Helen. She came to school with a severe obesity problem. At five feet six and 178 pounds she could not bring herself to believe that she could ever slow jog one mile. It almost threw her into a tailspin. Our goal is to work individually with each student who is working toward loss of fat, and one day I chose to go on the jogging track with Helen just to help her see that she could do it.

We started going around the track at more of a walk than a jog. Helen kept saying, "I can't do it," and I kept encouraging her by saying, "Slow to a walk and just keep going, just keep going, just keep going."

With continual encouragement, Helen covered the full mile that day, doing far more walking than jogging. She was so motivated by her achievement that she began to engage enthusiastically in our fat-loss program. After four and a half months she had lost forty pounds. She got so enthusiastic about jogging that she started overdoing it and had to stop running for a brief time because of sore muscles. She did not, however, significantly regain any of the forty pounds that she had lost. When she was able to resume her exercise program, she combined it with proper eating and soon was down to her ideal fat level. (By "ideal fat level" I mean a correct percentage of body fat. We'll look more at this on pp. 21–24.)

Helen, by the way, is a good example of the important fringe benefits in a fat-loss program. When she started, she was withdrawn, antisocial, and depressed. As she engaged in the program and achieved success, she became an exhilarated, joyful person.

Right about now you may be thinking, *Hurray for Helen. I've heard about these jogging freaks before. I just can't see jogging several miles a day. I don't have the time, and I really don't have the ambition. Furthermore, Helen was a college kid and I'm an adult. This aerobic stuff is okay for kids, but not for older types like me.*

Okay, I hear you, but remember, Helen started slowly—*very* slowly. For many days she walked more than she jogged. Actually she could have achieved the same results by *walking only.* It would have taken a little longer, but the results would have been the same.

Exercise and Nutrition

As for aerobics being "only for kids," nothing is further from the truth. People of *any age* can participate in the long, slow, endurance type of aerobic exercise at their own speed and in their own way.

So, the first word to emphasize is *exercise*—slow, easy, aerobic exercise. Healthy, sensible exercise must become a permanent part of your lifestyle. Control of weight and fat is a lifetime proposition. The joys of an active life-style with sensible diet make it more than worthwhile.

Still skeptical? I won't try to kid you or lie to you. Controlling weight and fat *permanently* takes effort, but anyone can do it at his or her own speed. To do so you need to understand some simple principles about what fat is and why it is so dangerous. In layman's terms, I can tell you how to have the right percentage of fat on your body and how aerobic exercise works to burn off unneeded fat and keep it off.

Read on—you may have a lot to lose!

WHAT IS FAT?

Fat is the oily, greasy substance that we all want to get rid of. People who are fat talk about their "weight problem" or "being a little heavy." Ironically, the heavy stuff on our frame is the good stuff—the muscle. Fat is light, not heavy, and that is one of the reasons I say the problem is not being *overweight;* with most of us it's being *overfat.*

Fat accumulates on your body predominantly in two places: just under the skin (subcutaneous fat) and in the muscles. You can't see the fat in your muscles, but it looks exactly like the fat in an ideal steak that is "marbled" with just enough streaks of fat to make it taste wonderful. (Too much marbled steak, by the way, is a tasty but surefire way to consume too much fat in your diet.)

Subcutaneous fat, on the other hand, settles just under the skin on your stomach, waist, hips, legs, and arms. It is easy to see but hard to get rid of.

That extra flab that we would like to see melt away from our stomach, waist, and hips is caused by our fat cells (adipocytes). We all have a certain number of fat cells that are established by the time we reach adolescence. Once that number of fat cells is reached, it stabilizes and we don't add anymore. Overeating does not increase the number of your fat cells; it merely increases the fat in the cells that you already have.

So, the bad news is that once we establish our number of fat cells, we have them for life. Fat people have 190 percent more fat cells than slender types. Flab fighters also have fat cells that are forty percent larger than the fat cells in slender people.

Now, I can hear some people saying, "Oh, that's it—that's my problem.

I have too many fat cells, and there's nothing I can do. I'll just have to be heavy and live with it. Please pass the pie."

Not so! The good news is that although you can't reduce *the number* of fat cells in your body, you can reduce *the size* of your fat cells. Your goal is to have "skinny" fat cells, and you reach that goal with aerobic exercise and a sensible diet.

Understandably, one way we all put on too much flab is by eating too much fat. Unfortunately, fat is found in many of the tasty snacks we love to munch. That's why it becomes such a problem in regard to our total intake of calories.

Keep in mind that one gram of fat has nine calories, while a gram of carbohydrate or protein has only four calories. This means that if you eat a pound of butter, which is practically 100 percent fat, you consume about 3,500 calories. It takes 3,500 calories to add one pound of body weight. Therefore, simple arithmetic says that if you eat a pound of butter and don't burn any of it off, you will put on a pound of fat. To lose one pound of fat you must either burn 3,500 calories or eat 3,500 fewer calories than your normal daily requirement.

Because fat has more than twice the calories contained in carbohydrate or protein, it is the most effective fuel your body can burn. The trick is to consume enough fat for your body to use as fuel, but not to eat too much and start storing it in your subcutaneous tissue or in your muscles. We can learn that secret, but our bodies need to be taught *how* to burn fat with the correct amount of aerobic exercise. We'll explore that subject on pages 54 to 58, when we discuss your body's "setpoint," and how you can "retrain your enzymes."

There's one other way to answer the question "What is fat?" It may sound dramatic but it is true: *Fat is a killer.* Being too fat can cause angina, high blood pressure, congestive heart failure, intermittent claudication (a form of pain in the lower extremities), varicose veins, intervertebral disc disease, osteoarthritis, gall bladder disease, diabetes, asthma, and hyperlipidemia (which is increased fat substances in the blood). All of these diseases and disorders can influence everything from disability to premature death.

In respect to the human body, then, fat is many things, and most of them are bad. It is true that we need some fat. In correct amounts fat is a useful food. In fact, if you get too little fat in your diet, this can also lead to problems. For example, women who have too low a fat intake fail to menstruate.

But for the vast majority of us the problem is too much fat in our bodies, not too little.

HOW FAT ARE YOU?

How fat are you? Because you live in today's mechanized society, chances are your percentage of body fat is higher than it ought to be. In precivilized times, it was necessary that the human organism store large amounts of fat in order for it to survive long seasons when food was not readily available. In the conditions of life today in industrialized countries, however, the accumulation of fat no longer serves any useful purpose. It is just something extra to carry around.

"So, how do I know I'm carrying a lot of extra flab?" you may ask. "How can I know just how 'overfat' I am?"

Dr. Covert Bailey, author of the excellent book *Fit or Fat?*, has done extensive studies with people of all ages and body structures.[1] He concludes that the ideal amount of body fat for an adult male is 15 percent; and for a female, 22 percent. According to other extensive research, the ideal body fat for an athlete in professional, or serious amateur, competition is 11 percent for males and 17 percent for women.

I'm not quite sure why nonathletes should be allowed a higher percentage of body fat than athletes. Perhaps ideal goals would be the 11 to 17 percent range for males and the 17 to 22 percent range for females.

Unfortunately, most people have body-fat percentages well above the recommended norms. Dr. Bailey's findings show that the average male has 24 percent body fat and the average female has 33 percent. Dr. Bailey believes that these figures are much too high, and anyone with 24 or 33 percent body fat or above is in the category of "sick," or at least facing high susceptibility to illness. For example, his findings show that males with body fat above 24 percent suffer from fat deposits in their arteries. Fat deposits in your arteries are what help cause high blood pressure, arterial sclerosis, and, in extreme cases, a myocardial infarction (heart attack).

If you are interested in trivia, the highest percentage of body fat ever measured on a human is 68 percent. You're probably well below that extreme, but you are also probably somewhere over the ideal norm of 11 to 17 percent for men and 17 to 22 percent for women.

How can you measure your percentage of body fat? There are two basic methods: underwater weighing, which is the most accurate; and skin-fold measurements.

Underwater weighing is best because you get a *total* estimate of the fat in your body. As I mentioned previously, fat accumulates in our muscles and in the subcutaneous tissue just under the skin. Because fat is light, it tends to float and can be measured quite accurately by underwater weighing, which takes special equipment. Ironically, the lighter you are under water, the more fat your body contains. Underwater weighing equipment is becoming available at some YMCAs, as well as in some fitness centers, physicians' clinics, and in some high schools and colleges.

A more available method of estimating body-fat percentage is skin-fold measurement, usually done with calipers that "pinch" (hold together lightly) the skin in spots where fat tends to form in the subcutaneous tissues. You may have heard of the simple "rule of thumb" test anyone can do. With your thumb and forefinger pinch the skin on your waist, just above your pelvic (hip) bone. If the fold of skin—and fat—exceeds one inch, you are carrying too much body fat.

In our fitness and health center at Oral Roberts University we measure with calipers, which are applied to the front of the upper arm (bicep area), behind the upper arm (tricep area), behind the shoulder blade, and at the waist just above the pelvic bone. After measuring with the calipers, we calculate body-fat percentage with a formula provided by the caliper manufacturer. If you are interested in trying this yourself, you can buy calipers and complete instructions for under twenty-five dollars. Or, it might be simpler to find a medical doctor, YMCA, or fitness center that uses caliper measurements. Another means of measurement available at some Ys and fitness centers is done with a caliper that includes an electronic device called "Skyndex," which requires no special calculations.

To summarize, the ideal way to measure body-fat percentage is with underwater weighing, which measures fat in the muscles and under the skin. Less accurate, but still fairly reliable, is skin-fold measurement of the fat under the skin, done with calipers or an automatically computing caliper like "Skyndex."

If you are at all serious about fighting flab and getting your percentage of body fat down to correct levels, get measured where and how you can. Whatever you do, don't depend on the old familiar height/weight tables to determine fatness. Until recent years these height/weight tables were the best information available and have been promoted by health and life insurance companies with the best of intentions. But today much better methods are available.

It is quite possible for some individuals to be heavily muscled and "overweight" according to the height/weight tables. Every so often we get someone in our center who has excellent muscle tone and muscle mass, but who is anywhere from ten to thirty pounds over what he is supposed to weigh at his height according to the tables.

A recent example is a young fellow I'll call Sam, who was among the new crop of students at ORU. At nineteen years of age, Sam was a good twenty pounds "overweight" according to the height/weight tables. Yet,

Sam's body was so firm and hard that we could not measure it with calipers.

"What was your sport in high school, Sam?" I asked.

Sam replied that he hadn't played any high-school sports, but he had been on the power-lifting team at the athletic center in his town. He added that he also did some jogging.

We measured Sam underwater and found that he had a body fat content of only 6 percent!

Granted, people like Sam are rare exceptions. The typical person has a higher fat percentage than what is desirable. To repeat Dr. Covert Bailey's research findings, desirable fat percentage in the male is around 15 percent and in the female, 22 percent. (My own personal estimates include a little broader range: 11 to 17 percent for males and 17 to 22 percent for females.) Bailey's studies also showed that the average male has a 24 percent fat content and the average female, 33 percent—much higher than desirable.

So, if your doctor or a technician at the Y or at a fitness center weighs or measures you, and you find that your fat content is too high, don't despair or think that you are one of the unusual few who are in this condition. All of the research and experience of those who are in the field of fitness and weight and fat control show that up to 50 million Americans are significantly overfat.

And don't forget that the height/weight guidelines do not give an accurate picture. Most of us would be far better off if we spent no time studying height/weight tables and became concerned only with our fat-percentage content. A person can be just the right weight for his height (according to the height/weight tables) and still be plagued with flab and a fat percentage that is too high.

An example of this is a girl I will call Gloria. At eighteen, Gloria was a college student who was driven by the need to maintain a "Twiggy-like figure." She dieted constantly and was always worried about "getting too fat." At five feet four inches and 105 pounds, Gloria looked quite slender, but when we examined her, we discovered that her body was surprisingly flabby. Caliper measurements revealed that she had a body fat content of 27 percent!

We urged Gloria to go into an aerobic program and to start eating sensibly. She did so and was soon making progress toward a much firmer body. She also got over her anxieties about gaining too much weight.

Gloria is a striking example of someone who seemed to be the right weight for her height. She even looked quite slender at first glance. But her body fat content was much too high. Other overfat people who come into our health center are easier to spot. They weigh in at what seems to be an acceptable figure for their height, but it is easy to see that they have quite a bit of flab in the usual spots—stomach, waist, arms, and legs. These same people often complain of a lack of energy and stamina. And it almost always follows that they have not been maintaining any kind of proper program of muscle activity.

Maintaining proper muscle activity (getting proper exercise) is the name of the game. If you don't play that game, you are most certainly in danger of getting fatter and fatter. True, you may be one of the blessed ones, who don't have as many fat cells or you may have the kind of metabolism that allows you to eat all you want and "never gain an ounce." But, if you are such a person, chances are you wouldn't even bother to read this book. You are reading this book because you are concerned about flab and how to get rid of it. Contrary to myths and clichés that we've all heard, fat is bad, never "healthy," "strong," or the source of a "jolly good fellow." In the following pages I'll explain why fat is so dangerous and why "thin is health."

WHY "FAT" IS SICK AND "THIN" IS HEALTH

One of the biggest challenges (and frustrations) I face in my work is convincing people how serious overfatness can be. Many people I talk to regard fat as a simple cosmetic problem. They come in wanting to drop a couple of dress sizes or lose a few inches from the waist. What I keep trying to tell them is—*fatness is a killer*. Obesity—even being "mildly overfat"—is a disease that requires attention and treatment.

I often hear the argument: "Why get so worked up over a few extra pounds and a few extra folds of skin? Everyone knows that as you get older the weight gets redistributed. So, I'm a little heavier than I'd like to be and my 'love handlebars' are easy to spot. A little dieting, a little working out and I'll be fine."

Not necessarily. Fatness seems to have what scientists call a "threshold." Even a few pounds above this threshold can cause all kinds of health hazards. There is a danger zone for weight and fatness, and many people are into that danger zone without realizing it. A goodly number of these same people develop serious problems, some of which could even be fatal. Following is a brief list of the hazards you are risking by carrying "those few (or quite a few) extra pounds":

- Fat people have higher levels of blood lipids, which are fats and oils in the blood that increase the risk of heart disease or stroke.
- Fat people have a much stronger tendency to have that "silent" problem—high blood pressure.

- Fat people suffer more often from coronary heart disease.
- Extra weight may bring on diabetes in persons susceptible to this disease.
- Fat women suffer more often from gynecological irregularities; obese pregnant women are more likely to have toxemia, which leads to serious complications.
- Fat people have more complications and problems during and after surgery.
- Also, carrying around a load of extra fat (even a few pounds) strains the bones and joints and can accentuate arthritis, especially in the knees, hips, and lower spine.
- Excess fat strains the muscles of the abdominal wall (belly), sometimes giving rise to formation of abdominal hernias.
- Increased and adverse amounts of fat in and around the muscles of the legs slows blood return through the veins to the heart, which is a factor in precipitating varicose veins.
- A fatty chest can cause difficulty in breathing.
- Gout is much more common in obese persons.
- There is even a marked increase in accidents among the severely obese.

The old concept of the happy fat person has been thoroughly disproved. In fact, fat people are much more susceptible to depression.

If all of the above problems were not enough, there are also well-known social, and even economic, disadvantages to being fat. A fat person: (1) is less likely to be sought after as a marriage partner; (2) pays higher insurance premiums; (3) meets discrimination when applying for a job; (4) cannot find attractive clothing as easily; (5) is limited in choice of sports and activities.

Nationwide, fat girls have only one-third the chance of being accepted into college that lean girls have. (I'm happy to say that at Oral Roberts University this is not the case.) Even during early childhood years, a fat youngster often suffers severe ridicule from classmates and the humiliation of being chosen last for games.

I could go on, but you get the point. Being fat is a *severe* handicap—physically, mentally, and emotionally. Our society, consciously or unconsciously, is becoming more and more punitive toward the fat person. For example, according to the studies of Dr. Jean Mayer, obese adolescent girls suffer from heightened sensitivity, obsessive concerns, passivity, and withdrawal. All of these traits are similar to those of minorities who are subjected to intense prejudice.

Studies done on our ORU campus also confirm the disadvantages of overfatness. As part of her work on a master's degree, Barbara C. O'Conner, a nurse practitioner, did research on the effects of body fat on the health of a group of ORU coeds. She conducted her study for one entire school year, approximately nine months, and carefully logged each student's health record and number of visits to the health clinic. Visits to the clinic were counted and classified in two categories: medical and athletically related.

At the beginning of the study all of the 357 freshmen women involved were measured for body-fat percentages by the skin-fold estimate method. Fifty-seven percent of the women had a body fat content above 26 percent. Forty-three percent had a body fat content below 26 percent. If you remember Dr. Covert Bailey's figures, the ideal body fat content for a typical woman is 22 percent, with very active female athletes having as little as 17 percent. For purposes of her study, Barbara O'Conner decided to give women in the 22 to 26 percent body-fat range the benefit of the doubt. Anyone above 26 percent of body fat, however, she termed "overfat" to a greater or lesser degree. This means that in the study of 357 coeds, 57 percent were in the overfat range with body fat of 26 percent or higher. In that overfat group approximately 70 of the women were measured at figures that Barbara chose to term as obese—anywhere from 30 to 42 percent body fat.

During the nine-month study, 76 percent of the students in the overfat group visited the Student Health Service Clinic. During that same period, only 58 percent of the women in the group with body fat under 26 percent visited the clinic. Barbara O'Conner also recorded that visits to the clinic for athletics-related injuries were significantly higher in the overfat group. Thirty-six percent of the overfat coeds made clinic visits for athletics-related injuries while only 19 percent of the students with less than 26 percent body fat made such clinic visits.

In summary, Barbara O'Conner's study showed a measurable correlation between percentage of body fat and health. Those students with a higher percentage of body fat were adversely affected. The overfat were significantly more ill than the underfat. In addition, the injuries and illnesses of the overfat population were more serious and more debilitating than those of the group who could be considered "normally fat."

Most significantly, women students with body fat of 30 percent and above were the least-healthy group.[2]

So far most of the news in this section has been bad. I wrote it this way to dramatize and underline one basic fact: Being overfat, or as many of us like to put it, "carrying a few extra pounds," is definitely unhealthy. The good news, however, is that obesity is always reversible. You don't have to stay fat. You can rid yourself of your fat before serious problems set in.

Once you get rid of your fat, you can look forward to just as long and healthy a life as the skinny types who never had to battle flab. Studies show that mortality rates are not any higher for people who were formerly fat than for those who were never fat.

Assuming you are convinced you have at least some fat to lose, the next question is obvious. What do you do about it? Most of the remainder of this section on flab deals with what might be called one basic physical law. Violate this law and flab will almost always form in ample amounts on your body.

You may have heard of Murphy's law: "If anything can go wrong it probably will." Krafft's physical law of aerobics states: "Fat accumulates in direct proportion to the amount of time spent moving jaws rather than legs and feet."

Some people like exercise; some can take it or leave it; and some hate it. But we *all* need it. Stick with me and I'll show you how to work out an exercise life-style you can live with—much longer.

HOW FAT GOES ON—AND COMES OFF

"I can't understand it. I eat like a bird and still can't lose an ounce."

You may have heard a complaint like that from a friend. Maybe you've muttered the same lament yourself. At the ORU Student Health Service I hear this kind of remark quite often. I smile understandingly and try to explain that all of us find it easy to fool ourselves. The hard truth is, fat accumulates when caloric intake exceeds calorie output. To put it another way, we get fat by eating more and exercising less.

In the pioneer days of our nation obesity was not a major problem. It's true that back then people didn't know as much about nutrition. They ate far too much fat. But for the most part men and women had to put in many hours of physical labor, which burned off the extra calories that they consumed. The big factor in keeping people fit and relatively thin was the healthful amount of physical activity they had to engage in each day.

As we have become more "civilized," we have lost many good things that a more natural life-style provided. A back-to-the-country, back-to-the-farm, back-to-nature type of life-style would automatically help us to exercise more intensively, and just as automatically we would solve a lot of obesity problems. But we enjoy our technological goodies too much. We jump into the automobile to go three blocks to the corner grocery store. We turn on the television set rather than enjoying a walk in the beauty of God's outdoors. And while we watch television, advertising bombards us every few minutes urging us to head for the refrigerator to get snacks and drinks in order to "enjoy the program more."

Calories do count, and they count up fast. Depending on your job and life-style, you need a certain minimum number of calories per day. In fact, we all burn a basic number of basal calories every day and night, no matter how much or little work we do. For men the basal number of calories is 1,600, for women it's 1,500.[3] Then, depending on how active we are, we burn additional calories per day as we walk about, dial the phone, yawn, take out the trash, yes, and even while we drive the car. (Naturally, a stick shift takes a few more calories than an automatic.)

According to the Food and Nutrition Board, National Research Council, the recommended calorie allowances per day for a 154-pound man are as follows:

Sedentary—2,500 calories
Moderately active—3,000 calories
Very active—3,500 calories

For a 123-pound woman the calorie allowance is:

Sedentary—2,100 calories
Moderately active—2,500 calories
Very active—3,000 calories[4]

(Note: For each decade over the age of twenty, these numbers should be reduced.)

For all of us weight and fat control is a simple matter of "energy in and energy out." All you have to do to gain a pound a week is simply fail to burn off 500 excess calories each day. By "excess" I mean calories over and above the amount you need acccording to your job and activity schedule. For example, that 154-pound man with a sedentary occupation needs 2,500 calories per day. If he continually puts away 3,000 per day and doesn't burn off that extra 500, it wouldn't be hard at all to gain 50 pounds in a year.

Most of us have a fairly good understanding of what I've covered above. We know that we should only take in so many calories per day and that when we "pig out," we gain weight. Just talk to anyone when they come back to work after vacation. They will usually tell you they gained five to ten pounds, because they ate so much more than usual while they "took it easy" (i.e., sat around).

Many of us go through the calendar year playing the dieting game. We overeat during vacation and then try to lose the weight gained. We overeat during Christmas season and then try to lose that. And so it goes. We struggle and struggle not to eat. We keep looking for the latest-and-best new diet or scheme or "miracle plan" to keep our weight under control.

Exercise and Nutrition

And it's true, you can lose weight and fat by dieting; many people do. But as I said earlier, the chances are good to excellent you will put that weight back on in the form of more fat than before. And, as I also said before—and will say again and again—the *only* way to take off fat and *keep it off* is through aerobic exercise.

The immediate question is, "Well then, what is aerobic exercise?" The word *aerobic* means "with oxygen," or "with air." During aerobic exercise the body burns up its fuel (calories) by utilizing oxygen taken in through the lungs. Aerobic exercise is long, slow, endurance type exercise. It means continuously exercising without pauses. This is crucial. That is why I have listed swimming, bicycling, running, jogging, and walking as excellent aerobic exercises.

The opposite of aerobic exercise is what is called anaerobic exercise, which is defined as "exercise not requiring oxygen." Short sprints and dashes, or brief, but mighty, efforts to lift weights are examples of anaerobic exercise. Yes, these activities take some oxygen, but the oxygen is not consumed by the aerobic-burning process inside the body's cells. To get your body into "aerobic gear," so to speak, you need the long, steady pumping of air through the lungs, which happens when you go for a brisk two-mile walk or a five-mile jog.

Anaerobic—short-term, overexertional—exercises do not contribute to weight loss and are much more likely to cause injury. Look in any book on aerobics and you will see that sports like tennis, handball, baseball, football, and even basketball are described as only fair aerobic activity. That's because all of these sports take short bursts of exertion, but then also include periods of stopping, standing, and in the case of baseball, even sitting between innings.

Any amount of exercise has some benefit, of course, but the really important exercise as far as losing fat is concerned is the continuous movement, where you *keep going*. It is right here where we labor with a common misconception. From earliest childhood many of us are admonished to run hard, go fast, get after it, get it over with quickly. This kind of mind-set actually works against us when we are attempting aerobic— long, slow, continuous—exercise to lose fat.

Hal Higdon, a friend of mine, is an outstanding author as well as a very active aerobic runner. In a recent article for a national publication Hal said this: "If you want to lose weight, the slower you run the better."[5] Hal's remark is a colorful way to underline what I've been trying to say. The body metabolizes (burns off) fat more efficiently during exercise done at slow speeds. *Gentle exercise*, whether running, swimming, cycling, or just walking, burns fat more efficiently than brief fast-paced exercise.

The key is to keep at it—for at least thirty minutes or more. Obviously, slow, gentle walking or jogging for thirty seconds isn't going to do you much good. Tests suggest that a jogger who is moving at a slow, submaximal pace obtains as much as 50 to 60 percent of his energy from body fat. So, the trick is to take it easy, or as one outstanding older runner has said, "Start slowly, then taper off."

I realize that if you are one of those people who hate exercise, the thought of any aerobic activity is not going to send thrills of anticipation up and down your spine. But without aerobic activity your battle against flab will continue to be a losing one and by "losing" I mean you will keep *gaining* fat instead of getting rid of it and keeping it off. That's why I keep emphasizing the idea that aerobic exercise can be gentle, easy, and slow. Exercise physiologists tell us that excellent benefits can be achieved by going slower—and without most of the strains that sometimes come with jogging and running.

In other words, you do not have to become a marathon runner to engage in pleasant, easy aerobic exercise. All you need to do is get your heart rate up a little higher than it beats while you are sitting in the car or leaning back in front of the TV set. This is good for your heart and also burns off fat. We'll look at how all this works next.

HOW YOUR HEART RATE HELPS YOU LOSE

In the preceding pages we talked about how and why aerobic exercise gets rid of fat. I stressed that aerobic exercise should be slow and easy, but it must be carried on long enough and hard enough to do the job. Your exercise intensity, or how hard you are working, is best determined by your pulse or heart rate. You need a target or training heart rate at which you should do your fat-losing exercises. Simply stated, it is best to exercise at an intensity of 70 to 85 percent of your maximum heart rate.

What is your maximum heart rate? You estimate your heart rate by subtracting your age from 220. At almost 60 years of age, I estimate my maximum heart rate at 220 minus 60 or 160 beats per minute—the rate at which my heart would beat if I were working at full capacity.

To determine my exercise or training heart rate I simply multiply my maximum heart rate by seven-tenths or 70 percent. Therefore, my training heart rate is 70 percent of 160 or 112 beats per minute. The estimate of 112 isn't a figure that has to be precise. It only has to be within a target range. The target range I'm after for a training heart rate is between 70 and 85 percent of my maximum, so I should exercise at somewhere between 112 to 136 beats per minute. A top figure of 136 beats is, of course, 85 percent of my theoretical maximum heart rate of 160.

What is the best way to count your heart rate? Taking a pulse is simple and easy for some persons, but a little more difficult for others. The best way is to reach with your left hand, palm side down, over to the thumb side of your right wrist and press down with three fingers. Just above the wrist you can feel the artery pumping in the groove between the bone of the thumb side and the tendon nearby. The sweep second hand on your wristwatch should be in plain view on your left wrist.

Once you have found your pulse, count it for only six seconds of that sweep second hand on your wristwatch. Six seconds will be ideal because you can simply add a zero to it to estimate your pulse rate.

To get a good idea of your training pulse rate (70 to 85 percent of maximum) walk or jog a block or two, then stop and immediately take your pulse. Suppose you are forty years old. That means you're looking for the pace that will produce 126 beats per minute. (Remember the formula: 220 minus 40 equals 180 times seven-tenths equals 126.)

Some persons can count while they are walking or running, but I can't; I have to stop. It is important, though, to count your pulse right away. Don't wait a minute or two until your heart slows down somewhat because then you would not have an accurate figure. Get the number of pulse beats per six seconds and add a zero. That figure is a good estimate of your training pulse rate.

Remember you are aiming for a range from 70 to 85 percent of your maximum heart rate, and it does not have to be an exact number. As you become used to checking your pulse you will find that you can estimate it readily in six seconds as you pause during or right after your walk, run, or whatever exercise you are doing.

Heart rate is the best indication of whether or not you are doing your exercise at the proper intensity. If you are significantly overfat, you will find that your pulse, even during a moderate walk, quickly reaches the training heart range of 70 to 85 percent of maximum. As you become trained and shed fat, the amount of effort necessary to get the pulse into the training range will gradually increase. Much later on you may even find you have to break into a jog to reach a heart rate in the training zone.

I dealt recently with a thirty-seven-year-old pastor who had returned to school to get a master's degree. He was typically out of shape, but nonetheless he tried to start his program by jogging immediately. But any amount of jogging sent his pulse rate to over 200, which was above his recommended maximum of 183 beats per minute (220 minus 37).

I told him firmly, *"Walk only* for the first few weeks. Jogging is out for you until you get in better shape." He did as I instructed and walked only for almost three weeks. Later on he started mixing a little jogging with the walking. Eventually he was jogging at a slow pace and enjoying his proper training rate, which was around 128 to 155 beats per minute.

So, now you see how aerobic exercise is easily measured by heart rate. Take 220 minus your age and then 70 to 85 percent of that number. If you exercise in this range and do not try to exceed it, you benefit in two crucial ways:

1. You will be exercising safely.
2. You will be exercising at the most effective level for getting rid of fat.

But some obvious questions remain. If you are like most of the people I deal with at the ORU Health Service, you are concerned about the time all this takes. How often should you exercise? How long or far should you walk, run, swim, or bike? Here is the good news. In less than fifteen minutes you can start burning off the fat forever!

HOW OFTEN AND HOW LONG?

Aerobic exercise must be continued long enough for the oxygen we breathe to burn excess food stores, particularly the fat on our bodies. In his book *Fit or Fat?* Covert Bailey estimates that twelve minutes is a minimum for continuous exercise to be effective. This is certainly not an ideal amount of time, but whenever you can exercise continuously for at least twelve minutes you will be into the range at which some fat loss can occur.

As to the "ideal" amount of time, most authorities say about thirty minutes five times a week should maintain and slowly improve fitness along with significantly resulting in the loss of fat—if you need to lose. Research shows that if you exercise fewer than three days a week, however, the fitness effect will regress.

From my work at the ORU Health Service, I believe the ideal schedule is one hour at least three times a week of endurance exercise and a shorter period—about thirty minutes—on three other days. My personal aerobic program includes a schedule of six days a week, and I usually alternate with one-hour and half-hour workouts.

I use a phrase with my students that is certainly true for me, and it may be true for you: "I am so extremely busy that I cannot afford to jog or walk *less* than one hour at least three times a week." I firmly believe this because of the mental-health benefits that are also important in aerobic exercise. I really need that full hour three or more days a week to regroup my attitudes and release my tensions.

Remember that with aerobic exercise the emphasis is on time, not distance or speed. If you want to shape up fast, exercise longer, not harder. To review, an aerobic exercise:

1. Lasts a minimum of twelve minutes
2. Maintains your heart rate at 70 to 85 percent of maximum for the entire time
3. Should be done a minimum of three days a week—and six is ideal
4. Is steady and nonstop

Covert Bailey states that if he were obese (as he once was), he would walk three to four hours per day to get the fat off.

If six days of exercise is good, is seven better? To be motivated enough to exercise seven days a week is commendable. However, our Lord rested one day during creation, and it is a good rule for us to do the same. Perhaps God set that example because He knew something that we didn't about "burn out."

To sum up, the absolute ideal for exercise is six days a week, scheduled at a specific time each day. That way it becomes a part of your life—something you genuinely look forward to each day six days a week.

The next question might be whether you need to continue exercising for six months or a full year. It's easy to answer that one. The program should become part of your life-style and should continue as long as you are in good health and strength. There is no age limit on aerobic exercise. The oldest person I worked with is a lady of sixty-seven. She ran her first marathon at the age of sixty-five. I know of several people in their seventies who run marathons. Let me remind you that a marathon is a little over twenty-six miles!

A healthful life-style means continuing effective aerobic exercise as long as one lives. And the whole idea behind aerobic exercise is to help you live longer and healthier. As I like to tell my students at the ORU Health Service, "Personally I want to die young, but as late in life as possible."

If you have stuck with me to this point, you may be ready to give aerobic exercise a try. (On the other hand, you may have already started or perhaps you have tried it, stopped for a while, and aren't sure if you want to try it again.) When should you begin? Well, how about right now?

WHEN DO I BEGIN?

If not right now, how about right after work tomorrow? Get out some comfortable clothes, tie on those supercushioned jogging shoes (or any good walking shoes) and go out the door!

Even this first time, be sure to keep going for at least twelve minutes, but don't push it. Your motto is "easy does it." Watch your pulse and don't get it over the limit of 70 to 85 percent of your maximum heart rate. Be extra careful and do not move too much or too fast this first time.

You may be wondering about the need for a doctor's physical exam. This is usually not necessary if you make a gentle beginning by simply walking. You should be having regular checkups by a physician already, with a complete exam at least every three years. Few doctors will forbid something as easy as walking; in fact, most doctors will encourage it. If your doctor says no and you believe you are healthy, you might get a second opinion from another physician. It always helps to find a doctor who walks or jogs himself. Unless you have a really serious problem, you should get the green light for participating in aerobic exercise on a sensible basis.

I often suggest to people that they begin their aerobic program in the evening after work to release tensions that have cropped up during the day. But any time is the right time of day to begin your exercise program. The important factor is that it's the right time for *you*. For homemakers, how about early-morning hours? It's inspiring to me to go out into the cool of early morning and see pairs of women briskly walking away the flab and building good muscle tone along with high self-esteem.

These women are living proof that walking is the number-one sport for just about anyone. All sorts of fancy and expensive "toys" are marketed as the latest answers to exercise and losing weight. Almost all of them are useless as far as fat-losing aerobics is concerned. Why bother with these gadgets? God gave us two marvelous appendages called feet. Walking is a delightful way to use those feet, especially if you can walk outdoors. As long as you make sure your heart doesn't race out of control, it is nearly impossible to overtrain or harm yourself by walking. Few of us do not have access to a surface upon which we can walk, and walking requires no specialized equipment.

If you can afford them, it is a good idea to buy a pair of well-cushioned jogging shoes that fit and support your feet correctly. Please don't use tennis shoes, "deck" shoes, or other "sneaker" types of footwear. The modern, well-developed jogging shoe is a great invention, and you will be amazed at the difference it makes, whether you are running or walking.

You may be wondering what I do for aerobic exercise. Running or walking? I admit to being a slow jogger, but the chief reason is that I have become too fit to get my heart rate up to the proper speed by walking. I must jog or run in order to reach 70 to 85 percent of maximum heart rate.

I particularly enjoy the fun of competing in distance races in a "noncompetitive" manner. I say noncompetitive because racing is just as much fun if I finish last.

A word of caution is in order about exercising in extreme heat. If you are beginning your program in hot weather (90 degrees or above), take your time and go only very short distances at first. Even though I am in excellent condition, when the thermometer registers over 100, I return to walking and still get to enjoy the outdoors even when the temperature is sizzling.

What happens if you enjoy and prefer walking but get into such good shape that you have a hard time getting your heart to training range? One answer is to use a backpack with gradually increasing loads. Another possibility is speed or race walking, which is appealing to a growing number of devotees. Always take care to watch your heart rate to ensure that you are not overdoing it but that you are getting into the training range.

If walking seems a bit tame for you, try other outstanding aerobic sports like bicycling, swimming, cross-country skiing, or aerobic dance. Granted, you can run into problems as you search for variety or something more exciting than walking. Snow is not always available for skiing. Many of us don't have access to a swimming pool on a daily basis. It is sometimes hard to find a path or road where you can bicycle for any distance in safety.

Rhythmic aerobics or aerobic dance is great, but there is usually too much bounce in this sport for the overfat person, at least in the beginning. Your best bet is to walk for a while and then try rhythmic aerobics and other challenging activities.

By the way, swimming is one of the best of sports for conditioning, and it is especially beneficial to people with orthopedic problems in their muscles, joints, or bones. Ironically, however, it is not the best activity for losing extra fat under the skin. Swimming takes fat out of your muscles, to be sure, but do not expect to readily note your fat loss by pinching skin if you are a swimmer. The body keeps a certain amount of subskin fat to protect it from cool water.

Joseph Moreno is a good example of what swimming can do. He came to us at 236 pounds, with a severe knee problem and 29.6 percent body fat, according to underwater weighing. He went into a swimming program that included one-half to one mile per day at a slow, steady, aerobic pace. By mid-term, underwater weighing registered his body fat at 23.8 percent, but his weight had only dropped one pound. By the end of the year, however, his weight had dropped to 215, and underwater weighing showed his body fat at 22 percent, a drop of 7.6 percent over nine months, which we consider excellent results.

At no time during the year did we try to estimate Joseph's body fat with skin calipers. He kept a typical swimmer's sleek appearance with the extra layer of fat under the skin. Where he lost the most body fat, however, was in his muscles. He left our obesity-level class and continued swimming on his own with a goal of getting his body fat below 20 percent.

Let me say once more that sports like golf, tennis, bowling, racquetball, and the like are all good, but they just do not qualify for the job of burning fat through aerobics. All of these sports have too much intermittency, that is, standing around between plays or action. These sports do not provide *continuous* activity. It's a good idea to walk or jog to get in shape *to* play these sports. But do not try to get in shape *by* playing golf, tennis, softball, and so forth.

Other ways to engage in aerobic activity include cycling on a stationary bike or running in place on a mini-trampoline. Many persons, including my beloved wife, LaVerne, find such aerobic activities just the thing. One attractive feature of stationary cycling or running in place on a trampoline is that they can be done in air-conditioned or heated comfort. To bike or jog in place would be boring for me—but to each his own. Any exercise that you enjoy which is continuous and uses large muscle groups will do the job. For most of us, especially those who are definitely obese, walking will usually be the ideal way to begin.

Therefore, if you are reasonably well physically, today is the best day to begin your program. If something comes up to frustrate you, don't berate yourself. To paraphrase the lead song from a hit musical, "Tomorrow's aerobics are just a day away!"

WHO SAID IT WAS QUICK AND EASY?

Not me, that's for sure. People who say that losing fat is quick and easy are telling an unmitigated untruth. It takes time and it takes continuous effort to lose fat and keep it lost.

Advertisements on TV, radio, and in newspapers and magazines tell us we can lose quickly and easily through special diets and devices like belts and massage machines and gadgets. All of this is just not true or is vastly overrated.

Yes, you can lose four or five pounds "overnight" by sweating out water or taking a diuretic that prompts your kidneys to get rid of the water in a hurry. But this has nothing to do with losing actual fat. As soon as you drink normal amounts of water again—which you should do just to stay healthy—that "lost" four or five pounds will be mysteriously found again. As for crash dieting, I have already pointed out that while you can lose weight, the odds are overwhelmingly in favor of your regaining it with a net gain in fat once you do put the lost pounds back on.

My own fat-loss program has extended over ten years. Admittedly, I was not completely out of control at the start, but at 206 pounds and body fat somewhere close to the 24 percent level, I was concerned enough to make some personal changes in my life-style. I began by walking and, as my conditioning improved, went to slow jogging for long distances. In less than a year I had dropped below 190 pounds and below 20 percent of body fat. After nine years of aerobic exercising, I am at 175 pounds with a body-fat percentage of 15 percent, which I consider ideal for me.

Your rate of progress may be faster or slower than mine. That is not important. What is important is that you commit yourself to getting rid of your extra flab and that you continue to work at it with regular aerobic exercise and sensible eating.

At Oral Roberts University our definition of "obesity level" is 24 percent body fat for males and 34 percent body fat for females. People above these body-fat percentages are usually anywhere from 30 to 100 or more pounds "overweight." I put quotes around the word *overweight* because I am referring to the height/weight tables, which most people understand and use as a frame of reference. We could call that gray area between the ideals (11 to 17 percent for males and 17 to 22 for females) and the obesity levels "somewhat" or "just a little" overfat.

As I said earlier, the height/weight tables are not really accurate. Your fat percentage is what counts, not your weight. With most people, of course, their weight goes down as their fat percentage drops. Because getting weighed underwater or measured with calipers for fat content is not convenient on a daily basis, we use loss of pounds as a rule of thumb in our programs at Oral Roberts University. We require obesity-level students to lose eight pounds (and 1 percent body fat) during each sixteen-week semester. This translates into one-half pound per week, which is not a great deal to ask of anyone.

As you get into your own program you can probably do a lot better than a half a pound a week. How much better should you try to do? Dropping as much as two pounds a week on the average, with variation from week to week, is the *most* that you should expect to lose in a program that is serious but sensible. For someone at obesity level, a loss of one pound per week, or about fifty pounds per year, is an excellent success story. Furthermore, if you lose from one-half to two pounds per week consistently with aerobic activity, it will be a permanent and genuine loss of fat. Fat will not return, but will be gone for good as long as you are faithful in aerobic-exercise activities.

In this book it may sound as though I were the one doing the day-to-day work with the overfat students. In reality my job is as advisor and consultant. During the last school year 100 ORU students were in the overfat group that we call the exercise and weight-control class. Through moderate regular exercise activities the miraculous result was that 91 of that 100 were successful! Credit for this fabulous record goes to the motivation of the students themselves, but Mrs. Sally Schollmeier, the faculty member who teaches, encourages, and leads this exercise and weight-control group, deserves much applause. We need each other.

Greg is a perfect example of how all this can work. A student at ORU, he entered our Health, Physical Education, and Recreation Program at the start of fall term at 313 pounds and body fat of 40 percent. Greg began with walking exercises four times a week. We also gave him plenty of individual counseling and carefully monitored his diet. His cooperation level was excellent.

Greg's enthusiasm mounted with each week. By Christmas his weight had dropped to 282 pounds, and his body fat was at 32.2 percent. By the end of the school year his body fat was 26.7 percent, and his weight was 265.

When Greg started the program, his dimensions included a fifty-inch waist and a twenty-and-a-half-inch collar. At year's end he bought a pair of slacks with a forty-inch waist, and his collar size was down to seventeen. He told us, "For the first time in my life, I've been able to buy clothes off the rack."

Greg's stress level dropped dramatically as well. His blood pressure went to 140 over 60. When he started the program, he was in a decidedly unhealthy range of 150 over 100.

Through our counseling, Greg discovered he was using food as a weapon to "get back at people." He began eating less at meals and cut out his between-meals snacks, which had featured frequent binges on sweets. At year's end he still had more fat and weight to lose, but he was well on his way and committed to a new life-style. His comment: "I control the eating, it doesn't control me. It's freedom."

You may have noted that Greg lost a total of forty-eight pounds over a school year of nine months. Most important, his body fat went from 40 percent to 26.7 percent. I mentioned that he began the program by walking, something we strongly advised due to his 313 pounds. After a few

Exercise and Nutrition

months he switched to slow jogging, and by year's end was doing thirty to sixty minutes of slow jogging four or five times a week.

Greg is a good model for anyone at severe obesity level to follow. Begin your aerobics with walking and aim for a weight loss of fifty pounds the first year. As you get into better condition, you can switch to jogging, biking, or other activities.

For most people, walking is usually fun to at least some degree, but I often get questions from joggers such as, "When does jogging or running start becoming fun?" I believe many people have been misled by those of us who are promoting exercise. The truth is *not every single minute of every workout is fun.*

My good friend Dr. Thaddeus Kostrubala is a San Diego psychiatrist who wrote the fine book *The Joy of Running*. But Tad was not entirely in agreement with his publishers when they gave his book that title. He says, "I thought the title would mislead people. If you approach running or any other fitness exercise with the idea that it always has to be fun, you are bound to be disappointed. Running is work. Painful work, *glorious* painful work, but it's still work."

Hal Higdon states, "The so-called runner's high may not exist for many people. The fun may come not during exercise, but afterwards, knowing that you are physically fit and more capable of coping with the stress of everyday life."[6]

My own experience is that a mildly vigorous jog becomes fun after the first two miles. If my time schedule permits a longer workout, slow jogging of five, six, or eight miles always proves to be fun during the last half. On days when I take only a shorter jog of maybe two to two-and-a-half miles, it's mostly work, and the joy comes during and after my shower, when I really feel good. For me the shorter workout is seldom fun, but it pays dividends in how good I feel about life afterward.

Keep in mind, however, that this is *not* a book on the joys of jogging or "reaching the runner's high." This is a book about losing fat through aerobic exercise and sensible eating habits. Jogging and running are only two forms of aerobic exercise. You may prefer biking, swimming, or walking, all of which are easier on the feet, knees, and other joints, while still giving you the heart rate you need to reach aerobic-activity levels.

As I have said several times, walking is something almost anyone can do. A brisk walk is usually enjoyable from the first step. That is not to say walking won't get you tired or that there won't be days when a brisk walk doesn't look half as enticing as a slow amble to the TV recliner. Those are the days when you will have to decide whether you want to be fit or fat.

No, aerobic exercise is not quick and it is not easy, but it can be tremendously rewarding. You can achieve the weight you want. You can rid yourself of those extra layers of unlovely fat by committing yourself to a lifetime of aerobic exercise and sensible eating.

I have mentioned "sensible eating" at several points. Maybe it's time we took a brief look at what sensible eating is all about.

WHY YOU SHOULD EAT SMART, NOT LESS

In a book like this it is easy to emphasize exercise to the point that it sounds as though it doesn't matter what or how much you eat. But that would be foolish. As I stressed at the beginning, exercise is the horse and diet is the cart. Exercise comes *first,* but diet has to be there also or you do not have a complete approach to fighting flab correctly.

I do have trouble, however, with that word *diet.* I'd like to throw the term *diet* out the window and promote the concept of "eating smart." We have preached diets and dieting so hard in our culture that the word has come to have mostly negative connotations. Mention the word *diet* around your friends or acquaintances and you do not see any smiles of joy and happiness. I've yet to see a book titled *The High of Dieting.* Eating sensibly sounds much more positive. To eat sensibly is a happy experience in every way, socially as well as psychologically and physiologically.

To talk about eating sensibly, we have to look at the various food groups and how much or how little we should have of each main group. You may be familiar with some of what follows, but I think it's important to go over it as review to show just how your eating habits should tie in with your exercise activities.

We have already mentioned the three major groupings of food: fats, carbohydrates, and protein. In a book on getting rid of fat it will come as no surprise that a good rule is to eat less fat. Americans eat an average of 42 percent of their daily calories in fatty foods, but the recommended amount is 30 percent. With a little effort you can easily identify most of the fatty foods. Fat intake slips up on us when we least expect it; it is found in food more than we think.

For example, butter and margarine are almost 100 percent fat, and both are used extensively in cooking. Another source of fat is meat. We think we are getting "pure" protein in steaks and high-quality ground beef. But in these types of meat, the more expensive cuts are usually the highest in fat. It's all right to eat steak or ground beef, but use small portions, especially of the marbled varieties that are streaked with fat for better taste.

You may have heard that, along with cutting down on fats, it's wise to go easy on the carbohydrates. Entire diets have been built around the

Exercise and Nutrition

cutting of carbohydrates to very low levels. An example of this type of diet is found in *Dr. Atkins' Diet Revolution*.[7] I believe carbohydrates have received unmerited "bad press" for years. It's true that we need to reduce our use of *refined carbohydrates,* like sugar and white flour, because they are high in calories and extremely low in nutritional value. But we need to *increase* our use of *complex carbohydrates,* which provide energy, fiber, vitamins, and minerals. Excellent sources of complex carbohydrates are vegetables, whole-grain breads and cereals, and fresh fruit.

Foods with complex carbohydrates provide a double bonus: (1) Many of them contain fiber, which helps with digestion and keeping the colon clear; and (2) some of these foods are quite low in calories.

Personally, I tossed out my calorie-counter books years ago, because I depend so directly on aerobic exercise for fat-and-weight control. Nonetheless, I realize many people are calorie conscious or try to be. So, early in your own fat-loss program, you may need to keep an eye on your calorie intake. After all, if you are trying to lose fat and want to burn more calories than you're taking in, why have a high-calorie dish when something else, with less than half the number of calories, is available?

For example, in the complex-carbohydrate family many vegetables like green beans, cauliflower, broccoli, and carrots are very low in calories. Be careful, however, with avocados (which are quite high in calories), and some of the fruits. For example, bananas, prunes, and raisins are "calorie dynamite." All these are good, but go easy.

Sometimes the calorie count rises according to how a food is prepared. Potatoes are often labeled as high in calories, but actually a medium-sized potato contains zero fat and about 125 calories. Turn that potato into French fries, however, and you can increase the fat content to 65 percent, and the calorie count jumps to several hundred.

Carbohydrates are quite likely the most misunderstood food group of all. A lot of people think they have to reduce carbohydrate intake, but in most cases people need to *increase* carbohydrate consumption to around 50 to 60 percent of their daily total. Just be sure you are getting the "good guys"—the complex carbohydrates I mentioned above.

Protein might be called the "glamour" food group. Protein is advertised as vitally important to the body and this is true, because it is the source of essential amino acids that are necessary for the building and maintenance of body cells and functions.

Good sources of protein are fish, poultry, and legumes. Three other high-protein sources are red meat, eggs, and cheese, but try to go easy on these. As I have already mentioned, red meat can be very high in fat; eggs and cheese increase cholesterol. Actually, in America we have an overabundance of good-quality protein. For the typical American family, protein intake of 12 percent of total calories is sufficient. Protein also comes in vegetables in the legume family—peas, dried beans, and lentils.

There is much debate about minerals and vitamins, and the subject is too broad to tackle in a brief book on how to lose fat. If you are interested in learning more, you can read about them in any number of good books that are available at health-food stores or your local bookshop. We do not have to get into the fine points of argument to realize that our bodies need all of the essential vitamins and minerals. I am not at all sure that the recommended daily allowances (RDA) are really enough, however, for persons exercising vigorously and regularly in an aerobic program. So, for instance, I take a simple multiple vitamin-and-mineral supplement. I also take moderate extra doses of vitamins C, E, and B complex. Whenever I get muscle aches, I also take some calcium.

There are physicians who may tell you that if you eat a well-balanced general diet, you will need no extra vitamins or minerals. No one really knows if this is right or wrong. As more and more data continue to come in, we are getting a better picture. But until all the evidence is gathered, why not be sure? A multiple vitamin-and-mineral supplement is a small investment in good nutritional insurance.

Be careful, however, not to overdose on vitamins, particularly vitamins C, A, D, and E. I recently treated a runner who had severe urinary bleeding until I convinced him to cut down from ten grams of vitamin C each day to one-half gram per day.

We have taken a look at the three basic food types: fats, carbohydrates, and protein. In order to get the balance and variety that is so important to your total diet, I suggest that you follow what is called the Four Basic Food Groups Plan. In these four basic food groups you can find adequate amounts of fat, carbohydrates, and protein.

The first group is the meat group, which provides proteins, minerals, fats, and B vitamins. Included here are red meats, fish, poultry, dried peas, beans, lentils, peanut butter, and nuts. There is a lot of talk today about the dangers of eating a great deal of red meat. Being an Oklahoman, I may get some calls from my friends in the cattle business, but I have to recommend cutting down on red meat. I have already covered the problems with "marbled steak," which is streaked with fat. Many people are switching to more fish and poultry instead of having their usual hamburgers, roast beef, steak, pork roast, and so forth. My own eating habits have changed over the last few years, and I now have beef only once or twice a week, while fish and chicken and some vegetarian meals have become staples in my diet.

The second major food group is fruit and vegetables, of which you should have four servings each day. Here is where you get vitamins A and C, minerals, and fiber. Included are foods like citrus fruits, melons, tomatoes, strawberries, broccoli, carrots, leafy greens, squashes, potatoes, and yams. As you pick from this group, be sure you include one green or yellow vegetable per day and one citrus fruit or medium-sized glass of citrus juice such as orange or grapefruit juice.

The third group is bread and cereal. You should eat four servings of these daily. Here's where you get carbohydrates, proteins, vitamins, and minerals. If you choose "natural cereals" like granola, oatmeal, cornmeal, and "seven grain" mixtures, you will get some of your requirement of fiber, which is so important to keeping your digestive tract clear. Try to get all the fiber you can. Another thing in its favor is that fiber fills you up without filling you out.

Still another excellent source of fiber is 100 percent whole wheat bread, particularly brands with bran added. Other good natural breads include those containing rye or rice. Go easy on the highly advertised "junk food" cereals. They have very little nutritional value and are loaded with sugar.

The fourth group is dairy products, which provide calcium, phosphorus, proteins, vitamin A, and riboflavin (a B vitamin). Included in the dairy-product group are milk, yogurt, cheese, and ice cream. You should have two or more servings of this group daily. Watch the dairy-product group carefully, however, to keep your fat intake down. You can control fat intake by drinking only nonfat milk and using low-calorie yogurt, or skim-milk cheese. Stay away from ice cream except for occasional splurges to give yourself a treat for normally being self-disciplined.

Don't think that fat is a problem only in the milk or dairy-product group. Watch all of the four groups for too much fat. Avoid high-calorie baked goods, deep-fried foods, cream products, solid fats, sauces, and gravies.

In the above paragraphs I have given only the barest sketch of the three basic food *types* (fats, carbohydrates, and proteins) and the four basic food *groups* (meat, fruit and vegetable, bread and cereal, milk and dairy products). If you want to learn more, I suggest that you pick up one or more diet or nutrition books and do a little reading to become familiar with what you are consuming daily in each basic food group and food type.[8] You will also quickly become an "expert" on calories and which foods have high-calorie and low-calorie counts.

Calories do count and they count up fast, especially when you eat fatty foods. Each of us has to work out his own eating plan to get the right amount of each food type and group, enough vitamins and minerals, and yet keep the daily calorie intake within reasonable levels. All of this is part of eating smart, or sensibly.

However, do not always nitpick about the number of calories you are eating. Just keep in mind that if you want to indulge yourself, it means that you need to do a little more walking or jogging to burn off the extra calories that the indulgence has added. My personal nemesis is the pie counter. I confess that my indiscretion occurs quite often, and I am well aware that I must burn an extra 300 or 400 calories on the jogging path every time I down a piece of pie.

Understand that I am not giving you license to commit this kind of folly as regularly as I do. If you are engaging faithfully in enough aerobic activity, however, you can work out your own system for having an occasional treat. The point is if you are having your daily walk or run or bike ride and eating sensibly, you do not have to worry about every calorie you consume. An occasional treat is easy to handle, but let me emphasize the word *occasional*. If you start gobbling up all the pie, cake, and ice cream in sight, while trying to mix in a little aerobic activity and a halfhearted attempt to eat sensibly, you are headed for disaster, and the fat will go right back on your body. If you are in any kind of weight and fatloss program, you should eat at least 1200 calories per day with a very balanced selection of foods.

If you start talking about nutrition and calories, some of your friends and acquaintances may start to kid you or even start to get irritated with your remarks. Don't be obnoxious, but at the same time don't back off out of embarrassment or timidity. Today, nutrition is recognized as an absolutely vital element in health care. In the Surgeon General's 1979 report on health promotion and disease prevention, entitled "Healthy People," the following suggestions were made concerning nutrition. Americans would be healthier as a whole if they consumed: (1) only sufficient calories to meet body needs and maintain desirable weight; (2) less saturated fat and cholesterol; (3) less salt; (4) less sugar; (5) relatively more complex carbohydrates such as whole grains, cereals, fruits, and vegetables; (6) relatively more fish, poultry, and legumes and less red meat.

In summary, there are three simple rules you can follow:

1. Cut down on fats. Try to eat only 30 percent of your daily calories in fat. Watch the junk food like French fries and the number of pats of butter that you can sneak into each meal without realizing it. A fairly good balance for a diet would include 30 percent in fats, 55 to 60 percent in complex carbohydrates, and 10 to 15 percent in high-quality protein.

Exercise and Nutrition

2. Eat a wide variety of foods (review the material on the four basic food groups). Most people could stand getting acquainted with a great many more fruits and vegetables. As I work with people at our Health Service, my main concern is that they use as much natural food as possible without having to go to undue expense at health-food stores. I recommend a "vegetarian type" of diet, with additions of fowl or fish and very little red meat.
3. Watch your calories but don't carry a calculator to every meal. Get a general idea of the amounts of calories in the basic foods that you like and consume daily and weekly. Then eat only the sufficient number of calories you need to keep up your strength and your aerobic activities.

All three of the above rules can be condensed into one: *Eat a good nutritional diet.* Don't waste your time on empty calories. As long as you are out there trying to burn away that fat with aerobic exercise, you might as well be filling your tank with the right fuel.

Yes, it's a little more trouble to watch what you eat and to be aware of food groups and food types, but it's more than worth it. Along with committing yourself to a life-style that includes aerobic exercise, commit yourself to a life-style that includes proper eating habits. And when I use the word *commit,* I am talking about saying, *"I will do this,"* not "I guess I'll try." The fight against flab is waged on the exercise track and at the table, but you win it or lose it in your head. For some tips on waging successful psychological warfare, see the next section.

YOU REALLY ARE WHAT YOU THINK!

"Attitude Decreases Fattitude" could be another title for this part. One counselor told me that two out of three persons who come to him have as their major problem inadequate self-esteem. Repeatedly, he sees living proof of the old saying: "You become or remain what you think you are."

The concept of "you are what you think" has obvious implications for fat people. Your layers of flab are *not* the real you, but if you think you can't lose and that you'll "just have to live with being heavy," you will be trapped in a fat body and quite likely suffer from low self-esteem.

But it doesn't have to be so. *Anyone who is able to walk does not have to be fat.* You can be sure that God doesn't make junk, and he does not want his beautiful creation enfolded in excess flab.

So, think thin! Move out slowly but surely into an active life-style.

Keep visualizing the slender you that you want to become. Stick with it and you will become thin. Remember that you are someone special. You can achieve whatever your mind conceives—*if you really want to.*

The power of what the mind can do is illustrated in the story of Lois. A few years ago my wife and I sought to help Lois as she struggled with trying to lose weight and fat. Lois came from a home in which she lived with her mother, grandmother, and aunt. All three of the older women weighed over 200 pounds. Lois' father had deserted the family when she was very young.

Lois' mother, grandmother, and aunt all gave her a great deal of love and attention. How did they express love? You guessed it: with food. Day after day Lois was programmed with one basic concept—caring means feeding.

For Lois to become slender, or even to desire a healthy slim body, she would have to undergo a reprogramming of her attitudes. She had a negative picture of men (due to her father's desertion), and she was totally dominated by the concept that a caring person is an obese woman who prepares and provides rich, fatty foods.

We tried diligently to alter Lois' basic thinking but we failed. Lois finally left school to return to the safe retreat of the all-feminine circle where love was expressed with food. She did not like being fat, but she found security in a situation where she could see herself only as a fat person receiving love from other fat people. Lois simply could not picture herself as thin.

Denise has a story with a much happier ending. When Denise began our program, she had a kidney problem that required her to be on a dialysis machine two or three times a week. With body fat of 35.4 percent Denise was definitely at obesity level. She stood a good five feet five inches and weighed 200 pounds. Her dress size was eighteen to twenty and she wore size eighteen jeans. As she started her program, which featured aerobic walking exercises, she focused on her clothes and began "picturing" herself in smaller sizes. By the end of the school year she was in a size eleven-twelve dress and her "Jordache look" was a size thirteen! Her body fat went down to 27.5 percent, and her weight dropped to 176 pounds. Even more important, she was able to decrease her visits to the kidney dialysis machine from two to three times a week to once a month.

Other improvements by Denise included an increase in her self-confidence and ability to relate to others. She showed a marked decrease in worry about what people thought of her and proved this by showing a marked increase in wanting to go to the store to buy clothes.

"I just kept seeing myself as a smaller person," Denise commented. "I prayed I wouldn't have to keep hiding by standing by the wall."

Denise's emotional improvements are typical of people who get into programs of regular exercise. Tom Lee, an R.N. on our ORU staff, recently did some fascinating research concerning the effect of aerobic exercise on depression. At the beginning of the fall term, he used the Taylor Johnson Temperament Analysis to test forty-four freshmen women who had never engaged in any form of continuing physical exercise. After taking the test, all of the women engaged in a gradually increasing exercise program of the same type that all first-year students are asked to follow at Oral Roberts University.

After six to nine months the women were brought back for retesting with the Taylor Johnson Temperament Analysis. All of the women who showed marked depression in their first TJTA test were significantly improved when retested.

The key to ridding yourself of depression or other negative emotional states like anxiety, worry, hostility, and so forth is to realize you are a very special person. As self-esteem goes up, problems like depression have to come down. One psychological tool that I often use with people trying to lose weight and fat is the idea of positive reward. Once you are into an aerobic exercise program and losing one to three pounds every week, you start to feel good about yourself. You know you are losing actual fat, because your clothes are fitting better or possibly even becoming a bit too large for you. Inches are melting away slowly but surely. That is the time to reward yourself by buying a new dress or perhaps a color-coordinated jogging outfit. (I always caution people not to buy the most expensive items, because they may be trimming away even more inches, and what they purchase may eventually become too big also.)

Of course there are many ways to reward yourself other than buying yourself something. Perhaps you can change the route for your aerobic workouts. Walk along the river or in the park instead of along the same old path through the neighborhood.

Reward yourself by switching to bicycling or roller skating instead of jogging each day. Boredom is a dangerous enemy of the person who has achieved some success in an aerobic program. Change the scenery or the type of activity and it will help with boredom.

Another kind of reward that I find most pleasant is taking a day to go fishing or backpacking. With backpacking, aerobic activity is built right into the enjoyment. Even fishing can be aerobic if there is a canoe to paddle or a boat to row.

Another thing you might want to do is skip a day of aerobics, or even two days (but absolutely no more than that). In the end, it will be a slight change in the routine, and you can take a couple of days just to relax and feel proud of yourself. Don't be surprised, however, if you are restless and anxious to get back on the jogging or walking trail. Once the aerobic exercise bug bites you, you find it difficult to stay away from exercise, and you feel "antsy" or sluggish if you don't get in your daily workout.

Another way to reward yourself is in what you eat. Perhaps you enjoy between-meal snacks. Indulge yourself, but as I said earlier, *eat smart!* Try whole wheat crackers and skim-milk cheese, or learn the realistic delights of carrot sticks or celery. The best approach to losing flab is to eat five or six *small* meals per day anyway. Just be aware of how many calories you are consuming, and keep your consumption of fats well under control. Have a between-meals snack now and then, but don't go off the deep end with continual munching and feeling justified by saying, "Well, I'm going to get in my workout later, so I can handle this."

If you are confident you can handle it, use dessert as a rare reward. From time to time have a dish of ice cream or a piece of pie. Just be sure that you really desire the dessert treat. Never eat a dessert you don't really want.

Remember that when you use desserts as a rare reward, the emphasis is on the word *rare*. You can't make desserts a twice-daily habit and expect to get much results. An occasional dessert will give you fat and carbohydrates that you can burn in your aerobic program. It's true that most Americans need to cut down on fat and sugar, but you don't have to cut them out completely if you are exercising regularly. Americans consume an average of 125 pounds of sugar per person per year, an almost obscene figure. There is no reason, however, why you can't handle sixty pounds per year, *if you are burning it off with aerobics.* Try to stay away from the soft drinks, however. They are a highly concentrated form of sugar that isn't good for anyone, even the most dedicated aerobics participant.

As you can see, there are many ways to "think yourself thin." Don't fail to use the psychology of positive reinforcement whenever and wherever you can. In whatever you do, use thought patterns and rewards that are meaningful to *you*. As the hair-color commercial puts it, "You're worth it!"

THE POWER OF SETTING GOALS

While it's true that you are, or you become, what you think, it's equally true that you have to do more than simply envision yourself as a slender person. The other side of the thinking-thin coin is to set some goals and plan how you are actually going to become thin.

Exercise and Nutrition 49

I always urge people in our weight-loss programs at ORU to set *long-term goals* and to have some intermediate expectations or subgoals that they can reach along the way. For example, losing fifty pounds in one year is an excellent goal for someone who is truly obese. For others, losing anywhere from ten to twenty pounds in a year would be a very realistic goal for one year's time.

Whatever you do, don't ever plan to lose more than two pounds a week. True, you may go into a program of dieting and exercise and suddenly drop several pounds in a few days. Much of this is water, and there will be no harm in this faster weight loss early in the program.

After you lose a few pounds, you usually reach a plateau where it becomes more difficult. For some weeks you might not drop another ounce. If there were some easy, quick way to measure flab daily, you could see that you are losing fat even though your weight remains unchanged. Remember that even when you aren't losing pounds, you are burning off fat if you are faithfully engaging in sufficient aerobic exercise and eating sensibly. And it's fat that you want to get rid of.

Your ultimate goal should be losing what jiggles and bulges where it's not supposed to. Another goal might be to lose a dress size or a couple of inches on belt size. Whatever goal you set, be realistic.

At the ORU Health Service we work hard to help everyone set realistic goals. Our fat-control program is positive, effective, and popular for the most part. An overwhelming majority of those who have participated have been helped toward a new life-style that is healthy and slender.

As I mentioned, our standards classify obesity level at 24 percent fat for male students and 34 percent fat for females. People at obesity levels are placed in special exercise and weight-control classes. Their goal is to lose eight pounds and at least 1 percent of body fat during a sixteen-week semester, an average loss of one-half pound per week. We have found that almost anyone can reach these goals if he or she is not bound or hampered by other problems.

Of course many students exceed the loss of eight pounds per semester. Some have dropped as much as twenty and thirty pounds during one semester. We always ask students to be careful over Christmas and summer vacations. These are critical periods to guard against regaining any of their lost weight and fat. Then they are asked to lose another eight pounds and additional percentages of body fat during the next semester. This routine continues until the students reach levels of fat percentage that are termed "below obesity."

Tina is a good example of someone who made excellent progress over the year. While she didn't lose quite as much body-fat percentage as needed, she did drop in weight according to her goals, and she held that figure through those critical Christmas vacation and summer vacation times. Tina came into our program at 44.5 percent body fat and at a weight of 209 pounds. By Christmas she had dropped to 42.1 percent body fat and she weighed 196. By year's end her weight was at 191—a total loss of 18 pounds over the year—and her body fat was at 39.6 percent. She held those numbers over the summer and came back the next fall to continue working hard in the program with new resolve to reach her coveted body-fat-percentage level of under 34 percent.

Obviously most of the readers of this book will not have the benefit of the Oral Roberts University HPER weight-loss program. You're probably going to have to do it on your own. If you have no significant physical problems (other than excess flab), here is an outline of how to proceed. You can plug into the following steps at any point, depending on how much weight and fat you need to lose:

1. If you are in the "high obesity" range (anywhere from 50 to 100 pounds or more overweight), make your goal the loss of 50 pounds per year until you reach a level below 34 percent body fat (women) or below 24 percent body fat (men). You will, of course have to establish your body-fat percentage to begin with. You can do this with underwater weighing or some form of skin-fold estimate.
2. Once you drop out of high-obesity range (above 34 percent body fat for women and 24 percent body fat for men) you are in what I call "low obesity" level or "overfat." Your fat percentage will be around 20 to 24 percent for men and 30 to 34 percent for women. You will still want to work on losing fat and weight and at this level a loss of twenty pounds per year is realistic. Your body-fat percentage will drop accordingly.
3. As you drop below 20 percent body-fat percentage for men or 30 percent body-fat percentage for women, you are approaching your final goal. You will recall that previously I gave a range of "ideal body-fat percentages": 11 to 17 percent for men and 17 to 22 percent for women. As you work toward your ideal weight and percentage of body fat you should aim for a loss of around ten pounds per year. At this stage don't be in a hurry; your body will be in much better condition and will be taking its time about losing those last pounds and percentages. Shoot for a slow, steady decrease in skin-fold thickness over several years of time.

One more word about measuring percentages of body fat: At the ORU Health Service we have found that the only accurate way to measure

Exercise and Nutrition 51

people in high-obesity levels is with underwater weighing. Skin-fold calipers just aren't reliable because in a highly obese person the skin is pulled too tight to allow for the correct amount of "pinching" of the skin. Once you are in the low-obesity range, however, calipers do the job quite well. You may get so interested in your new "flabless" life-style that you will want to buy your own set of calipers. On the other hand, you may be content to get measured by your physician, or at a local Y or fitness center.

As you set your goals and work toward them, remember one thing: Losing fat permanently is a slow and steady process. Put out of your mind forever the psychology and reasoning of people who push crash diets, losing a few pounds in order to get into next summer's swimsuit, and so forth. If you try to lose fat rapidly, you may succeed temporarily, but it will just come back, usually worse than before.

By faithful use of aerobic exercise, you can reach your "perfect" fat and weight levels. *Once you are there, however, don't stop your aerobic-exercise program.* If you do, all your work will be lost and the flab will return. You will have to maintain workouts at least three or four times a week to stay at the level where you want to be.

Sincere flab fighters are sentenced to life on the aerobic road. You can walk it, jog it, run it, bike it, or swim it, but you *can never get off*. Interestingly enough, you won't want to. You'll be hooked on being thin, happy—and healthy!

WHY WALKING IS A "PERFECT" EXERCISE

Up to this point I have emphasized over and over that engaging in aerobic exercise *does not* mean that you have to become a world-class Olympic athlete. Many people equate aerobics with jogging or running, covering three to ten miles a day at brisk paces like eight minutes per mile, or less. We read constantly of marathons (a distance of over twenty-six miles) or "ten K" runs (approximately six miles). All of this is there for you only if you get into great condition and want to participate. If running or jogging is not your bag, however, you can always walk your way to victory over flab.

As my good friend Charlie emphasizes, the key is not outstanding athletic accomplishment; the key is learning to be active at a pace that is pleasant and easy for you. Charlie's full name is Dr. Charles T. Kuntzleman, and he is one of the leading health and fitness experts in the country today. While an executive at the national level in the YMCA, Charlie has developed three national YMCA fitness programs. He has also written more than a dozen books on health and fitness along with conducting over 100 fitness and weight-loss workshops across the United States and Canada during the last few years. He is a national director of Living Well, Inc.

In one of his books, *Your Active Way to Weight Control,* Charlie makes some excellent suggestions for developing an active life-style that will result in a slender, healthful you. One of his chapters is titled, "Walking, the Perfect Exercise." Here he quotes a study by Dr. Michael Pollock of Mount Sinai Hospital, Milwaukee, Wisconsin. Dr. Pollock used a group of healthy, yet sedentary, men between the ages of forty and fifty-six. After twenty weeks of walking two and one-half to three miles a day, at least four days a week, the transformation in the physical condition of these middle-aged men was fantastic. Following is a lengthy excerpt from Charlie's book that gives you his reasoning and enthusiastic endorsement for walking as an aerobic exercise:

> Naturally, for walking to be aerobic, you need to "walk with authority." If you shuffle a few steps, stop and smell the roses, and then shuffle a few more, it probably won't increase your heart rate more than ten beats. Instead, step out. Swing your arms. Hold your head up high and walk with pride. Move just fast enough to make you breathe deeply. You will soon discover walking can keep you at your target heart rate, burning those calories and fat away.
>
> It's safe. Unlike most recreational sports there is no one to bump into, no fast ball to dodge, no tackler to avoid, no apparatus to fall from, and no barbell to drop on your toes. When you leave your house for a walk, you are engaging in a safe, yet healthy, exercise. Walking is an exercise that spans all age groups. It is a great exercise to do together. What better way to enjoy fitness than as a family.
>
> Remember, the key to any exercise, including walking, is your pulse rate and personal feeling. Your walk should also be painless. If you experience any chest pain, jaw, or neck pain, slow down. If that doesn't stop the pain, see your doctor and describe what happened.
>
> The minimum of twenty minutes is recommended. Six days per week is your ultimate goal. If you take more than two days off, you will lose the benefits from your walking program.
>
> Build walking into your life. Here's where the fun comes. And creativity. As you begin to examine your life-style, you will find innumerable ways to program more activity into your daily routine. You can turn those idle moments into pleasurable, fat-burning walking. Here are some suggestions:

1) Never drive less than one mile. Think of the number of trips you make that are less than one mile, to church, to the post office, to school. Make a pact with yourself, that from this day forward I will walk instead of drive whenever the trip is less than a mile. You will save gas and burn a few calories with each trip.
2) Park in the good spots. You may need to reconsider what good means. The really good parking spots are the ones that no one else wants, farthest away from the entrance to the store, factory, or office, but you never have to fight to get one. You can pull into your spot, get out, and take a brisk walk to your destination and still probably get there faster than the people driving around in circles looking for a spot up front.
3) Have a walking lunch. Instead of standing in line at the fast food counter or waiting in a crowded restaurant for the waitress to bring you your order, carry a whole wheat sandwich and some fruit, or a thermos of soup, and walk to a park bench. Enjoy your lunch. Then spend the remainder of your lunch break walking. Great nutrition and great exercise.
4) Take a short walk just before supper. The usual routine for a person who works is to walk through the door, grab the newspaper and a drink, then sit down until dinner. This type of break, however, is hazardous for the health-conscious. Drinking a beer or a mixed drink increases calories and elevates your appetite. Consequently, you end up eating more for supper and feel like doing nothing more than returning to the easy chair and an evening of television. The end result is an evening of sitting and eating. A pleasant ten- or fifteen-minute walk can be effective in reducing the job tension from your day, and often exercise tends to curb your appetite. In the end you win out by dealing with tension and fatigue in a positive way, probably consuming fewer calories, and getting in a little extra walking.
5) Avoid elevators and escalators. It sounds simple, but in exercise every little bit helps. Besides, you usually get there quicker this way since there are no waiting lines.

Walking may not be perfect, but it's the closest to perfect as an exercise suited for anyone, anytime, and any place. It burns up calories to help you lose weight and it produces positive changes in your cardiovascular system, and walking is as close as your front door.[9]

While I'm a jogger myself, I agree completely with everything Charlie says in the above paragraphs. He makes a convincing case for walking as the "perfect" approach to aerobic exercise. Even though I jog long distances for the most part, I still do a great deal of walking as well. Furthermore, I see additional living proof of the benefits of walking in Peggy, who is now a nurse on our department staff at ORU. You might say she walked her way into the job.

Peggy came to school to work on a B.S. degree in nursing. Because she was at 35.5 percent body fat and 178 pounds, she got into our program to reduce high-level obesity. By year's end she was down to 166 pounds, a bit short of our goal of eight pounds per semester. But her body-fat percentage was down to 28 percent, which was excellent progress.

The change in Peggy's self-image and confidence level was also extremely noticeable. I believe it is safe to say that she never would have had the courage to ask for a job in our department if she hadn't participated in the aerobic program.

She continues to work on her weight and fat percentage. I see her every day at work, of course, but more encouraging is seeing her after hours walking up a storm on our track for thirty to sixty minutes five or six times a week. She's looking better all the time.

Walking does work. My suggestion is to get out there and try it. Most of us had to crawl before we could walk. Many of us need to walk before we jog or run. The good news is that walking is all we need. So, go for a walk—right now!

WHAT YOU SHOULD KNOW ABOUT THE "SETPOINT THEORY"

All along I have been loudly insisting that exercise is the key to losing flab and keeping it lost. A relatively new concept called the "setpoint theory" lends further weight to the case for continued exercise. In their new book, *The Dieter's Dilemma,* Dr. William Bennett and coauthor Joel Gurin describe scientific research that strongly suggests we are all programmed genetically to have a certain level of fatness.[10] This genetically determined internal control system, or "setpoint," originates somewhere in the brain. Your setpoint acts like a sort of thermostat that tells the body how much fat it should carry. Some of us come with a high setting on our "fat thermostats" and others have a lower one. We get that setting at birth; it is the luck of the genetic draw.

As I mentioned earlier, we all have our permanent number of fat cells by the time we are in late adolescence. The setpoint theory says we inherit that number of cells and there's nothing we can do about it. Other theories say we develop our fat cells throughout childhood and if we overeat as children, we wind up with more and larger cells than we should. All the scientific evidence is not in yet, but I believe both theories probably apply. We are genetically programmed at birth with a "setpoint" of fat cells. If we overeat as children and as early adolescents, that setpoint can be raised even higher.

Once the setpoint is established, it is almost impossible to change it through dieting only. The setpoint theory says that when you go on a diet—particularly a crash diet with a very low calorie intake—your body rebels. You see, your body doesn't know the difference between a crash diet and starving to death. Your setpoint "thermostat" starts working overtime to do two things:

1. The setpoint mechanism sends signals to your metabolic system that say in essence, "The body is starving! Slow down—don't burn the calories so fast."
2. The setpoint system sends signals to your appetite control center that say, "You're hungry! Eat more to get the body back up to its proper level."

While it is still an unproven theory, the setpoint concept provides an excellent explanation for why many—if not most—people who try to lose fat and weight by dieting only almost always regain what they lose. Their setpoint always counters the weight loss and sooner or later (usually in less than six months and sometimes in a few weeks) they are right back up where they were. Their setpoint keeps them in a certain range, and they can't go below that range for very long.

Not only that, but if you're not careful, you can *raise your setpoint still higher* by eating too much rich food that is high in fat, and particularly sweets. And as if that isn't bad enough, even artificial sweeteners, which have no calories to speak of, can drive your setpoint up![11]

In an interview with *Executive Fitness Newsletter,* Joel Gurin, coauthor of *The Dieter's Dilemma,* explained that the absence of calories in artificial sweeteners doesn't really help because the taste of the sweetener acts on the brain in such a way that it raises the setpoint and makes the body want to store more fat.[12]

All of this seems to send us back to square one. Those of us with a high setpoint are predestined to have a certain percentage of fat and a certain weight. Is there nothing we can do? Actually there are several ways to turn down your fat thermostat. Brain or intestinal-bypass surgery are options, but not very attractive or advisable. Bennett and Gurin also believe that the use of chemicals, such as those in diet pills, can turn down the setpoint—as long as you keep taking the pills. Nicotine also seems to affect the setpoint and many smokers can testify that when they give up smoking they gain weight.

None of the above are very healthy approaches to the problem, however. That leaves—you guessed it—*exercise*. Bennett and Gurin believe that aerobic exercise acts like a handle to crank down your setpoint.[13] As long as you maintain an adequate exercise program (at least thirty minutes of aerobic activity four or five times a week), you can eat normally and maintain your lower setpoint. Stop the exercise program, however, and your setpoint creeps right back up again to its old level.

One major reason aerobic exercise effectively lowers your setpoint is that it increases your metabolic rate. You have probably heard (or used) the typical argument given by people who are overfat: "It's my metabolism—it's just slow." We also hear over and over that skinny people eat more than Mr. and Mrs. Flab, but the skinny ones never gain an ounce. And for the most part this is true. The startling but proven fact is that fat persons, on an average, eat *less* than slender ones!

It is true that sometimes the slender person can thank his lucky genetic stars that he can eat all he wants but never gain weight. But all slender people aren't necessarily programmed from birth to be that way. Through an active life-style and exercise, they have changed their metabolism to include a predominance of fat-burning enzymes.

Enzymes act as catalysts in your body to stimulate the fat-burning process. Your body is like a factory that burns two kinds of fuel: sugar and fat. Without going into a short course on biochemistry, it is essentially accurate to say that people who are overfat have a predominance of sugar (glucose) burning enzymes; people who are fit and in the ideal range of body fat have a predominance of fat (fatty acid) burning enzymes.

To come back to the comparison of your body to a factory, remember that we eat three basic kinds of food: fat, carbohydrates, and proteins. Your "factory" converts all three of these foods into body-building materials and fuel. The fuel is produced in two forms: fatty acids and glucose. When you eat fat (a lot of butter, for example) little conversion is necessary, and the butter becomes fatty-acid fuel. When you eat protein (for example, eggs) or carbohydrates (for example, bread), your body's conversion machinery breaks these foods down into glucose (a fancy word for sugar).

What happens, then, if your daily routine is not very active? (Remember, by "active" I mean some form of aerobic exercise for at least twelve minutes at a time.) If you are not active, your body burns little or none of the fatty-acid fuel. Instead, it burns primarily the glucose (sugar). If you overeat even a little bit, the chances are good that your body's boilers will not burn all the glucose. At this point another conversion process takes place in your cells. Any excess unburned glucose is *converted to fat* and stored as flab—on your tummy, arms, legs, or other embarrassing locations. And, needless to say, if you have also eaten a certain amount of fat, the fatty-acid fuel never gets burned at all and it, too, gets stored as more flab.

But when you become more active, particularly with some kind of aerobic exercise, you gain two tremendous benefits:

1. You have more muscles, which you build through the exercise, and your muscles consume more fuel (calories). Your muscles are like motors in your body that burn your fuels—the fats and the glucose.
2. By consistently participating in aerobic exercise, the enzymes in your muscles, where your metabolism takes place, literally shift from the type that function primarily to burn glucose (made from carbohydrates or protein) to the kind that burn fat as the main fuel.

This shift from sugar-burning to fat-burning enzymes that occurs through exercise is why a world-class runner like Frank Shorter (winner of the gold medal in the marathon at the Munich Olympics) burns as much as 80 percent fat as fuel while he is just sitting down. Through his extensive running and training programs he has built a slender yet muscular physique that promotes the burning of fat.

Keep remembering that the key to having all of this work for you is to *stay with your aerobic exercise program.* If you go on it for a while, then quit for a while, and then try to go back on it, you will have disappointing results. It seems that the fat-burning enzymes are unstable. Your body soon switches back to the sugar-burning enzymes if you sit around for very long. But even gentle running or brisk walking will at least keep you with 50 percent fat-burning enzymes and only 50 percent sugar-burning enzymes.

Quit your aerobic exercise program, however, and the percentages will go more into the 70 to 90 percent sugar-burning and only 10 to 30 percent fat-burning enzymes. And, of course, as you allow your body "factory" to convert over to burning more sugar than fat, your setpoint acts accordingly and puts more fat back on your body—back to that genetically predetermined range that keeps you anywhere from a little too flabby to a great deal overweight.

Most of what I have said above is a very simplistic explanation of the many complex activities that go on in your body all the time. If you want to know more, I highly recommend Covert Bailey's excellent book *Fit or Fat?* Bailey's nontechnical writing and clear diagramming will give a good picture of how your "factory" operates. But if you have had enough talk about enzymes and fuel conversion just remember one basic fact: *Fit persons are fatty-acid burners and fat persons are sugar burners.* You can change from an overfat person to a fit person by exercising and building the kind of enzymes that burn fat rather than sugar. Over a period of time, aerobic exercises will literally change your metabolism and make you a more efficient fat user. You get a higher metabolic rate with consistent exercise.

As I said earlier in this chapter, the setpoint theory is unproven. Some people call it pure speculation, and others even label it quasiscientific nonsense. Nonetheless, evidence from scientific studies (described in great detail by Bennett and Gurin in *The Dieter's Dilemma*) is piling up. And regardless of what you might think of this setpoint theory, there is overwhelming evidence that continued aerobic exercise reduces fat content in your body and brings your weight down as well. There's also overwhelming evidence that trying to lose fat and weight by diet only is a difficult, if not hopeless, task.

If you aren't so sure you agree with the setpoint theory of Bennett and Gurin, I offer you the "exercise level theory" of Jim Krafft, which simply says: Fat content (flab) accumulates or disappears in direct proportion to the amount of aerobic activity engaged in.

I have seen it work in my own life; I have seen it work in the lives of hundreds of people here at Oral Roberts University. And it can work for you—if you are willing to do just a little work yourself!

WHY BEING WELL INCLUDES MORE THAN LOW FAT PERCENTAGE

Earlier in this book I stated that any percentage of body fat above 24 percent for men and 34 percent for women is in the category of "sick," or disease producing. The opposite of sickness is wellness, and one of the major goals of this book is to promote wellness to anyone who will listen.

Fortunately wellness is an increasingly important concept in our thinking in America. A priority item for me is serving on the board of directors of the Organization of Wellness Networks, a group of experts and specialists who come from many disciplines that have to do with health and fitness. This group meets annually to exchange information and discuss methods of promoting wellness among the general public.

In the last few years I have observed that when I talk about wellness, people are much more apt to listen. Medical care is costing more than we as a nation can afford. The alternative to medical care is the prevention of illness, and it's a far more attractive alternative emotionally as well as economically. None of us desires illness, yet our life-styles continually cause us to be ill. We spend billions of dollars annually to fight illness and bring ourselves back to point zero—not being sick. Not being sick is often referred to erroneously as "health," but recovery from disease is far from a total state of health. Our birthright as human beings is creative well-being, or moving into what I call "positive wellness." Helping people achieve creative or positive wellness is my purpose in life.

Wellness includes a lot of things. It encompasses stress management, job satisfaction, the environment, social relationships, and other factors, but none of these is central to who a person really is. I believe man lives in a body, but he is essentially a spirit with intellect, will, and emotions. Wellness of the spirit is the hub about which every other facet of wellness revolves. You can be totally free of excess fat, but if you are in the midst of a spiritual desert you are in a far worse state than many obese people. Personally, I believe the human spirit is only well when it is properly related to God. The vital first step in wellness is faith.

Bruce Larson has written the book *There's a Lot More to Health Than Not Being Sick*. The title of Bruce's book rings true. I strongly recommend that you read it. You should be well in every aspect of your being, not merely your fat percentage.

If wellness becomes a cult of physical health only, it has badly missed its purpose. A human being is a whole person with many facets. The body is important, but it is not primary. If the advice in this book produces an active slender person who is nevertheless miserable, I have failed.

God has created a marvelous physical house in which we can live, and we have the opportunity to assist Him in its care. I believe we honor God when we do all we can to keep that house—the body—well and healthy.

It is not too surprising that depression is one of the major illnesses in America. More than 50 percent of our population experiences significant depression at some time during life. Many of these depressed people are fat. Since the most widely documented help for depression is walking, slow jogging, or other aerobic activity, we are able to treat effectively two conditions at once: being overfat and being depressed.

I have personal knowledge of both conditions. When I was in my late forties, my first wife died of cancer, and I went through a period of typical depression. Also, I had periodic bouts with tension and anxiety that built up through job pressures.

My own passion for jogging comes from a multiplicity of reasons. I began around age fifty, largely because I felt something could be done about some minor electrocardiogram changes, which I discovered when I was examined at the Kenneth Cooper Aerobics Institute. At that time I had a body fat content of almost 24 percent and weighed 206 pounds. In addition I was suffering from an arthritic condition that developed after I was exposed to dysentery on a trip to Mexico. My rheumatologist told me that I couldn't do any walking or jogging for at least six months, but after a brief stay in the hospital, I started anyway. The first year of walking and jogging was difficult, but I stayed motivated because I wanted to become more fit and healthy.

Now I run slow and long, purely for fun. I find that jogging is the best method for releasing tension and emotional pressure. Even now, on some rare days, I will have a run that is totally uncomfortable and even painful, but I have learned the difference between harming myself and going through a certain amount of beneficial pain. In some mysterious way even those occasional runs of drudgery have a quality of joy.

Many times, but not always, I have experienced a mystical, almost unbelievable, breakthrough experience. This usually occurs about forty minutes into a jog. Now I much prefer jogging or running to competitive sports like racquetball or tennis. In fact, I now regularly give up opportunities for racquetball or tennis because I find these somewhat boring as compared to a slow, relaxing run.

I am not enthusiastic about competition, but I still enter long distance races purely for the comradery and excitement of being with others. Even though I finished last in my first marathon (26.2 miles), I enjoyed a tremendous sense of accomplishment, completeness, and exhilaration. I have now completed six marathons.

I still battle anxiety and tension, which are the precursors of depression. That's why I usually do my jogging after work, when I am able to regain my equilibrium and feelings of well-being. I find it difficult to explain clearly my passion for jogging. Perhaps the most important point for me is that in my daily exercise experiences I find myself genuinely close to God.

My aerobic activities have provided many direct physical benefits. My arthritis is gone and my electrocardiogram reads perfectly. But even without the specific physical results, I believe I would continue jogging just for the relaxation, clearing of the mind, and the outstanding spiritual rewards.

I have written this work with the sole purpose of trying to convince you to start aerobics or to keep going in what you may have started already. I firmly believe the key to wellness is aerobic exercise.

A FINAL WORD ON THE FIRST WORD

The message of this work was epitomized when one of my colleagues, Dr. Lynn M. Nichols, was checking over my manuscript. He was reviewing the section, "The First Word Is Not *Diet*," and remarked, "Isn't this a mistake? You are saying that the essence of losing fat is exercise. I thought the essence of losing weight was a sensible diet."

To correct that kind of misconception is precisely why I wrote this. It has been so engrained in us that diet is the way to lose fat that it is extremely hard to get across that the real way to lose fat is by regular endurance exercise.

I will say it one more time. *Dieting is helpful, but the way to lose weight, the way to lose fat and keep it off, is through exercise.* And by exercise I mean aerobic activity, carried out regularly for the rest of your life. Aerobic exercise is slow, easy, and continuous and it builds the fat-losing, or fat-burning, enzymes. As Covert Bailey has said, "You become a better butter burner." Exercise increases your metabolism.

Losing weight and fat is not done through restrictive dieting. It is done by having fun through regular, sustained, enjoyable exercise. So burn that butter, Baby! And while you burn it, have fun and get slim.

God bless you as you become a winner at the losing game!

Source Notes

1. Dr. Bailey's fine book makes an excellent companion to the present volume. See Covert Bailey, *Fit or Fat?* (Boston: Houghton Mifflin Co., 1978).
2. Barbara C. O'Conner, "Body Fat and Its Effects on the Health of a Group of College Coeds As Shown by an Investigation of Their Visits to the Health Clinic," a thesis prepared in partial completion of a master's degree in public health, 1980.
3. Donald Cooley, *How to Lose Weight* (New York: Random House, 1956), p. 13.
4. Cooley, *How to Lose Weight,* p. 12.
5. Hal Higdon, "Slow Down," *Parade* (August 30, 1981).
6. Hal Higdon, "Ten Most Asked Questions About Exercise," *The Physician and Sportsmedicine* (September 1980), p. 112.
7. Robert Atkins, *Dr. Atkins' Diet Revolution* (New York: Bantam Books, Inc., 1981).
8. See, for example, Covert Bailey, *Fit or Fat?* chapters 23 and 24.
    Another excellent little book is *Eating Smart* by Judith Stern, Sc.D., nutrition consultant to Campbell Soup Company's Turnaround Program, and R. V. Denenberg. Box 8688, Clinton, Iowa 52736.
9. Charles T. Kuntzleman, Ed.D., *Your Active Way to Weight Control* (Spring Arbor, Mich.: Fitness Finders, 1980).
10. William Bennett, M.D., and Joel Gurin, *The Dieter's Dilemma: Eating Less and Weighing More* (New York: Basic Books, Inc., 1982). In chapter one, "Fat and Fate," Bennett and Gurin present the thesis that reducing diets are not effective for weight control because of the body's predetermined setpoint, which dictates how much fat one should carry.
11. Bennett and Gurin, *The Dieter's Dilemma,* p. 100.
12. "On Losing Weight: Is Fat Fate?", *Executive Fitness Newsletter,* vol. 13, no. 20 (October 2, 1982), Rodale Press, Inc.
13. Bennett and Gurin, *The Dieter's Dilemma,* p. 7.

2
Fitness
Cecil B. Murphey

BE A BETTER YOU!

Remember when you wore a size eight and you prided yourself on your tiny waistline?

Remember when Mom said you had a bottomless pit for a stomach, because you ate constantly but didn't gain weight? When older folks kept trying to fatten you up?

Do you sigh, recalling those bygone days, silently wishing you could be thin, healthy looking, and in shape once again?

You can be.

Would you like to run up a flight of stairs or chase the kids across the yard and not pant for breath? How would you like to get back into those clothes you wore in high school?

You can do it.

How would you feel if someone who hadn't seen you for ten years said, "Why, I hardly recognized you. You look so young—and in such good shape"?

It can happen to you!

How would you like to feel good—really good—about yourself? Wouldn't it be great not to wear your clothes loose to cover blobs of fat? Wouldn't you like to peek at your reflection in store windows, smile, and think, *I look great?*

You can do it.

That's the purpose of this book—to help you become a better you.

Exercise and Nutrition

Don't take my word for it. Ask others who have shaped up. They'll give you wonderful physical reports—
  lowered blood pressure
  less anxiety
  steadier heart rhythm
  healthier-looking skin
  lower cholesterol levels.
Here's what Edna said eight months later:
  "My posture has improved.
  I have less stiffness in my joints.
  I don't suffer from chronic fatigue the way I used to."
"What do you get out of physical exercise?"
I asked this of several friends as well as members of the American Fitness Center, in Jonesboro, Georgia.
Here is a sampling of their replies:

- "I've got more energy."
- "Greater self-esteem."
- "I'm more optimistic about life."
- "I'm not as tense as I used to be."
- "I've lost weight and inches around my middle."
- "I fall asleep quicker."
- "I don't need as much sleep as I used to."

Consistent and regular exercise makes these changes!
Many of us adults are out of shape. But we haven't always been flabby, tired, and achy.
Think back. Remember your childhood days.
As children we didn't need to be urged to exercise. We did it naturally.
Unfortunately, we tend to decrease our physical activity after the age of twenty-five.
Then the results of soft living hit us:

- Flab develops.
- Muscle tone decreases and muscles atrophy.
- This causes more flab.
- The muscle tone decreases . . . and the cycle goes on.

Most people not only decrease or stop their exercise at twenty-five, they also fail to cut down on their food intake—eating as much at forty as they did twenty years earlier, when they were more physically active.

Once we reach thirty, we need fewer calories every year!
That's not all . . .
Instead of continued physical activity and lower caloric intake, we stretch out on a comfortable sofa. We put only the same small group of muscles through repetitive patterns of action. Day after day, year after year.

Yet . . .
        we have more than 600 muscles and 200 bones.
Putting it into practical terms, to stay firm, strong, and flexible:
   We   **need**   **exercise.**

> Exercise strengthens while inactivity wastes.
>
> HIPPOCRATES

THE SHAPE-UP CRAZE

Did you know that *today*—or any day—more than 70 million Americans will practice some form of physical exercise? That's half our adult population. And yet, according to the November 2, 1981 issue of *Time* magazine, only about one-fourth of the population exercised regularly in 1961.

Jogging, for instance, has been growing in popularity for more than a decade. The Peachtree Road race, run annually in Atlanta on July 4, has had to *limit* entrants to the first 25,000. The Boston Marathon, because of its increased popularity, now is limited to those who can meet certain standards of performance.

Football players of the Los Angeles Rams attended jazzercise classes twice weekly in the spring of 1982 in an attempt to stay in shape and keep limber during their off-season.

The Serious Athletes

Statistics indicate that Americans have become serious about physical fitness. Consider these figures as estimated by experts in the field. America now has:

- More than 20 million runners
- 6 million (mostly women) jazzercisers, dancercisers, or aerobic dancers
- 13 million biceps builders
- 20 million on a diet right now.

We're also listening to warnings about too much sugar, too much salt, the addition of preservatives and, additives to our food, and we're learning to eat balanced meals.

We now read package labels in the supermarket as we search for artificial ingredients and hidden poisons, and we love the word *natural*.

Books such as James Fixx's *The Complete Book of Running* and *Jane Brody's Nutrition Book* have hit and stayed on the best-seller lists for months.

Fitness-conscious Americans can recite information about vitamins and minerals and are moving toward more simplified meals avoiding heavy starches, and rich desserts, and are moderating in the amount of red meat and whole milk products we use.

Even the fast-food chains now offer salad bars, and we're eating more green and yellow vegetables, whole grains, and fruits.

We have rediscovered miller's bran (the residue from the production of white flour) which not only aids in bowel regulation but possibly is beneficial in preventing diverticulitis and cancer of the colon.

THE EXPERTS SPEAK

Recognizing the fitness boom in our country, a question-and-answer column in *Better Living* (June, 1982) asked, "What do you do to keep in shape?"

Top cardiologists answered the question, each urging people to get involved in a personal fitness program. All but one spoke of his own fitness program (and most of them listed jogging).

One expert pleaded for people to stay in motion with what he called nonstructured exercises, such as standing instead of sitting, moving around frequently, and taking stairs instead of elevators.

Nicholas Kounovsky, author of *The Joy of Feeling Fit,* and vocal exponent of physical fitness, has served as consultant to national and international organizations, foundations, and publications. He says, "Fitness makes for joy in living."

Eleanor Metheny writes in *Connotations of Movement in Sport and Dance:*

> We [women] play tennis for the same reason that men paint pictures, sing, play musical instruments, devise and solve algebraic equations, and fly aeroplanes ... because it satisfies our human need to use our human abilities, to experience ourselves as significant, creative, and, therefore, personalized beings in an impersonal world.

Kathryn Lance, author of several books on fitness, including *Running for Health and Beauty* and *Getting Strong,* said she was a 120-pound weakling. After getting into a fitness program that included weightlifting, she felt much stronger after only twelve weeks. "I had also improved my figure and general well-being. Best of all, I was able to maintain my new level of strength by exercising only once or twice a week. The exercises, which had been difficult at first, became easier and more pleasant week by week."

Katherine Switzer, the first woman to run in the Boston Marathon, said in an interview, "Sports are as natural—and as good—for women as they are for men."

GETTING PSYCHED UP

Before I try to get you psyched up, I want to tell you how I psyched up myself.

"You need to exercise," I told my flabby reflection in the mirror.

My reflection agreed.

Unfortunately, I made one tactical error. I said, "I'll start a serious program next week."

Within a week my commitment to physical shaping up had died like hundreds of other ideas for self-improvement.

Exercise and Nutrition

Two years later, I said, "I'll run—starting today." *And* I followed through.

First, I measured one mile with the car—half a mile out and half a mile back.

Then, in sloppy clothes and walking shoes (not knowing much about running shoes) I started out.

I burst into full speed—and for at least ten seconds I felt great. I didn't even reach a quarter of a mile before I stopped, fell to the ground and panted. Minutes later, I huffed as I walked back home.

During the following year I would start a shape-up program and stay with it for a couple of weeks; then I'd miss a day. Once I started to miss exercise days, I was ready to quit again.

> Then, tired of my flab,
> > scared of my soaring blood pressure
> > concerned because of my lack of energy

I prayed.

> "God, I'm going to shape up. I'll do everything I can. Help me stick with it. Don't let me give up."

That was eight years ago. I'm still at it.

It happened like this: Howard, a thirty-five-year-old and the victim of a heart attack, worked out three times a week at a health spa.

He invited me to go with him. I joined the first day.

"I want a program to get me into shape and tone up my muscles," I told an instructor at the spa.

The instructor gave me a list of exercises that took about twenty minutes. (Most of these exercises could have been done at home without any special equipment.)

That's how I got started.

Others have psyched themselves up differently.

Wilma and three friends get together five mornings a week for a lengthy walk. They've been doing it for three years.

Two businessmen go into the equipment room at lunch and do calisthenics together for ten minutes each workday.

My daughter Cecile got into running by reading books and magazines on the subject.

A friend said, "Everyone in my neighborhood started trimming down and shaping up. Whenever we had neighborhood gatherings, fitness became the central topic of conversation. I started exercising and joined a racquetball club so that I could feel part of our community again."

If you're not already involved in a shape-up program, do something to get yourself enthused.

Such as . . . Read books on health.
Subscribe to fitness magazines.
Ask friends.

Check on programs and courses on getting into shape offered by recreation centers, the "Y," your local college, or the office or factory where you work.

We all notice people who are in good physical shape, often staring in envy not only at their body contours but their graceful walk, their sense of well-being, and their look of self-assurance.

Do you know someone like that? She may be a co-worker, someone who attends the same church you do—maybe a neighbor. Select such a person and start a conversation:

"You look as though you're in great shape,"
you say. "How do you do it?"

Most people who walked the flabby road, and left it by shaping up, become wildly enthusiastic when asked such a question. They'll often give you all kinds of hints. (They might even agree to help you get started.)

Try this:
Each morning, stand naked in front of your mirror.
Stare at yourself.
Say aloud,
"God made this body.
I'm responsible for taking care of it
and keeping it in shape."

Here's another tip.
Think of yourself as a house owned by someone else, in which you're the tenant.

"You're responsible for doing repairs, cutting the grass, and whatever needs doing, but you pay no rent," the owner says.

How would the owner respond to seeing the yard overgrown with weeds, garbage on the back steps, and windows broken?

Apply that idea to yourself. "What can I do to this body to show God I want to take care of it?"

Exercise and Nutrition

Read everything you can about physical fitness *and* disease. Learn about hypertension, emphysema and other respiratory ailments, heart disease, diabetes. This is not to frighten but to inform—*and* as a reinforcement to get your body into shape.

Join a biking club or one devoted to bikers and joggers. In most metropolitan areas, the local newspaper lists weekly sports activities. Take up a sport—but make sure it's one that requires constant motion. Racquetball, squash racquets, running, walking, and swimming have good overall benefits. Tennis requires a lot of movement for poor players. (The better you get, the less you move!) What about an aerobic-dancing class? Take up clogging or square dancing.

Many of the above involve participating with others. For some people, that's the only way to get psyched up to begin.
Most important,

SET A GOAL FOR YOURSELF.
Make it a realistic one.

For instance, it may be as simple as, "In three months I will walk two full miles, four times a week."

    Write out your goal.
    Display your goal on the refrigerator.
        Tape it to your mirror.
        Put a copy on the dashboard of your car.
        Why not take one copy to work? Tape it just inside
            a drawer you open several times a day.

                Stop right now. Write down your goal:

                _____
                _____
                _____

Find ways to remind yourself of this goal.

Tell your friends. Urge them to ask you each week for a progress report.

My wife found that putting up slogans and cartoons in the kitchen helped her stay away from excess food and reminded her of her goal to get into shape.

    GOD DOESN'T WANT ME
        TO BE FAT.
                                        TASTE MAKES WAIST

A friend has this over her sink.

>DON'T BE A HUMAN
>GARBAGE CAN

Next to the scales, at a local health spa, they have an enlarged colored photo of a glob of fat with the caption:

>This is what five pounds of extra fat
>looks like.

Try *imaging*.
Imaging, a technique that has come into wide use in the last decade, works like this.
Look at yourself frequently in a mirror or a glass window. In your mind, however, envision yourself the way you'd *like* to be.
Keep this image before you daily—every time you catch a reflection of yourself.
This constant input of positive self-imaging can help motivate you to act out your imaging.

Try prayer.
God cares about you because He created you. Ask His help in your proposed program. Ask Him to help you discipline yourself.
P.S., Also, forgive yourself in those instances when you neglect your exercise program for a few days or blow your diet.

FOUR PROBLEMS

Since I've become addicted to fitness, I talk to people about shaping up. I've heard dozens of excuses, reasons, and problems.
The four problem areas most commonly mentioned are:

1. "I don't have time."
Wrong. We have time for what we believe is important. If concern for our health and general well-being become important to us, we will find time. We all do the things we consider important. As long as we complain, "I don't have time," we're actually saying, "Fitness isn't that important."
2. "I don't have the energy."
We hear people say, "When I get home from work, I'm so tired, I just want to collapse."

Exercise and Nutrition

Or, "By the time I get the kids to bed, I'm too worn out for anything physical."

That's the time to get into shape. If you were in good shape, you wouldn't be that tired out.

Further, the tiredness probably has not come from physical activity *but from the lack of it.*

3. *"Women who train look like amazons and lose their femininity."*

Actually, it's the opposite. Women who lift weights, for example, develop *firm* muscles, but because of their thicker subcutaneous layer of fat, they don't bulge the way men do.

More important, the female body retains its contours. Muscular development of the chest improves the bust line. The thighs and hips, the real trouble spots, are s-l-i-m-m-e-d by exercise.

4. *"But I . . ."*

This covers any other problems you have that prevent your getting into shape.

But if you want to *look* your best, *feel* your best, have more energy, and retard aging, you'll realize that instead of problems, you have a great opportunity. You can even say, "I'm going to get into shape, starting today."

TO DIET, TO DIET

For most people, getting in shape means that horrid word: *diet.*

Whether they feel the need to round off an inch at the hips, and two at the waist, or for an overall slimming program, they continue to face the starkness of the word.

A friend recently said, "Is it an accident that the word *die* is there? When I try to lose pounds, I feel as though that's what I'm going to do—die!"

To diet . . . to diet . . .

But before thinking about specific diets, let's look at food.

Food—we all need it. Among other reasons, because it supplies our energy.

Experts long ago classified four basic food groups to help us in getting a well-balanced diet every day:

    milk and dairy products
    meat and other high-protein foods such as fish and eggs
    fruits and vegetables
    grains (as in bread) and cereals

All diets revolve around these four food groups, restricting some, forbidding others, insisting on a few, and suggesting additional portions.

Body weight follows a simple rule. When we eat more food than we need to meet the demands of our body, we store the excess in our body as fat. And we gain weight.

If we eat less than our body demands, we take energy from those fat deposits and burn them up. We lose weight.

Before you rush out to try a newly published diet, here are a few things to bear in mind:

Jane Brody, in *Jane Brody's Nutrition Book,* emphasizes that no one diet fits everyone's problem. We're all different with different needs. She also acknowledges that some people need a "higher authority" to tell them what to avoid and what to eat.

For such people,
> a structured diet may be the answer.

But no matter what diet you choose, bear in mind these three things:

1. There's no shortcut to thinness.
2. You probably took years to put on your excess weight. Be willing to take a year to get it back off, especially if you're 20 percent, or more, overweight.
3. The real answer for keeping off pounds isn't a perpetual diet, but devising a new life-style—a life-style of eating *and* exercising that keeps you healthy, provides nutritionally balanced meals, doesn't deprive you of the pleasures of food.

HOW DENSE ARE YOU?

Did you know that your weight could increase from 150 pounds to 160 and yet not affect your actual size?

Or your dress size could go from a twelve to a ten, and yet the scales still show you at the same weight?

How can that be?

The answer: *body density.*

Outward appearance (such as dress or shirt size) doesn't accurately indicate weight. We also need to consider the body density.

Low body density occurs when you don't use up the food energy you absorb. Instead you store it in the form of fatty deposits in your tissues. This initially increases *size,* not weight. People with low density have a tendency to be less healthy, even malnourished. Their bodies burn calories less efficiently. Fatty tissues are larger than other body tissues.

Exercise and Nutrition 75

High body density occurs when you burn up more food energy than you absorb and have to use stored energy to keep you going. This converts the fatty contents of your tissues into muscles (firms your muscles). Muscle tissue is heavier than fat tissue. That means weight can rise while dimensions remain the same.

Stable body density means that you use the same amount of food energy that you absorb, and the density of your body remains the same.

Body density changes in all of us.

If, for instance, you become extremely active, you will have a high body density. You can eat larger-than-normal meals and your weight will stay the same or might even increase by as much as ten pounds, while your measurements remain the same.

When thinking about density, here's the rule:

> The higher the density,
> the fitter you are.

Fat-free tissues yield more energy and work with less strain. If you want to get the most from your food and to achieve the greatest freedom of movement, high density is your goal.

ISOMETRIC, ISOTONIC, AND THOSE OTHER STRANGE WORDS

For the past decade, physical-fitness experts have tossed certain terms around for us to absorb.

Here are a few of the common ones:

Exercises characterized as *aerobic* (*aero* means air) are those that require the increased and steady use of oxygen for a significant period of time—usually at least twenty minutes. Using sufficient oxygen to meet the demands of these exercises that require endurance and stamina is thought to be beneficial to the cardiovascular system.

> Examples of such rhythmic, sustained exercise are continuous running, bicycling, and swimming.

Anaerobic exercise results in bursts of energy production from short spurts of explosive activity. Rather than depending on oxygen for energy, fuel for this type of exercise is the carbohydrate glycogen stored in muscle fiber and released with the start of activity.

An example of anaerobic activity would be the game of racquetball. It is characterized by quickness rather than endurance.

Isometric exercises came into prominence a few years ago with the promise that men could double their muscle strength and bulk in six minutes a day by performing exercises that required approximately six seconds each.

These exercises involve contracting a muscle and holding it in a static position for a few seconds.

> Example: Press your arm against a wall. The muscle is contracting, but it isn't going anywhere.

Isometrics work. Those using the exercise do build bigger, stronger muscles. *But* the muscles work best only in the position in which the exercise is being performed. That is, if you press against a wall with your arms for ten seconds a day, your muscle will become much stronger—but mostly when it performs an action similar to that of pushing against the wall. It does gain some strength throughout its entire range of motion.

Isokinetic exercises are performed on machines that provide constant resistance against the muscles as they go through the whole range of motion. The Nautilus is the best known isokinetic machine; it promises to produce greatly increased strength in a short period of time.

> The disadvantage is that you need machines that are expensive and very large. You will probably have to join a health club to get the use of them.

Isotonic exercises are those in which you raise or lower a weight through the range of motion of a muscle. Most of life's activities are done with isotonic muscular contractions. Every time you pick up a box of cereal, you are doing an isotonic movement because your muscles are moving the weight of your body.

> The best examples of isotonic exercises are calisthenics and weight lifting. Calisthenics includes such exercises as pull-ups and sit-ups, in which the weight of your body acts as a resistance to your muscles.

TOES IN THE WATER

The first time my Dad took me swimming, I was six. My older brother and one of my sisters dashed into the water and paddled around, laughing and enjoying themselves.

I wanted to get into the water, too. But I didn't know how. I remember standing on the riverbank, sticking my toes in the cool water. My sister kept calling, "Come on in!"

"I'm scared," I called back, but I did put both feet in the water. Then I took a few steps until my knees were submerged. Each step I took was harder than the one before.

Without my expecting it, Dad came from behind, grabbed me, dunked me, and then after I paddled wildly for a few seconds, pulled me back out. He didn't let me flounder alone.

"Get back into the water and start paddling, or you'll never learn," he said.

I was afraid to try. But I didn't want another dunking. I got back into the water and inched away from him.

My brother grabbed an arm, and I had my first swimming lesson. I felt awkward and paddled stiffly, but I got into the water.

That's how exercise works, too. Just sticking a toe in the water isn't enough. You have to take a plunge and commit yourself if you're going to get into shape.

Plunging in doesn't mean setting up a three-hour daily routine. It does mean a commitment to physical fitness *and* jumping in by actually doing it!

So now you're *committed.* You're psyched up. How do you get from sticking in your toe to taking a deep plunge?

1. Be sure you're convinced of the value of and need for physical fitness.

> We find time to do anything we want. When we know shaping up is important for ourselves, then we're ready to jump in.

2. Remind yourself that even though you sweat, grunt, and it tires you the first few times, you're going to feel better about yourself after you've established the habit of physical fitness.

> Ask former flabbies. Let them tell you how much better they feel about themselves and about life. This matter of physical fitness reaches into all areas of life. For example, more than one psychiatrist now realizes that a crucial step in rehabilitation for psychiatric patients involves their seeing themselves as effective human beings. These doctors have put their patients on a physical fitness program

and have noted that they learn to feel good about their bodies and about themselves.

3. Enjoy your exercise program.

   You won't stick with any program unless you enjoy it. In devising your own fitness program, make it as much fun as possible. Especially incorporate "cheating" exercises (*see* pp. 84–90). And give yourself at least a three-month trial to make it a vital part of your life.

4. Get positive reinforcement.

   Ask for reinforcement if you have to. Tell two or three cheerful types (avoid the pessimists) that you plan to get into shape. Explain your need for encouragement. Ask them to tell you every time they see any improvement in your appearance or attitude.

5. Begin today.

   Don't wait for a better time. (There never is a better time.) Don't wait until you can join a health club. You can do most exercises in normal clothing, in any place. Schedule exercises into your daily pattern. If you can't find twenty minutes at a single period, break it up: Five minutes in the morning, five at noon, and another five before or after the evening meal. That's fifteen minutes squeezed into your day.

6. Encourage yourself.

   Each day as you start your exercises, encourage yourself by saying aloud such statements as:

   > "I will stick to my program."
   > "I'm going to be a better me."
   > "I'm going to become physically fit."

Most of us believe what we hear repeated frequently. Say your own words of self-encouragement, speaking positively of your goals and determination. You'll learn to believe that voice!

BEFORE YOU DO YOUR FIRST EXERCISE

Choose a time based on personal preference and daily schedule—one that you can keep *regularly*.

Exercise and Nutrition

Regular activity is more beneficial—and healthy—than sporadic work. A four-hour Saturday session is too harsh on your system, and one day a week doesn't do enough. Plan some form of exercise for a minimum of three times a week.

Have a set schedule of exercises for yourself. (You may vary or change them later.)

Forming the habit of same-time-same-place-same-activity helps assure you of continuing with your exercise program. Don't rush. Relax when you exercise. This is time set aside just for you.

Learn to breathe properly in doing exercises.

Exhale through your mouth with lips half-closed; inhale through your nose, nostrils wide open. If you need additional air, open the windows.

Choose exercises that involve all parts of the body, separately as well as together.

Don't be too ambitious.

Proceed carefully and slowly. Don't overtax yourself, especially in the beginning. Begin by performing a small number of exercises in a minimum number of repetitions. Increase this gradually but never to the point of fatigue. Moderation is your key to successful exercise and fitness.

Exercises become easier with practice.

It takes time and patience to learn new skills (remember when you learned how to drive?). Exercising becomes easier as you practice. Once you begin an exercise program and stay with it, it becomes increasingly easier.

Make at least a three-month commitment to yourself.

It often takes three months for people to establish the habit. (In running, we say it takes up to three months until people become addicted!) If you persist, exercise will become a natural part of your life. You'll find it one of the highlights of your day.

Look your best when exercising.

Sound strange? A valuable secret of successful exercise involves looking as attractive as possible at all times. The way you dress improves what you see in the mirror. Wear leotards or practice shorts that look good on *you*.

Even if you have flabby curves, you want to keep reminding yourself that they'll go away in time. Say aloud, "I'm going to be a happier, more attractive me."

Your workout clothes will help!

Do your exercises smoothly and rhythmically.

Each motion in an exercise can be learned and performed in a graceful and efficient way, without strain and without using excessive energy. Make certain you carefully follow instructions on all exercises. Follow the rhythm indicated, not in jerky motions, but in a smooth flowing count. Keep your toes pointed in the direction of the movement, hands and arms graceful. Keep your face pleasant and avoid a tense look or a grimace or labored breathing and puffing. If you have to puff to do an exercise, you are working too hard!

Plan your program carefully.

Many factors go into determining how much exercise you need. Experts base programs on your calendar age and your physical age, as well as the length of time since you last engaged in vigorous physical activity.

Calendar age is important but physical age more so. You can be old at thirty, still young at sixty—it depends on your health, your attitude, and your fitness.

If you have any question about physical exercise, talk to your doctor first.

If you're taking any regular medication, don't even put your toe into the water until you've been assured that it's okay.

And finally . . .

Don't strain.
Don't overdo—especially in the beginning.
When you get tired, *stop*.

A WORD ABOUT BREATHING

Don't hold your breath during exercise.
Holding your breath causes muscle contraction that closes the glottis (opening between the vocal cords in the larynx) which increases the

Exercise and Nutrition

pressure inside the chest cage. This action decreases the amount of blood returning to the heart, resulting in a loss of oxygen when most needed.

Improper breathing can also cause tightness in the neck, dizziness, and headaches.

Breathing freely is better for anyone—but especially for those with lung or heart disease.

For example:

> In push-ups, exhale during the pushing up, inhale while lowering your body.
>
> When running, exhale every other time your right foot strikes the ground.

During heavy exercise, if your breathing rate *exceeds* fifteen times in fifteen seconds, this is a signal to slow down or decrease the exercise.

SHAPE-UP EXERCISES

How do I shape up?

How do I maintain physical fitness without large amounts of time and heavy energy drain?

Here we describe conventional exercises that affect every part of the body. Do them regularly. Once you've mastered them, you may want to add, change, or even modify them to fit your individual needs.

> Time: At least fifteen minutes, three times a week. Twenty minutes daily is ideal.
>
> Place: Anywhere you're comfortable, but as much as possible, make it the same place each time. (We're all creatures of habit and most of us are sensitive to our surroundings.)

Be sure to incorporate suggestions from section on cheating exercises.

Warm-up Exercises

1. Jumping Jack. Stand with arms at side. Jump. Spread the feet to the side, and simultaneously swing the arms overhead on count of one. Then swing the arms down and jump back to the starting position on count of two. Try to do it rhythmically and at a moderate cadence.

For beginners, no more than fifteen repetitions.

2. *Deep breathing.* Stand with feet comfortably apart. Slowly swing your arms forward and upward, raise up on the toes, and inhale deeply until the arms are in an overhead position. Swing the arms down, drop to the heels, and exhale as the arms are returned to the starting position.
   Repeat five times.

3. *Side Twister.* Stand with feet comfortably apart, arms extended out to the sides, palms down. Slowly twist to the side as far as you can, bob gently once, and repeat to the other side. To relieve strain on the knees, turn the far foot slightly in as you twist.
   Do five on each side.

4. *Knee Bends.* Men, stand with feet comfortably apart; women, with legs together, hands on hips. Bend the legs to just short of a ninety degree angle, extending the arms forward for balance as you go down, then return and repeat in a slow to moderate cadence.
   Do this ten times.

5. *Slow Jog.* Stand in place with the arms in a running position. Slowly jog in place or in a small circle for fifty counts (count only as your left foot strikes the ground).

6. *Waist Stretch.* Stand with your legs apart, arms at shoulder level, elbows bent. Twist your body to the right, keeping your hips immobile. Twist your body to the left, exhale as you twist, inhale as you straighten up.
   Repeat six times.

7. *Waist and Back Balance.* Sit on the floor with your knees bent, feet off the floor, arms forward. Slowly extend one leg and then bend it. Extend the other leg, bend it, and continue for ten times, alternating legs.

8. *Hip Bump.* (For women only.) Sit on the floor, legs extended in front, lean back, arms at an angle, the weight on your palms. Lift your hips and twist your body to the left, then bump your hips on the floor. Lift hips again, twist your body to the right, and bump the floor again.
   Repeat twenty-five times each side.

Top-to-Bottom Exercises

1. *Toe Touch.* In each of the following four positions, bend down and touch the toes and then return to your starting position.
   a. With feet apart at shoulder width
   b. With feet together
   c. With legs crossed at the knees—first with right over left
   d. And then with left over right
   Repeat four times in each position.

2. Sprinter's Drive. Place hands on the floor at shoulder width and lean forward with your right leg well up under the chest, with the left fully extended to the rear. Alternate leg positions in a two-count rhythm as follows: (a) shift positions (b) return to the starting position.

Do this ten times.

3. Push-Ups. Women, keep the knees in contact with the floor throughout the movement. Lie flat on the floor with hands directly under the shoulder joints, fingers pointing straight ahead. Straighten the arms and raise the body in a straight line from head to heels for men (from head to knees for women) to a fully extended position supported by the arms and toes (knees for women). Lower the body in a straight line by bending the arms until the chest comes to within an inch of the floor.

Repeat in a moderate rhythm up to ten times.

4. Sitting Stretch. Sit with feet together, hands at the sides. Without bending the legs, bend the trunk forward, tuck the head in, reach forward as far as possible, and grasp firmly around the legs, ankles, or feet, according to the extent of your reach. Hold for the count of six, relax, and return to the starting position.

Do five times.

5. Side Leg Lifts. Lie on one side with the legs together, the head supported by the elbow and hand, and the other hand on the floor in front of the body for balance. With the leg straight, lift it as far as possible and return to the starting position.

Do ten on each side.

These basic exercises help shape up all parts of your body.

1. Master all of the exercises.
2. Do them regularly—at least twice a week.
3. Then eliminate or add exercises.

You can do them all.
    You have only 8 warm-up exercises
          +
           5 top-to-bottom exercises
           ―――――
           13 separate exercises

Best of all, you can do them all in about fifteen minutes!

If any of the exercises seem difficult at first, perform only a part of it, such as a slight knee bend instead of a full bend, *but* progress until you can eventually do the full exercise.

After you can do all the exercises the suggested number of times without undue fatigue, increase the repetitions slowly by one or two a week.

DON'T-JUST-SIT-THERE EXERCISES

Even if you're sitting all day at a desk, or too tired to move from your easy chair in the evening, *you can exercise.*

And you can exercise while you're sitting!

1. Sit at edge of chair, arms crossed, feet flat on floor. Lean back slowly. Stop just before your upper back touches chair back and hold. Slowly return to sitting position. Repeat four times.
2. Sit at edge of chair, back resting against chair back, knees together and feet flat. Keeping legs tightly together and with knees bent, slowly lift legs as high as you can, keeping your back against chair back. Hold, lower, and repeat.
3. Stretch arms up to ceiling as high as you can and hold. Then stretch arms out to side, fingers pointed upward, and push out as hard as you can and hold.
4. Sitting with feet flat on floor, arms raised, and chin tucked to chest, slowly lean forward as far as you can, trying to touch forehead to knees. Slowly curl back up and repeat.
5. Sitting straight with legs stretched out, lift one leg up to at least seat level. Keeping leg lifted, flex foot toward you as far as you can and hold. Point foot as far as you can and hold. Circle foot from ankle slowly around. Reverse directions. Then circle entire leg from hip, toe pointed. Reverse directions. Repeat as many times as you can with each leg.
6. Sit straight in chair, legs stretched out, feet flexed. Keeping legs straight, slowly lift both legs as high as possible, but at least level with seat. While holding legs in air, spread them as wide as possible, then close slowly and open again, repeating as many times as you can.

CHEATING EXERCISES

I heard one doctor say, "Calisthenics are fun. But they are of no real value unless they're done continuously and vigorously enough for at least ten minutes."

Exercise and Nutrition

Maybe he's right.

But I hate doing calisthenics (even though I do them six days a week). For me, they're boring.

I persist with calisthenics because I need them. I like getting them finished so that I can do exercises I enjoy, especially running.

If you find calisthenics boring, don't despair. You can "cheat"! And you can do it fairly, too.

Sensible dieters long ago learned to cheat fairly by substituting artificial sweetener for sugar and skim milk for whole. They've learned other tricks, which help them in their weight-control problems yet appear not to demand sacrifice.

The same thing can happen when getting into shape. You can cheat—and cheat fairly!

BUT, like creative dieting, it still demands discipline, commitment, and a basic fitness plan.

Here's how I got into creative cheating.

It began during the first years of our marriage. I taught school in those days, and it meant a dress shirt five days a week and another on Sunday—at least six every week. Because this was before the days of permanent press, it meant those six shirts had to be ironed every week.

Shirley and I shared the ironing. When she started to press the first shirt, she timed herself. It took ten minutes plus a few seconds. I did my first one in slightly under ten minutes.

From then on, we played a game. We determined that the quality of the ironing must be as good as a ten-minute job. We would work to reduce the time.

Over the next few years we cut that time down to slightly under five minutes. We not only accomplished our task (ironing my dress shirts) but had fun doing it. *The game took the chore out of the work.*

Then, thirty pounds and four waist inches ago, I embarked on a fitness program. I didn't intend to look like Arnold Schwarzenegger or a member of the United States weight lifting team. I wanted to feel good and look fit.

I tried all the conventional exercise programs. Boring! I kept at the exercises with some degree of faithfulness. But each morning it was an I-guess-I'd-better-have-my-punishment-now attitude.

Then I remembered the game Shirley and I had played with ironing. But, instead of cutting off minutes, I decided to find ways to force exercise on myself that wouldn't look or feel like exercise.

And I did! So have a lot of other people!

Let's look at some of them. After you've read through the list, perhaps you can think of your own creative ways to cheat fairly. Make it a game for yourself.

Cheating While Shopping

1. When you drive to a mall to shop, park your car as far away from the stores as possible. It's an exciting alternative to cruising up and down the lanes near the buildings, trying to find a spot closer to the store entrance.
2. Make extra trips back to your car. After you've made one or two purchases, instead of carrying several bags around, walk out to your car, put them in the trunk, and return to the mall.
3. When you buy groceries and push the cart out to your car, return the cart—not to the areas marked for that purpose, but all the way back to the store itself.
4. In the grocery store, instead of standing in front of the cereal, stand at least two feet away, forcing yourself to reach and/or bend to pick up the box you want.
5. Leave your shopping cart at the end of an aisle, go up the aisle, and as you pick up each item, return it to the cart and go on to the next item.
6. Extend your park-and-walk idea. Leave your car a full block from the cleaners. Why not walk a quarter of a mile to your dentist's office?

Inside Buildings

1. Don't ride elevators. Use the stairs. I decided that I would walk or run up steps to a maximum of six floors. If I have to visit the ninth floor, I walk my maximum and then take the elevator.
2. I go down the stairs for up to ten floors. Going down requires less energy. You might want to start initially with simply going down two flights and walking up one. Increase your floors over a course of months.
3. If you do ride the elevator, be creative. For instance, when I'm the sole passenger, I bend over and touch my toes as the elevator zooms upward. Or I do simple stretching exercises. When others ride with me, I do isometric exercises, such as leaning against the elevator wall and push, hold, relax; push, hold, relax. Sometimes I raise myself up and down on my toes or my heels. Occasionally I bend first to the left and then to right, assuming other passengers (if they pay any attention) will think my back is stiff and I'm loosening up a little.
4. Avoid escalators. Whenever possible, take the steps. If you're in a situation where you see no steps, then walk up the escalator. If you can't

Exercise and Nutrition

move ahead because of other people, do things such as turning around three or four times, as though wanting to look back where you came from. Or shift your weight from one leg to the other. How about carrying your briefcase instead of putting it on the moving steps? The two extra pounds shifted frequently from one arm to the other (even as you walk) provides a neat little exercise.

At Work

1. Exercise when you talk on the phone.
I receive lengthy calls every day. I have a long cord in my office (and a twenty-foot cord at home). As I listen, I move around, trying not to sit still during these lengthy conversations.

Try variations:
    a. Do knee bends or side bends—the kind of exercises that don't distract your mind from listening attentively.
    b. Grip the phone with your right hand, press hard, release, and then repeat. Change hands and start the exercise again.
    c. Sit in your chair, back straight and tailbone against the back of the chair. Lift both legs until they are parallel with the seat of the chair. Then raise the right leg slowly as far as you can, return it slowly. Repeat using the left leg.
    d. Sit straight and pull in your stomach muscles, hold a few seconds, release, and then repeat the process.
2. Don't buzz an extension. Instead, walk to that other department. Stand at the person's desk when you talk, instead of sitting.
3. Look for opportunities to carry small items. Offer to help co-workers move heavy objects. Don't scoot chairs, but lift and carry. Those few seconds of physical effort strengthen muscles most of us seldom use.
4. Bend to open drawers or file cabinets. When I open a file drawer, I stand far enough away that I have to bend. Bend from the waist, keeping legs straight.
5. Lunch breaks. If you brown bag it, go for a walk while eating, if necessary, or at least immediately afterward. Plan for at least five minutes of continuous movement before returning to work. Your afternoon will go better, and you'll have more energy.
6. Wear comfortable shoes. One way to keep moving is to wear shoes that don't make you miserable when you walk. Buy shoes that give you ease of movement and don't make your calves ache after being on them for fifteen minutes.
7. Take an exercise break every hour.
    Prolonged sitting weakens muscles in the legs and can interfere with

circulation. At least once an hour, *move*. Stand up and stretch. Walk down the hall for a drink of water. Open a window or close one.

8. Don't ask for anything to be brought to you. Get it yourself. People not only appreciate your coming for files or objects, but you get the added benefit of another opportunity to exercise.

9. When talking in a group, stand when you speak, or pace the room.

At Home

1. Plan a minimum of five minutes of exercise. As soon as you get home from work, shopping, dinner, or merely visiting the neighbors, take five minutes for physical activity. Play with the cat. Crawl with the baby, on your hands and knees. Put on a record and waltz or skip around the room. Put the dog on a leash and walk the animal for at least five minutes.

2. If you have more than one level in your house or apartment, keep your coat or purse on a different level from the front door. If you're on a single level, keep the purse or coat in a room as far from the door as possible, giving you the excuse to move that much more.

3. Get dressed creatively. Exaggerate your motions. Bend over to put on a shoe (never sit), or balance yourself on one foot as you put the shoe on the other. When putting on a shirt or blouse over your head, stretch. Stand on your tiptoes as you comb your hair.

4. Walk across the room, taking ten steps holding your abdomen in. Relax. Do it a second time.

5. When you leave the house and go to the car or the mailbox, hold in your abdominal muscles. Find ways to do this on short walks you do regularly, and it'll soon become a habit.

6. In the kitchen, it may take longer to prepare meals, but you can cheat by making every motion separate. Don't keep the salt at the back of the stovetop. Place it far enough away that you have to twist your body to reach it and twist a second time to return it. When setting the table, don't grab plates, glasses, and silverware at one time. Make the plates a trip, return for the glasses, and then the silverware.

7. In the bathroom:

   a. When brushing your teeth, jiggle to the count of fifteen as you brush your uppers. Then fifteen as you brush your lowers.

   b. As you comb your hair, jiggle up and down. Swing your hips. Play the radio or sing, and move your body in time to the music.

   c. Keep your cosmetics far enough away from the sink that you force yourself to reach for them. Stretch as far as you can for the deodorant or other items.

   d. When you finish with your facecloth, twist it as hard as you can,

Exercise and Nutrition

wringing out the water. Hold that tension a few seconds. Then twist it as hard as you can in the opposite direction.

e. Hold the cloth against your chest and then, pulling with both arms, you stretch an entirely different set of muscles than those mentioned above.

f. Do knee bends in the shower.

g. When you dry off, lift your legs high, bend forward when you towel off your back. Stretch upward and even stand on your tiptoes when you dry off your arms.

8. Make the laundry a fun thing.

At our home I do the laundry every week. First I carry the clothes hamper down the steps and dump all the clothes on the floor. Then I pick up each item separately and put it in its proper pile. This causes me to bend a lot. When loading the machine, I pick up each piece, one at a time, place it in the washer, then bend down to pick up the next.

9. Try it with dishwashing. If you use an automatic washer or do your dishes in the sink, discover ways to bend, stretch, or move. One woman told me that she does a simple kind of soft-shoe dance at the sink.

10. Avoid time-saving and effort-saving gadgets.

You don't need to go back to the hand lawnmower (although that's great exercise!), but don't use push buttons for opening garage doors. Instead, think of the great opportunity to reach down, pull up the garage door (which means lifting a heavy object), and then later closing it by pulling it all the way to the floor again.

Don't use remote control for television. This gadget only encourages you to sit longer. When you do change channels, jump up! If you're not too embarrassed with others around (or you're alone), why not get on your hands and knees and crawl to the set, change channels, and crawl back?

11. Commercial breaks during TV time can be more than moving to and from the refrigerator. Instead, make each break (or at least each half hour) an opportunity for exercise.

a. Jog in place. March in place.

b. Do knee bends.

c. Place a broom handle (or any long stick) across your shoulders, with your arms grasping either end. Stand straight, bend to the right, without moving your hips or legs. Then to the left.

d. If you have a stationary bicycle, do your pedaling then.

e. Stand straight, then lean over and place your hands on the back of the sofa, and swing your waist and hips.

f. Jump rope.

Now it's your turn:
   Follow these cheating exercises.
      Discover your own ways to cheat fairly.

Some bright person set up three rules for attaining physical fitness:
1. Don't lie down when you can sit.
   2. Don't sit when you can stand.
      3. Don't stand when you can move.

STICK WITH IT

If you're like most people, you'll want to give up your exercise program after one or two weeks. That's the time to say, "I'm going to stick with it."

The most common reason for giving up? *Boredom.*

The first few times it probably will be boring—from the time you learn the routine until you've made exercise a firmly ingrained habit. You become aware of the effort and repetition involved, and your brain might interpret all that as boredom. It may also be in your attitude. If you expect it to be dreary, you'll probably find it so. However, trying to psych yourself up by saying, "I'll enjoy every minute of it," won't work either.

If you can keep in mind the *purpose* of your shape-up program, you'll be able to stick with it. You're working to improve your overall appearance, to enhance your health, not merely to fill in ten minutes a day with activity.

Here's good news, though: The longer you work out regularly, and the longer you continue to exercise, the less you're aware of boredom. As physical exercise becomes a part of your life, your body actually looks forward to doing it—you become addicted.

You also get better at the exercises, and that increases your sense of accomplishment. Your muscles start to feel good and exercise seems natural.

But . . .
   how long does it take for exercise programs to begin to feel good?

It varies from person to person. I always urge people to stick with a program for three months. By then they're hooked.

But, until your exercise has become a firmly ingrained habit, you'll probably have to exert extra willpower to do your workouts.

If you find yourself avoiding the exercise program, ask yourself *why.* Is it boredom? That will go away. Pain? Pain from exertion is transitory and slight—some people even find this kind of pain pleasurable. Examine your reasons—and then do your shape-up anyway.

Yet even after exercise has become firmly established, you'll find days

Exercise and Nutrition

when you won't feel like exercising or when exercise sessions will be unpleasant.

Most people who work out regularly have down days. To help get you past that, I have a few suggestions.

1. Distract yourself. Work out to music. When I run, I find memorization helpful—Bible verses or poetry. A few years ago, my wife and I ran with small, homemade cards that fit into our palms—she studied Spanish, and I worked on Greek.
2. Listen to the radio—especially an all-news station. You can buy transistor radios you can carry on your body while you shape up.
3. Vary your routine of exercises. Change the place you work out for a few days.
4. Keep a record. Jot down your daily workout, including the exercises, the number of repetitions, and time spent. When I first started doing calisthenics, this kept me going—because I had to give account to myself. Some prefer a loose-leaf notebook with details noted of how they felt, alongside information on daily weight and body measurements. Whatever log or journal you decide on, keep it faithfully.
5. Trick yourself. When I've started to work out and don't feel like completing my exercises, I say to myself, "I'll only do one-third of them today," to get myself started, allowing myself to quit if I need to. Usually, however, once I get into the motion of exercise, I find I can keep going.
6. Remind yourself constantly of the positive results of shaping up.

>"I'll look better."
>"I'll age slower" (which we know is true).
>"I'll fit into my clothes better."
>"I'll have more strength . . . more energy."

7. After you've exercised, remind yourself of how good you feel. Most people have a great sense of well-being afterward.
8. If all else fails, plan to write a book on the subject. Then you'll have to shape up—*and stay in shape!*

AN ADDED BONUS: SHARPER MINDS!

Doctors at San Diego State University tested the reaction times of sixty-four men and women, ages twenty-three to fifty-nine. Half were runners, the others were sedentary. The test measured how fast each participant could react to either of two lights by releasing either the right or left index finger from a switch.

Results: The nonexercisers showed a gradual increase in reaction time, coinciding with their increase in age.

Runners, however, showed no lengthened reaction time! The oldsters proved every bit as quick as the youngsters.

Conclusion: Exercise seems to force the same kind of adaptations on brain cells as it does on muscles. It has to do with enzyme activity and blood flow.

If reaction time seems a crude measure of mental aging, the researchers argued, "it provides an excellent indication of how effectively and efficiently the processes of the central nervous system are working." They also use the same device to measure degrees of senility.

MISCELLANEOUS FITNESS TIPS

1. Exercise alone isn't enough for fitness. When you combine a physical regimen with healthy dietary habits, you can then expect to get in shape—and stay there. Someone said, "Exercising without obeying the rules of health is like swallowing two pills—the first makes you feel great, the second counteracts it."
2. The slogan of the American Health Foundation is: Die young as late as possible! Keeping physically fit helps make that slogan a reality.
3. Before you get into an exercise program, especially if you have been inactive for a long time, *start slowly*. Don't overdo—especially in the beginning.
4. The best time to exercise: regularly. Whatever time of day you prefer, aim for a schedule that keeps you exercising at least three times a week.
5. A set schedule is the easiest way to be faithful to a fitness program. Know when you will exercise and for how long. Don't rush into your exercises.
6. Breathing: Exhale through your mouth, lips half-closed, inhale through your nose, nostrils remaining wide open. If indoors, you may also want to open windows for additional air.
7. Begin by performing a few repetitions. Increase this number gradually, but never to the point of fatigue. Moderation leads to successful exercise as well as fitness.
8. Sleep: The amount you need depends on your age, habits, and needs. Some require only four or five hours; others as many as nine. The most restful (or deep) sleep usually occurs just after the first hour of slumber and then slowly lessens until you awaken.
9. Try napping! If you can take a ten-to-twenty-minute rest, you can recharge your batteries and start out fresh again.
10. Stick with it! You'll probably be tempted to quit after the first week or two. Commit yourself to stay with your fitness program for *at least three months*.

Exercise and Nutrition

11. If you lack the personal discipline to set up your program and stick with it, then consider (a) recruiting one or two others to get into shape with you or (b) joining a health spa or community center that offers physical exercise.

FINALLY . . .

At the beginning I explained how I got into physical fitness. After nearly a decade, I'm more committed to keeping my body in shape than ever before.

I'm not trying to win any prizes. I'll never look like a professional athlete. I exercise regularly and stay in shape for myself.

And for God.

Perhaps those last three words sound strange, but

God made my body and I'm responsible for caring for it.

3
Junk Food
Virginia and Norman Rohrer

PREFACE

Ever since food processors began to denature food and substitute chemicals for nutrients, junk food has been a part of the "civilized" diet. This greasy, breaded, fried, salty, spicy, heavily sweetened, chemically treated, and additive-laden food is characteristic of the fast-food phenomenon in America today. The industry dangles temptingly before our appetites hot dogs, French fries, doughnuts, frozen desserts, thick shakes, and soft drinks as children grow fat, teeth decay, resilience softens, and muscles grow flabby.

"Convenience" food was introduced in the 1940s when mom needed something quick in order to get back to the factory during World War II, while her soldier husband on the front lines was eating Spam and other artificial rations. In the 1950s hamburgers, fried chicken, and other specialties in quick-service restaurants and take-out shops became popular.

Convenience foods were heralded as a major step forward. With less time needed for simmering and basting, the frozen foods in disposable tins seemed like blessings. Children's lunches were also easier. Thanks to modern food technology, mom no longer needed to braise the brisket for sandwiches. She simply popped in those prepackaged chips. Soon youngsters discovered the delights of putting luncheon meats between white bread and munching the soft dough. The brown bread was for peasants or those strange vegetarians down the street who didn't know any better or who were so lacking in culture that they had not taken the step toward refinement.

Exercise and Nutrition 95

Twinkies, Oreo cookies, and other such tasties became available when commerce and science joined forces to distribute the nation's food. At the same time, Americans were moving from farms to cities, and family life in the United States was undergoing drastic changes. The automobile gave young people mobility, and convenience foods went hand-in-hand with the revolution.

In the sixties, waves of young Americans "dropped out" of American society to create a kind of counterculture. They expressed their dissatisfaction with what President Eisenhower had called the military-industrial complex, let their hair grow long, and put big-business food chains on their "hit list." They formed rural communes and began to grow and raise their own food "naturally" or "organically," that is, without the use of synthetic fertilizers, pesticides, fungicides, or growth hormones. Others became vegetarians and devotees of raw foods, or of yogurt and honey, wheat germ, and alfalfa sprouts with natural vitamin therapy. American society tolerantly dubbed this group "the granola generation."

Big business, ever watchful of the market, jumped on the bandwagon. Next to the sugar-coated corn, rice, and other refined cereals stood boxes of products labeled "everything natural, nothing artificial."

Still, the phenomenon of the fat teenager is a serious problem in America today. How can we lure young people away from the empty calories, grease, salt, and sugar that play havoc with body and soul? Remember: Love is not equal to the amount of food your child eats. Love sometimes grows more with less.

Let's make a start.

THE MAD CHEMISTS

No one in that dreadful winter of 1609 in the Virginia Colony spoke of "junk food" or "health food." They spoke rather of possible starvation.

No pioneer breaking virgin soil in Kentucky in 1790 even dreamed of "instant" foods prepared in a minute by adding water or heating.

No sodbuster on the Great Plains in 1880 ever gave any thought to whether or not his crops were organically produced, although of course they were.

Until 1897, all the food—vittles, chow, grub, mess, or chuck—that Americans ate was naturally grown and processed. Jerky, strips of smoked or sun-dried venison or other game meat, was a gift from the Indians. The German (Pennsylvania Dutch) settlers learned how to dry apples for their schnitz. New Englanders "corned" their beef, and Southerners smoke-cured hams, bacon, and other hog-butchered cuts. Some vegetables were preserved by pickling; cabbage became sauerkraut; root cellars held vegetables like potatoes, onions, beets, carrots, turnips, parsnips, and rutabagas all winter.

A heat-sealing process for canning that killed bacteria was introduced in the early 1800s by a Frenchman named Nicolas Appert to provide healthful foods for Napoleon's soldiers. The Civil War in the United States (1861-65) hastened the production of foods in tin cans such as tomatoes, pork and beans, sauerkraut, and fruit.

Canned evaporated milk appeared in the mid-1800s and was popularized by Gail Borden, a man whose name was used by a large dairy. City dwellers without cows could now enjoy milk that was safe and tasty. Pasteurization (heating fresh milk to kill harmful bacteria) was introduced in the late 1890s.

Railroad refrigerator cars and the household icebox (forerunner of the modern automatic electric refrigerator) revolutionized the food-processing and distribution industries of the country.

In 1897 scientists in a lab produced a shimmering, colorful gelatin-based mass that soon found a place on every American shelf and was considered to be wholesome and healthful—the perfect dessert for children, dieters, invalids—everybody! Actually, such desserts are less than nutritionally adequate. High in refined sugar and synthetic additives, they tend to contain only 10 percent gelatin, which offers a poor quality protein at best.

Americans eagerly bought the tinted-sugar formula in the early 1900s. Coal-tar-dye-colored, imitation-fruit-flavored commodities, powdered and liquid soft drinks and confections quickly followed the new dessert into the stomachs of the brave sons of the New World.

The process of freezing food was introduced by Brooklyn-born inventor Clarence Birdseye. He noticed during a trip to Labrador in the early 1900s that fish drawn from the sea in subfreezing temperatures and quickly frozen by nature tasted as delicious as fresh fish when thawed and cooked. Flash freezing mechanically, he discovered, kept the tissues of meat and vegetables from breaking down. He patented the process in 1920 and launched the modern frozen-food industry.

Canning, refrigeration, freezing—all splendid advances for the food industry—led naturally to synthetic and artificial substitutes for nature's best. In 1897 the chemists might have put on the label, "everything artificial, nothing natural," and Americans would have applauded the catch line. But we've had the piper to pay for our sins.

There is, however, the rumbling of drumbeats across the land. The call back to "live" foods and national health has begun. An apron is the banner of this marching army, kitchen cutlery, its weapons as the army of

Exercise and Nutrition

ex-junkies marches against bankrupt foods that are weakening and killing this generation.

Join the revolution! The results of yesterday's bad habits can't be totally remedied, but all who are willing to change should be prepared for some happy surprises.

HOW KIDS GET TRAPPED

Americans consume 125 to 130 pounds of refined sugar every year, 55 pounds of fat, 300 cans or bottles of soda pop, 200 sticks of chewing gum, more than 20 gallons of ice cream, 18 pounds of candy, 5 pounds of potato chips, a couple more pounds of pretzels and corn chips, 63 dozen doughnuts, and some 50 pounds of cookies and cakes—each loving every empty calorie, tempting malnutrition, reducing energy levels, and inviting the syndrome of low blood sugar (hypoglycemia) and diabetes.

Taste Buds Rule the Head

Why do junkies enjoy their addiction and make no effort to break their habit even when told of the dangers? From birth, we learn to prefer foods that taste sweet. The first nourishment that passes through our mouths is milk—mother's or cow's—which contains lactose, one of nature's basic sugars.

"The primary function of taste sensitivity [is to] determine which parts of the environment contain substances suitable as food and which do not," explains Dr. R. J. Watson of the Department of Nutrition at the University of London. "Of the four basic taste sensations—sweet, salty, sour, bitter—the first two [are associated] with the possible presence of food and the last two indicate the use of possible harmful substances."

Flavor, say the behavioral psychologists, is probably the most important characteristic in satisfying the instinctive craving that is common to all. Experience determines which flavors are acceptable. The palate does not necessarily select those foods that make up a well-balanced, nutritious diet. The brainwashing of advertising lures us into the sweetened, oily, and salted fare whose flavors dance delightfully on the tongue.

Children are taught to look upon sweets as rewards. No clean plate—no dessert is the common admonition. So dinner is endured and dessert becomes a reward.

Hidden sugars in presweetened breakfast cereals with up to 68 percent refined sugar are the most successful in fostering the junk-food habit.

"Refined sugar is an incomplete food," says William Dufty, author of *Sugar Blues*. "All nutrients have been processed out. Incomplete foods are addicting. If a body is nourished, it has a cutoff point for foods it has obtained enough of, a natural reaction. But with incomplete foods such as refined sugar, the body is fooled and continually demands more and more. It can't get its fill."

Literature supports the contention that anything sweet is good. Shakespeare writes in *Hamlet,* "Sweets to the sweet, farewell!" Samson, in the Old Testament of the Bible, proclaims, "Out of the eater came forth meat, and out of the strong came forth sweetness." Parents say, "Be nice to your sister; you'll get more with honey than with vinegar."

Western civilization gets the message and gags on it. Radio and TV ads bombard our ears, and our heart responds to the tongue's demands. Impressionable, growing children sink deeper and deeper into the morass.

ADDING UP THE ADDITIVES

Junk-food catchwords include *additive, artificial,* and *chemical.* Americans once welcomed such laboratory discoveries as saccharin and heralded them as beneficial. Today they are seen as detrimental because time has uncovered the dangers to the human body of a number of synthetic substances added to food.

The highly toxic dyes developed in the mid-1800s gave luster to the new civilized foods. Brightly colored candies appealed to the eye, as well as the taste, of children. Federal food laws were passed in 1906 because of spoiled beef sold during the Spanish-American War. This situation uncovered scandalous conditions in the meat-packing plants. Other harmful, impure, and polluted food products surfaced until the sweeping Food, Drug, and Cosmetic Act was passed in 1938 to fight such outrages as "raspberry jam" consisting of gelatinous sugar mixtures with hayseeds!

The shelves of a supermarket today offer some 3,000 additives. Their strengths, hazards, and potential damage cause widespread confusion not only for the consumer but also for the Food and Drug Administration. The FDA can authorize or prohibit the use of an additive. The chemicals and preservatives added *since* 1958 (when the Food Additives Amendment was passed by Congress) are assumed to be safe after adequate testing by their sponsors. Those on the market *before* 1958 were not pretested. These were lumped by the FDA into a middle category commonly called GRAS (generally recognized as safe) to await testing at a later date. Of the approximately 600 or so pre-1958 additives, only about half have been reviewed so far. Most have been stamped "safe," but not all.

Long-term effects and the interaction of additives with other chemicals make the testing process tedious. Laboratory experiments cannot tell the full story. To be safe, more and more people are avoiding additive-laden foods—even the ones branded "safe."

Artificial Versus Natural

Is a natural substance from plants more safe than the chemical combinations from a laboratory? Is molasses extract from sugar used for coloring safe? How about gelatin from bones used for thickening? They're natural, so why aren't they totally safe?

The answer is: because all natural substances aren't totally safe. Caffeine and quinine are good examples of natural substances that can harm the body. Caffeine destroys vitamin B_1 and makes the body jittery. Coffee consumption is now implicated in cancer of the bladder. The gum tragacanth taken from plants and used as a stabilizer in salad dressings can cause swelling of tissues and breathing difficulty in the allergic individual. So can excessive use of sugar, mustard, and pepper along with many other spices, herbs, and extracts.

Keep in mind that numerous additives taken from natural sources, such as vegetable gums, milk casein, and hydrolyzed vegetables are doctored with laboratory compounds in the process of manufacturing them. The consumer cannot always separate the natural from the artificial and cannot always label one good and the other bad. *Natural* bacteria, yeasts, and fungi can poison and kill. Sodium benzoate, on the other hand, is a laboratory chemical that can retard food spoilage and prevent illness and death.

Few Americans can dine on fresh foods daily, so additives will be part of our food supply for a long time. It's a trade off. But it's still wise to bake and freeze your own bread to avoid benzoated sodas as much as possible. It's still wise to avoid sodium *nitrate* and sodium *nitrite* in cured meats and fish (frankfurters, bologna, salami, corned beef, bacon, and ham). These chemicals retard spoilage and stop the growth of deadly botulism bacteria. They also give these foods the red coloring and flavor to which our taste has become accustomed. However, in the stomach, nitrates and nitrites are converted into nitrosamines, which have caused cancer in laboratory animals. Bacon is a high-risk food because the high-heat cooking period results in increased bodily concentration of nitrosamines. To all this is added the high salt content of cured meats, making them items to leave off the shopping list.

Synthetic additives do more than prevent spoilage. They add color, flavor, leavening agents (baking soda, baking powder), and bleaching agents (for whitened flour) and thicken, stabilize, emulsify, and tantalize the hungry eye.

Purists tend to reject foods fortified artificially with the B vitamins, iron, calcium, and vitamins A and D, which are added commercially to many cereals and dairy products. Unfortunately, manufacturers advertise products "fortified" with synthetic vitamins and minerals as "abundantly nutritious" because they are "enriched." The consumer would be far ahead to gain these nutrients in pure fruit juices, whole grains, and fresh fruits rather than in the food to which they have been artificially added in smaller amounts.

Cheap ingredients such as gums and emulsifiers that artificially color or flavor or make creamy are additional dangers because they can be substituted for egg whites or cream and thus result in a bigger profit while shortchanging the customer nutritionally and economically.

The culprits Red Dye No. 2 and Red Dye No. 4 have been stricken from the safe list, but others are still being served that are potentially dangerous. One is Red Dye No. 40, which is carcinogenic in animals, and another is Yellow Dye No. 5, which is allergenic to humans. Food processors do not always comply with orders to eliminate banned dyes and often continue to use them to our detriment. It's best, therefore, to avoid all foods containing artificial coloring as much as possible.

Astutely avoid also such additives as BHT (butylated hydroxytoluene). These antioxidants are added to prevent rancidity in fat-containing products like potato chips, corn chips, and salad oils. They serve also to maintain freshness and extend shelf life in dry cereals, cake mixes, chewing gums, and candies.

Yet another culprit among additives is BVO (brominated vegetable oil). This emulsifier is put into citrus-flavored soft drinks to disperse the cloudy citrus portion throughout the beverage. Its residue is poisonous and can be stored in body tissues.

An additive that is difficult to avoid is MSG (monosodium glutamate), an effective flavor enhancer occurring naturally in seaweed, soybeans, and sugar beets. Asians have used it for years, but it has only been used commercially in the United States since the early 1900s. MSG spices up the flavor of factory-prepared soups, sauces, stews, and seasoning mixtures. It makes meat and poultry dishes taste more "beefy" or "chickeny" than they really are. Chinese food often contains heavy doses. MSG can cause dizziness and/or headaches. Some people suffer a numbness in the head, neck, chest, and arms after ingesting it.

Adults can tolerate MSG better than children, throwing off the aftereffects in about an hour or two. However, the public cried out angrily when tests showed that MSG damaged brain cells in baby mice. It was banned from baby foods, but MSG is still on the GRAS list for many foods that young children eat. Some foods like mayonnaise and salad dressings

Exercise and Nutrition

contain MSG without the requirement that it be named on the ingredients label.

Additives in Whole Food

Restaurant fare and processed foods carry the most additives, but growers, raisers, packers, and distributors have so tampered with edibles that even whole food is tainted by additives.

DDT, in the 1940s, was hailed as the miracle substance that would save vast amounts of crops from destruction by hungry insects. But by the time the testing laboratories caught up with the hazards, residues of DDT had built up in soil, water, plants, animals, and humans. Chemicals called PCBs (polychlorinated biphenyls) have also invaded, leaving minute toxic deposits in plant life, sea life, and in the tissues of animal and human body fat.

Add to these the dozens of pesticides, fungicides, herbicides, and synthetic fertilizers, and the contaminants become even more widespread. Some ranchers medicate their poultry and cattle with tranquilizers and antibiotics for maximum weight at the marketplace, but those chemicals tend to concentrate in the fatty tissues and livers of the animals that eat them. Then they are passed on in cumulative amounts to meat-eating humans.

There are more contaminants in our "silent spring": gases, dyes, and waxes used on fruits and vegetables to make them more attractive to the consumer who likes food that is glossy and vividly colored (just as in the magazine and TV ads). Tomatoes picked green far away and reddened en route to market by ethylene gas have fewer vitamins. Green oranges are colored artificially with Citrus Red No. 2 (suspected of being carcinogenic). The dye doesn't leak into the pulp, but some manufacturers use that same dye-soaked rind in marmalade, baking, or other cooking, and that's what is harmful. Industry caucuses rose up and successfully demanded an end to the "color added" label on the rind.

Labels With Missing Ingredients

Whole foods should contain information about the dyes, waxes, gases, and other spoilage retardants and cosmetic enhancers added, but most often they do not. The FDA reasons that these conform to its "standard of identity" for that product. That means, if a jar of mayonnaise contains a certain amount of vegetable oil, plus lemon juice or vinegar, and egg yolks, it can be labeled simply "mayonnaise" (although MSG is probably among its flavor enhancers with salt, sugar, and spices).

When manufacturers began substituting more and more additives and fake ingredients, a movement was started to take some processed foods out of the "assumed" category. Ice cream is an example. This cool smoothy lost its "standard of identity" status in July 1979. Thereafter, manufacturers were required to list all ingredients on the label (except artificial coloring). The powerful dairy industry forced the government to back off on requirements concerning artificial coloring.

A Discouraging Word

The overall picture of contaminated food intake in America can be discouraging: Cola-guzzling children wandering on caffeine highs; adults with headaches from Chinese restaurant syndrome (MSG); breakfast bacon with cancer-causing preservatives sizzling in the pan; potato chips loaded with BHT; soda pop with BVO; orange skins dyed with dangerous artificial coloring; once-edible apples coated with wax—all this while the cumbersome governmental regulatory red tape, the testing inadequacies, and the threat of business loss threatens to make improvement slowly, if ever, realized.

The Escape

Try to avoid as much additive-laden processed foods as possible. Whole foods are best. Seek food that has traveled the shortest distance from farm to market with the fewest intermediate agents. Eat in-season fruits and vegetables from farm stands and products from local egg and dairy farms.

When supermarket fruits and vegetables are bought, scrub edible skins with a brush and a nontoxic liquid cleanser. No residue will be left as might be the case when using a detergent. Leafy vegetables can be rinsed in salt water for cleansing and to float out the tiny bugs from down in the leaves.

Eat in fast-food restaurants less frequently. Resist the temptation to consume junk "just this once." It's always harder to resist the next time.

Failure to take action, could be regrettable.

THE MEDIA BLITZ

Ever since 1868 when George Mortimer Pullman designed a dining car for speeding trains, Americans have been eating on the go. Kids today are eating not only on the go but also on the run.

Michael S. Lasky, in his book *The Complete Junk Food Book,* refers to junk food made and sold expressly for children as "kiddie litter." The manufacturers of sodas, cereals, and candy blanket schoolyards with free literature, which nutritionists brand as downright lies.

Exercise and Nutrition

One of these booklets distributed by the National Confectioners' Association to some 60,000 students and teachers makes the following claims:

- Candy is vital for weight watchers. "To reduce, eat candy before and/or after each meal. We can promise you it works!"
- Candy plays a decisive role as a fever fighter and actually prevents vomiting, diarrhea, and convulsions.
- Cavities in your teeth are caused by "the lack of use of the teeth in hard chewing." Candy is passed off as only a minor source of dental decay.

The National Soft Drink Association tells youngsters that soda is "a good source of water." In that case, replies Dr. Michael Jacobson, codirector of the Center for Science in the Public Interest, "it would be better to drink water."

Dr. Jean Mayer, popular columnist on nutrition for major newspapers across the nation, maintains that the literature on "kiddie litter" is "outrageous, misleading, and contrary to fact."

General Foods, manufacturers of Post cereals, once launched a multimillion-dollar advertising program in which the company offered to donate gym equipment to schools that collected specified numbers of Post cereal box tops. Their letters lamented that in the current money crunch much-needed physical education equipment could not be obtained by cost-cutting school boards. Here was a free way to get it. The school principals were put in the position of having to endorse certain cereals to get the box tops in order to get the gym equipment, and many did so enthusiastically.

TV Lure

Television is still the direct line to a child's imagination. The "box" lures them relentlessly to partake of sugary sweet foods. The Broadcast Advertisers Report says that the young TV viewer is hit an average of twenty times an hour with invitations to enjoy some sugary sweet food. This compares to seven to nine commercials an hour on prime-time adult programming. Each commercial is targeted toward the impressionable child.

Robert B. Choate, a critic of TV ads for youngsters, told the Senate Subcommittee on the Consumer (which was investigating TV advertising to children): "When you take a child who sits and watches television from the age of two to ten or eleven and sits in front of the Saturday morning TV box and listens to sugar, sugar, sugar, sweetness, sweetness, sweetness, chocolate, chocolate, chocolate, that child picks up a habit which is going to continue through life."

A contingent of outraged teachers and parents formed the Action for Children's Television in the early 1970s and formally complained to the Federal Communications Commission and the Federal Trade Commission. In one of their petitions to the FTC, Action for Children's Television (ACT) documented the misinformation and false ideals that kiddie-litter commercials provided for American youngsters.

A chief complaint of ACT was that parental advice was pitted against TV ads that "come fast and furious." The group noted that cereal, one of the hallowed "basics"—a food TV tells them is part of a balanced diet—is advertised only on the merits of being "super sweet." The youngsters are taught to equate eating the "goodies" with basic human values.

The Surgeon General's Scientific Advisory Committee on TV and Social Behavior studied children subjected to television's barrage. It found that the junk-food products advertised on TV are more frequently requested by the child than other products.

The Cereal Institute, a public-relations wing of the cereal-processing industry, estimated that 1 billion "backsides" are shown to Americans each year—that's like half a million billboards by space. Most of the backs of packages carry hype on toy premiums or free items that are sent in exchange for boxtops. (Note: Four of the major cereal manufacturers now own toy companies.)

JUNK FOOD AND BEHAVIOR

The whole thrust of junk food and behavior was the focus of the First Annual Convention of the Feingold Association of the United States held in Washington, D.C. The sponsor was Dr. Benjamin F. Feingold, a physician long associated with the Kaiser-Permanente Health Care Program in San Francisco.

The diet that Dr. Feingold sets forth for children who are hyperkinetic eliminates all foods containing artificial coloring or flavoring, and all salicylates (substances found in artificial form in most headache pills and in natural form in certain fruits and vegetables—chiefly apples, peaches, oranges, cucumbers, and tomatoes).

Each parent at the Feingold convention had experienced heartbreaking episodes with their out-of-control children. Each, after a change of diet for the child, had seen dramatic changes for the better. Some referred to the change as a miracle.

The New York State United Teachers Association, with 2,000 delegates present, passed a resolution accepting Dr. Feingold's theory on food additives and the bad effect additives have on the hyperactive children. They even went on record opposing food additives for children *and* teachers!

One elementary school has instructed teachers to show children how to read labels. Anything with the word *artificial* cannot be brought into classrooms of that school.

A dietitian in another school ordered the kitchen to bake all the breads, cakes, and cookies it served. The official gave the order to serve only white cheeses with no colorings or additives. Chocolate milk and soft drinks were banned.

The national Feingold organization seeks to persuade food manufacturers to provide more complete and detailed labeling on products for sale. One processor correctly labeled his food "pure," but children were still reacting after ingesting it. The reason was quickly discovered: The package in which the food was sold had been treated with chemicals. These were absorbed into the food and set hyperkinetic children on a tirade.

The University of California at Los Angeles, with its vast biomedical research facilities, has taken an interest in children and their diets. In a "Child Study Program" UCLA studied hyperactive boys aged nine to twelve who are now receiving methylphenidate (Ritalin) medication to keep them emotionally and physically stable. Harvard and Yale Universities, smaller colleges, and increasing numbers of medical facilities are budgeting for research in this vital area, as more and more ex-junkies want to kick the habit and make their bodies (and emotions) stronger.

"We can do without food colorings," says the PsychoPharmacological Bulletin of April 1978, "but we can't do away with additives."

The elimination of additives used as preservatives would indeed limit our choices of food. But what is more important: our national health or tickling our taste buds? The motive, in the last analysis, is commercial profit.

Problem children in America often are suffering from the malnutrition of affluence, which manifests itself as psychoses. Because of the heavy onslaught of refined grain and sugar, an unstable blood sugar is often a result and a cause of emotional instability.

Doctors Gilles Lortie and Dean M. Laird, psychiatrists at the Worcester State Hospital in Massachusetts, have noted that such emotional instability includes the "inability to speak properly, purposeless movements, incoordination, silliness, negativism, twitching, incoherence, and mental dullness."

The physicians noted also that these symptoms have at times been improperly diagnosed as epilepsy, alcoholism, brain tumor, anxiety neurosis, hysteria, and psychosis.

Researchers have known for many years that psychological disturbances are one of the characteristic signs of nutritional deficiencies. A study titled *Disadvantaged Children* tells of severely ill youngsters who seemed to lose their natural curiosity. These cases, invariably, were those of severe protein-calorie malnutrition. The malnutrition of affluence does not necessarily cause protein-calorie deficiency, but it does bring on other problems that have just as striking an effect on behavior.

These behavioral studies, related to diet, ranged from observations on schizophrenia to alcoholism.

Dr. Josef Brozek, a prominent psychologist, is quoted in the book *Food Power: Nutrition and Your Child's Behavior* by Dr. Hugh Powers and James Presley, as saying: "Deficiency of all of the major nutrients, including water, eventually affects behavior even though the mechanisms involved will vary."

Dr. Ben Feingold in *Why Your Child Is Hyperactive* substantiates his claim that behavioral disturbances and learning disabilities often originate in the artificial food flavors and colors that are so much a part of junk food and food items not generally considered harmful.

Alexander Schauss, director of the Institute for Biosocial Research, is convinced that criminals commit crimes not because they are born bad but because they *feel* bad. A criminal, he states in his book *Diet, Crime and Delinquency*, doesn't break the law because his mother didn't love him. "He is bad because he *feels* bad," Dr. Schauss insists.

Heroin addicts in Harlem were able to kick their habit faster when they first got off a diet of fast foods, colas, and refined sugar. Physical exercise was also an excellent treatment for relaxing the addicts' need for drugs. When they were able to throw off the dual sins of junk food and drugs, their appetites increased notably. Pale, thin junkies became healthy, happy, ruddy-faced men and women.

Barbara Reed, chief probation officer, Cuyahoga Falls Municipal Probation Department in Ohio, told the United States Senate Select Committee on Nutrition and Human Needs about her experiences with 318 offenders. Of these, she said, "Two hundred fifty-two required attention as to their diet and vitamin needs." Mrs. Reed added: "We have not had one single person back in court for trouble who has maintained and stayed on the nutritional diet."

One senator challenged her finding: "I wonder," he said, "how many of these success stories are because of diet and how many are because they may have been receiving special attention, someone cared about their rehabilitation."

Mrs. Reed replied, "I have been in this field for fourteen years. I was giving people a lot of loving attention before without nearly the results as now. The two work hand in hand . . . but, I just don't think kids on probation heard what we were talking about when they were so disconnected with reality that they couldn't remember what had been said. Now they do remember and it makes a big difference."

In conclusion, at the Senate hearing Mrs. Reed said: "Never before has the court had such a tool for working with the many ill people who find themselves in trouble. We wonder what the results would be if this method of treatment could also be applied to all those sentenced to jail."

The Reverend Benard Mason of Glendale, California, founder and director of the Hypoglycemia Research Fellowship of Southern California, is convinced that "junk food has given rise to all kinds of mental problems—problems which generate all kinds of behavior problems leading to senseless violent crimes."

Alcoholism, food allergies, and many excesses—how much of these among the 12 million arrests of children each year are the result of what is put into the stomach? The subject is worth all the attention we can give it—at home, at school, at work, and at play.

WHAT A PARENT CAN DO

Good nutrition can be taught in creative ways to the delight of children. If correct habits have not been established early, the problem is more difficult but not overwhelming.

A child learns by example and experience what foods to eat. Dad is more influential than mother at mealtime. Mother is *supposed* to like the food, because she prepared it. If the child sees the father relishing his vegetables, the enthusiasm is contagious.

Variety is another key. A child who grows up eating only a small variety of foods has a higher risk of being deficient in some food nutrients.

Parents need to refrain from passing on their prejudices. A woman who was forced to eat spinach when she was a child and learned to hate it, told this to a neighbor at lunch in front of her toddler. She gave a clear signal to the little boy that a certain food was undesirable.

The ages from birth to six years set the stage for a lifetime of eating preferences. Environment is important. If a child begins his years programmed to eat lean meats, fruits, vegetables, and an assortment of dairy products, he might not discover his sweet tooth until late in his childhood. Such a situation keeps health and figure intact.

Dr. George Owen and Mrs. Kathryn Kram of the Ohio State University Pediatrics Department have prepared a study on the eating habits of youngsters from one to six from all over the nation. The survey showed that 77 percent of those studied were willing to try new foods between the ages of one and two. By the time they were in the two-to-four category, their willingness dropped by 10 percent. In the year of their fourth anniversary their adventuresome spirit dropped by another 7 percent.

There is a direct link, the researchers found, between a child's lack of eating and his mother's degree of interest in preparing the food.

Social Research, Inc., an agency that has studied a thousand homemakers, concludes: Housewives are blissfully unaware of their families' nutritional needs. The sight of pale, anemic, listless youngsters or children tearing around trying desperately to outrun their sugar "crazies" is enough to make sad the hearts of those whose eyes have been opened to the bountiful blessings of wholesome food. What a legacy to leave a loved one!

An honest physician will admit: Medical schools teach a student doctor how to practice medicine. They offer one diet for diabetics . . . one diet for weight watchers . . . and one diet for heart patients. To the honest seekers for nutritional advice the doctors, in turn, offer a shrug. As for vitamin supplements: "They can't hurt you," or "It's your money, if you want to waste it."

To find out how to get children off junk food and into the nutrition scene, a homemaker is well advised to take a good look within her own kitchen. The trouble doesn't come from economy. Americans spend a hundred billion dollars every year for food. They are eating well but not wisely. Every year consumer habits grow worse. Half the American population, states the United States Department of Agriculture, do not eat a balanced diet. Substandard nutrition does not follow class, cultural, or economic lines.

Among the most neglected foods on American tables are: yellow and green vegetables, citrus fruits, and milk. The meal most often skipped is breakfast. Bodies are most likely to be deficient in vitamin A, vitamin C, calcium, and iron.

In days gone by, the dinner hour in the evening was a time for wrapping up the day together. Since one-third of all dinners now are eaten outside the home, this time for closely knit family fun and sharing is limited. Today dinner can be at any hour, sandwiched in between frenetic work and leisure.

A study of 3,500 high school students in Massachusetts showed that 11 percent of the boys and 19 percent of the girls ignored breakfast habitually. Those who did stop in the kitchen long enough to eat grabbed the first bit of fast food available and sped off to meet the day.

"At school," said Lendon Smith, a pediatrician speaking in La Canada,

California, "we should ask the students which had breakfast. We should send home the ones who didn't because they don't have a brain anyhow."

Researchers at the University of Iowa discovered that collegians who skipped breakfast required longer time to make decisions ... were less steady ... didn't produce as much work as the students who did stop to refuel.

"Small children," says Harvard University nutritionist Dr. Jean Mayer, "cannot last without a meal as long as adults because their metabolism is much faster. They burn things much more rapidly ... so that small children cannot ... function all morning if they have had no breakfast."

A survey of teen snack preferences showed that girls and boys put soft drinks, potato chips, pies, cakes, pastry, and cookies at the top.

"All advertising," Dr. Mayer lamented, "or just about all, is on the worthless foods. There is very little advertising for fruits and vegetables ... advertising represents well over a billion dollars of expenditures, and it's all directed at the less useful foods. ..."

A nutritional revolution has begun, turning our nation back to health. Won't you join, for the sake of the next generation?

A GIFT OF LOVE

While strolling through the famous Huntington Art Gallery of Pasadena, California, we were smitten by the beauty of oil paintings dating to the eighteenth and nineteenth centuries. *Blue Boy* by Gainsborough, *Pinkie* by Sir Thomas Lawrence, *Lady with a Plume* by Rembrandt, and many other paintings silently attested to the skill of the artists.

How magnificent it would be, we thought, *to leave behind a legacy like that! What are we giving to succeeding generations as a result of our short pilgrimage?*

Then it struck us. Involved as we are with natural food, we realized that we are orchestrating the kitchen to create enduring health in our children. With the spatula as our brush and the breadboard as our palette, we are painting cheeks pink, putting sparkle into eyes and strength into bones, teeth, and muscle. The image of our children might never hang on a museum's wall or be printed in a collection of art, but they would give to their children and to their children's children a heritage that money cannot buy: glowing health.

Join us by leaving to your family this gift of love. Whether you are young or old, male or female, consider adopting the following resolutions and letting them be your special legacy:

1. Establish early a reverence for food as a beautiful gift from a loving Creator.
2. Expose children to a great variety of wholesome food. Let them experience and enjoy all types of flavors and textures of food.
3. Let them see mother and dad relish natural food. Fathers have more influence upon a child's taste preference than mothers. Encourage adults to be mature and to keep quiet about their own prejudices. Discourage criticism of wholesome food.
4. Do not give food as a reward or withhold it as punishment. Rather, accept it each day as a sacred gift necessary for good health.
5. Spend quality time in the kitchen and teach that cooking is a loving art not a drudgery. Emphasize both the beauty in food and their ultimate source of health and vitality.
6. If a person has genuinely tried to enjoy a food, but the body seems to reject it, accept that as valid—at least for the time being.
7. Major on natural and raw foods and minor on the synthetic, artificial, and factory-processed food.
8. Refrain from purchasing food that is of no nutritional value.
9. Consider the use of supplemental vitamins to assure adequate supplies of nutrients for maximum health.

There may be answers in this book to questions you have never asked. We hope that your consciousness has been raised, that you will find the will to practice what we've suggested, and that your rewards will be abundant.

Eat right and feel great. It's the answer.

4
Vitamins

Virginia and Norman Rohrer

WHO NEEDS VITAMINS?

Every body needs vitamins. Without them the body would soon die. They are the essence of life.

A vitamin is an unseen chain of atoms, which forms a molecule. You can't see vitamins, but you can read the body for clues about which ones may be missing from a regular diet.

"Every cell in our body requires vitamins to carry on the business of life," writes Robert J. Benowicz in *Vitamins and You*. "A life without these essential compounds is soon no life at all. Because of its extraordinary biochemical resilience, our metabolism can maintain itself—albeit at minimal levels of effectiveness—so long as small quantities of all the different vitamins are supplied to it."

Vitamins are not drugs, stimulants, or alien chemicals. Vitamins are nutrients, available in foods, that must be consumed every day. Vitamins are not indestructible. They are quite fragile and can easily be destroyed by excessive water, steam, heat, or freezing. Some vitamins are lost when food is chopped and exposed to air.

Vitamins don't replace food, but complement and complete what is lacking. Food is needed to assimilate and metabolize the vitamin supplements. If taken on an empty stomach, vitamins can cause nausea or dizziness.

Scientists disagree about a definition for the vitamin but they agree on the characteristics vitamins share. Like proteins, carbohydrates, and fats, vitamins are organic molecules composed of carbon, hydrogen, and oxygen. Unlike inorganic minerals, which are found in the ground, vitamins must be manufactured from raw food materials by plants or animals before the body can use them. But like their mineral counterparts, they are essential, in minute quantities, for *all* life.

Your body was designed to perform the metabolic process efficiently, taking vitamins from food and making them a part of you. Because of the intricate life processes at work, nutrients pass from the ground into plants and eventually wind up in the soup. The vitamins and minerals you eat help the brain to think, the eyes to see, the heart to pump, the ears to hear, the tongue to taste, the nose to smell, and all the rest of the incredible parts to work together twenty-four hours of every day for life.

What can a tiny nutrient do? British sailors learned long ago that the vitamin C in the limes that they took along on sea voyages prevented scurvy. The fruit gave them the nickname "Limeys."

In the early sixties a patient was admitted to a New York psychiatric hospital. During his worst days of disorientation, he accidentally discovered that vitamin B_3 (niacinamide) offered dramatic relief from a troubled mental state. His doctor labeled it a fixation, however, and immediately prohibited this "imagined cure." The man quickly lost ground, but he eventually fought his way out of that hospital. He began taking supplemental doses of that one vitamin and wrote a book about his dramatic mental healing.

A woman in her early fifties began suffering menopausal hot spells that awoke her at night. A gynecologist prescribed a dosage of 800 I.U. of vitamin E taken at bedtime. (It's a good idea to take vitamin E separately from other vitamins and minerals as it can intererfere with the absorption of iron.) Result: A single little vitamin supplement banished the discomfort, and allowed the woman entire nights of peaceful sleep free from hot spells.

The USRDAs (United States Recommended Daily Allowances) were created by the Food and Drug Administration to establish the standards for listing nutrients on food labels. These lists tell you what percentage of the nutrient is contained per serving. Ten nutrients, and calories, must be listed on food labels: vitamin A, vitamin C, thiamin, riboflavin, niacin, calcium, iron, protein, fat, and carbohydrates.

Most nutrition specialists believe these recommendations are below what they have found to produce optimal health.

These USRDAs are only estimates of the amount of vitamins and minerals necessary to keep the body alive and well. They start with a perfect body and assume that all food eaten is fresh and unrefined, taken from ground properly enriched with necessary growing ingredients, and cooked correctly.

Exercise and Nutrition

United States Recommended Daily Allowances

Vitamin A	5,000 I.U.	Vitamin C. (ascorbic acid)	60 mg
Vitamin D	400 I.U.	Vitamin E	30 I.U.
Vitamin B_1	1.5 mg	Calcium	1 g.
Vitamin B_2	1.7 mg	Magnesium	400 mg
Vitamin B_3 (niacin)	20 mg	Phosphorus	1 g.
Vitamin B_6 (pyridoxine)	2 mg	Iron	18 mg
Vitamin B_{12}	6 mcg	Zinc	15 mg
Pantothenic Acid	10 mg	Copper	2 mg
Folic Acid	0.4 mg	Iodine	150 mcg
Biotin	0.3 mg		

Source: This listing of USRDAs has been adapted by the FDA from the Recommended Daily Allowances (RDAs) of the Food and Nutrition Board of the National Academy of Sciences-National Research Council. This replaces the former MDR (Minimum Daily Requirements).

When all these factors are in place, the Recommended Daily Allowances are satisfactory guides. But if a particular food has been cooked to death ... if no raw foods are eaten ... if a person is ill ... if a wide variety of food is not eaten ... if a person is enduring severe emotional or physical stress (such as worrying, recuperating from surgery, smoking, drinking, and ingesting illegal drugs) ... or if a person is allergic to certain foods high in a required vitamin, then the picture changes. Requirements vary from person to person and for the individual from time to time.

Dr. Roger J. Williams is a brilliant scientist who was director of the Clayton Foundation Biochemical Institute in Texas from 1941 to 1963, a time when more vitamins and their variants were discovered there than in any laboratory in the world. He formulated a high-potency vitamin and mineral "insurance" supplement, which appears on page 114.

Since 1900 the life span of Americans has lengthened, but the quality of health of the human species has degenerated. Merely living a long life does not necessarily indicate good health.

Many practitioners of medicine have not developed skills in helping to prevent ills. The holistic approach is neglected. It is easier to prescribe drugs than to get to know the patient. More and more pills are prescribed for coping with life and handling the vicissitudes that affect our health. As Americans take more medication in all forms—from prescriptions to over-the-counter drugs—they jeopardize the complicated chemical relationships in their bodies. When the body is given drugs, it often cannot properly absorb and utilize nutrients from food. The composition of food is not the only factor. How those nutrients are processed in the intestines is of vital importance. It is better to eat plant foods with iron along with animal protein for better absorption, for example.

High-pressure advertising and fad diets add to the problem of eating properly. Vitamin interrelationships are dependent upon the presence of many nutrients. If metabolic pathways are blocked because of drug-nutrient interactions, the body will suffer deprivation.

Fortified Vitamin and Mineral Insurance Formula

A daily dosage of six tablets provides:

A (palmitate)	15,000 I.U.
D (cholecalciferol)	400 I.U.
E (alpha tocopherol as DL-alpha tocopheryl acetate)	400 I.U.
K (phylloquinone)	100 mcg
C (ascorbic acid)	2,500 mg
B_1 (thiamine mononitrate)	20 mg
B_2 (riboflavin)	20 mg
B_6 (pyridoxine hydrochloride)	30 mg
B_{12} (cobalamin concentrate)	90 mcg
Niacinamide	200 mg
Pantothenic Acid (D-calcium pantothenate)	150 mg
Biotin	3,000 mcg
Folic Acid	400 mcg
Choline	500 mg
Inositol	500 mg
Rutin	200 mg
Para-Aminobenzoic Acid	30 mg
Calcium (calcium phosphate)	250 mg
Phosphorus	250 mg
Magnesium	200 mg
Iron	30 mg
Zinc	30 mg
Copper	2 mg
Iodine	0.15 mg
Manganese	10 mg
Molybdenum	200 mcg
Chromium	200 mcg
Selenium	100 mcg

Source: This specially formulated high potency multivitamin and mineral supplement was designed by Dr. Roger J. Williams, of the Clayton Foundation Biochemical Institute, University of Texas, Austin. It provides the completeness of all the vitamins and minerals in the original Insurance Formula in higher amounts. It is manufactured by Bronson Pharmaceuticals, a direct-mail-order firm.

WHAT VITAMINS CAN DO

Your body is an efficient chemical factory. It makes most of the thousands of different chemical compounds it needs out of the food it swal-

Exercise and Nutrition

lows. It takes food apart and recombines the various compounds in the stomach before dispatching them to combat stations throughout the body.

The nutrients that are vital to sustaining life are proteins, carbohydrates, fats, enzymes, vitamins and minerals, and water. In this section we are focusing on vitamins, although minerals are listed along with their sources. A word about protein is in order here because every cell contains it. Protein is built by the essential amino acids ingested as food. Those eight vital amino acids are: isoleucine, leucine, lysine, methionine, phenylalanine, threonine, tryptophan, and valine.

Since the body isn't a perfect chemist, some of what it uses must be ready-made from foods. This includes the essential amino acids mentioned above, which the body utilizes in building protein. It must also have ready-made vitamins. A vitamin is something the body needs in small amounts but can't manufacture.

Vitamin A comes ready-made, for example, from animal products like liver, milk, or eggs. If it doesn't get these, the body can manufacture the vitamin by using substances found in dark green and deep yellow fruits and vegetables. Sweet potatoes, melons, pumpkin, squash, carrots, cantaloupes, and apricots get their yellow color from a substance called carotene, the "provitamin" of Vitamin A. A provitamin is a precursor of a vitamin, convertible in the body to a vitamin. In dark green vegetables like broccoli and spinach, carotene is contained in green chlorophyll pigment.

If an animal eats the plant, it converts carotene into vitamin A. Thus milk offers a ready-made source of instantly usable vitamin A.

The B vitamin niacin is manufactured only if it has enough of the essential amino acid tryptophan—a substance left over after the making of protein. There is enough tryptophan in two cups of milk to allow the body to produce 25 percent of a person's daily need for niacin.

That's your marvelous body chemistry at work!

THE VITAMIN ALPHABET

Fifteen vitamins have been isolated and studied. There are probably more to be discovered.

Following are guides showing what each vitamin is, where you can find it, what it does for you, and finally, our suggestions for supplements.

VITAMIN A
(retinol, carotene)

What it is

A is the anti-infection vitamin. Fat-soluble, this first of the vitamin alphabet is a product of plant and animal life. It needs fats and minerals to be adequately absorbed into the body.

When A comes from animal sources it is called retinol, and when it comes from plants it is called carotene. This vitamin is mobilized from liver stores and transported in plasma in the form of the lipid alcohol retinol, bound to a specific transport protein, retinol-binding protein.

Vitamin A is one that can be directly obtained from a specific source—fish liver oils. If a person is sensitive to oils or has an acne problem, he or she may choose to take the vitamin in the palmitate form, which is water-soluble rather than fat-soluble.

Where to find it

Apricots, cantaloupes, broccoli, carrots, eggs, fish liver oil, sweet potatoes, dark green vegetables, yellow squash, milk, butter, cheese, and yogurt contain substantial quantities of vitamin A.

What it does for you

- Needed for bone growth
- Helps maintain healthy skin and mucous membranes
- Prevents night blindness and is prescribed for certain eye disorders
- Protects the body from bacterial and viral infections
- Is thought to be of value in retarding cancer growth

Rx for daily supplemental doses

10,000 International Units (I.U.). However, those persons of greater weight and those who endure chronic infections might find increased amounts, such as 20,000 to 50,000 I.U., effective. (These higher doses should be taken only under supervision of a physician.)

Results of deficiencies

- Eye problems
- Night blindness
- Chronic infections

Exercise and Nutrition

VITAMIN B₁
(thiamin)

What it is

Thiamin was the first B vitamin to be discovered. It is found mostly in plant life and is water-soluble.

Where to find it

Whole grain cereals and breads, wheat germ, dried yeast, milk, oatmeal, fresh pork, vegetables, soybeans, and peanuts all are rich sources of vitamin B_1.

What it does for you

- Promotes a healthy nervous system
- Controls aerobic metabolism
- Necessary for growth and appetite
- Aids in the functioning of the digestive tract

Rx for daily supplemental doses

50 mg. This amount must be taken along with the entire B family of vitamins so that the body can best synthesize it and utilize its value. Vitamins B_2 and B_6 in the same amounts as B_1 especially are needed.

Results of deficiencies

- Beriberi
- Stunted growth
- Irritability

VITAMIN B₂
(riboflavin)

What it is

Riboflavin provides biochemical reactions necessary for the cells to live. It is water-soluble and must be ingested daily.

Where to find it

Brewer's yeast, chicken liver, fish, milk, cheese, eggs, beans, nuts, green leafy vegetables, plums, and prunes offer the body riboflavin.

What it does for you

- Helps to convert dietary protein into energy
- With vitamin A, maintains mucous membranes lining the respira-

tory, digestive, circulatory, and excretory tracts
- Fosters health in the nervous system, skin, and eyes
- Helps to control the development of the fetus

Rx for daily supplemental doses

50 mg

Results of deficiencies
- Sensitivity of eyes to light
- Digestive disturbances
- Lesions of the lips, mouth, eyes, skin, and genitals

VITAMIN B_3
(niacin, niacinamide, nicotinic acid, nicotinamide)

What it is

This vitamin results from the interaction of intestinal flora with the amino acid tryptophan.

Where to find it

Foods yielding B_3 include beef liver, chicken, pork, lamb, veal, roasted peanuts, swordfish, tuna, halibut, and yeast.

What it does for you
- Forms a coenzyme essential for metabolizing carbohydrates, fats, and proteins in all cells
- Necessary for normal liver function
- Promotes normal functioning of nervous system and digestive tract

Rx for daily supplemental doses

300 mg

Exercise and Nutrition

Results of deficiencies
- Pellagra, a deficiency disease resulting in a skin rash, dementia, and severe diarrhea
- Irritability, headaches, loss of memory, appetite suppression

VITAMIN B$_6$
(pyridoxine, pyridoxal, pyridoxamine)

What it is

Vitamin B$_6$ is essential for the metabolism of amino acid proteins.

Where to find it

Bananas are a good source of pyridoxine, along with beef liver, chicken, pork, brewer's yeast, peanuts, herring, mackerel, salmon, soybeans, and walnuts. The heat of cooking is especially destructive of this vitamin.

What it does for you
- Serves as a coenzyme in all cells and is necessary for their metabolism of protein and fats
- Assists in formation of red blood cells
- Needed for central nervous system activity

Rx for daily supplemental doses
50 mg

Results of deficiencies
- Sores of the skin, lips, and tongue
- Anemia
- Convulsions

VITAMIN B_{12}
(cobalamin, cyanocobalamin)

What it is

Cobalamin is essential for the normal functioning of all body cells—particularly those in the bone marrow, the nervous system, and the gastrointestinal tract.

Where to find it

The clinical source is the intestinal flora. In food it is found in liver and kidney of lamb, pork, beef, and veal, egg yolk, crab, salmon, sardines, herring, and oysters. Heat, light, and oxygen (in the processing of commercial food) tend to destroy vitamin B_{12}.

What it does for you
- Cobalamin synthesizes nucleic acids (DNA and RNA), proteins, and fats from dietary raw materials.
- With folic acid, it regulates the formation of red blood cells and genetic materials.
- Maintains the health of nerve-cell membranes, tissue membranes, the intestinal tract, bone marrow, and growth hormones

Rx for daily supplemental doses

100 mcg

Results of deficiencies
- Pernicious anemia
- Retarded growth
- Degeneration of the nerves and spinal cord
- Nervous symptoms

FOLIC ACID (B COMPLEX)
(folacin, folate)

What it is

Small amounts of this vitamin are synthesized by intestinal bacteria.

Where to find it

The name is derived from the word *foliage* because it is found in green-leaved vegetation. The principal sources are kidneys, liver, the heart of beef, lamb, pork, and chicken, asparagus, bran, tuna, yeast, and spinach.

What it does for you
- As a coenzyme in all cells, folic acid participates in the synthesis of nucleic acids (DNA and RNA), choline, and enzymes necessary for all cell divisions.
- Maintains the nervous system, intestinal tract, sex organs, white blood cells, and normal patterns of growth

Rx for daily supplemental doses
0.4 mg (400 mcg)

Results of deficiencies
- Disruption of cell and tissue functions
- Pernicious anemia and other anemias

(The use of oral contraceptives increase the body's need for the vitamin. Women who cease taking "the pill" because they desire conception are advised to have adequate folate stores before becoming pregnant. Maternal undernutrition may result in a greater deprivation to the fetus than has previously been believed.)

PANTOTHENIC ACID (VITAMIN B_5)

What it is
This B vitamin has been termed by the Food and Nutrition Board, "the highest of biological importance."

Where to find it
Sources rich in pantothenic acid include brewer's yeast, beef, pork, lamb, chicken liver, eggs, herring, raw peanuts, and bran. It is a major constituent of the honey bee's "royal jelly."

What it does for you
- Along with pyridoxine, pantothenic acid is vital for the body's defenses against infectious diseases.

- Protects against stress
- Serves as a coenzyme needed for carbohydrate, protein, and fat metabolism in all cells
- A requirement for the body to synthesize essential body fats from basic fatty acids

Rx for daily supplemental doses

100 mg

Results of deficiencies
- Susceptibility to infection
- Digestive disorders

VITAMIN H (B COMPLEX)
(biotin)

What it is

Biotin is a common vitamin found in many foods, but it is no less important than any other.

Where to find it

As is the case with most of the B complex vitamins, biotin is synthesized by intestinal bacteria. In the diet it comes from egg yolks, yeast, pork liver, wheat, corn, mushrooms, salmon, green vegetables, oysters, and chicken. The heat, light, and oxygen used to refine food tends to destroy biotin.

What it does for you
- Monitors the metabolism of fatty acids and helps in the synthesis of body protein, carbohydrates, and fat
- Keeps sweat glands, nerve tissue, bone marrow, sex glands, blood cells, skin tone, and hair in a healthy state

Rx for daily supplemental doses

0.4 mg (400 mcg)

Results of deficiencies

No specific disease is traced to a depletion of biotin. Deprivation, however, is known to prolong the effects of some protozoan infections.

CHOLINE (B COMPLEX)

What it is

The Food and Nutrition Board considers choline a vitamin but lacks sufficient evidence to recommend an RDA.

Where to find it

Some biochemical synthesis of choline occurs within the body. It is present also in beef liver, brewer's yeast, eggs, lecithin, peanuts, and wheat germ.

What it does for you

- Synthesizes fatty compounds that eventually become parts of cell and tissue membranes
- Is required for the synthesis of acetylcholine, which transmits impulses from one nerve to another
- Needed for kidney and liver function

Rx for daily supplemental doses

500 mg

Results of deficiencies

Tests on at least ten species of animals showed that choline deficiency leads to fatty infiltrations of the liver and severe hemorrhages in kidney tissue. Similar disorders in man include cirrhosis, liver steatosis, and chronic hepatic disease. The evidence that choline supplements relieve these human conditions is only circumstantial.

VITAMIN C
(ascorbic acid, sodium ascorbate)

What it is

Vitamin C strengthens blood vessels and helps hold the body's cells together.

Where to find it

Cantaloupes, cherries, citrus fruits (whole are best), tomatoes, parsley, green peppers, cabbage, guava, broccoli, Brussels sprouts, strawberries, and potatoes are the chief sources of vitamin C.

What it does for you

- Regulates amino acid metabolism
- As an antioxidant, it protects other vitamins and body tissues (membranes in particular) from injury caused by poisons and pollution.
- Promotes healing of wounds and helps to alleviate shock
- Helps the body to absorb iron
- Helps the body to form and maintain bones, teeth, connective tissue, and capillaries
- Assists the adrenal glands and ovaries to produce various hormones
- Regulates normal body growth
- May block formation of cancer-causing nitrosamines
- Increases resistance to viral and bacterial infections as well as to other infectious diseases

Rx for daily supplemental doses

60 mg (We suggest 1 to 3 grams daily, depending on your stress levels, environmental pollution, and exposure to diseases.)

Results of deficiencies

- Poor wound healing
- Weakening of the fibers that maintain capillary integrity
- Easy bruising, hemorrhaging, and tissue swelling
- Lethargy and general malaise
- Aching joints

VITAMIN D
(calciferol, ergosterol, viosterol)

Exercise and Nutrition 125

What it is

A fat-soluble substance, vitamin D is called the "sunshine" vitamin. When sunlight strikes the skin, it interacts with body oils and produces vitamin D, which is absorbed by the body.

Where to find it

Fish (cod liver) oils, seafood such as tuna, salmon, and herring all contain abundant quantities of vitamin D. So do milk, cheese, and yogurt.

What it does for you

- Builds strong bones and teeth
- Operates with parathyroid hormones to maintain proper mineral balance of calcium and phosphorus in body fluids and tissues

Rx for daily supplemental doses

400 I.U.

Results of deficiencies

- Skeletal malformations
- Retarded growth in children (rickets)
- Softening of bones and teeth in adults
- Imbalance of calcium and phosphorus in body tissues

VITAMIN E
(Tocopherol)

What it is

The technical name for vitamin E—tocopherol—comes from *tokos,* the Greek word for "childbirth"; *pherein,* meaning, "bring forth"; and *ol* for "oil"—the "oil of fertility." The name was given to E because its absence, researchers discovered, led to reproductive failure in rats by resorption of the fetus.

Where to find it

Fresh, whole-grain wheat products are the best sources of vitamin E. It is also found in many vegetable oils (corn, soybean, safflower oils, but not olive oil), especially when the oils have not been heated to extreme temperatures.

There is also some vitamin E in liver, beans and peas, butter, eggs, and leafy green vegetables.

What it does for you
- Needed for normal growth and fertility
- Protects Vitamin A and fatty acids from oxidation
- Maintenance of vascular and central nervous systems
- Promotes normal muscle metabolism

Rx for daily supplemental doses
400 I.U.

With vitamin E, it is important to buy only a formula that contains natural d-Alpha Tocopherol, which is 100 percent biologically active. Other tocopherols may be added, such as D-Beta, D-Gamma, and D-Delta.

Results of deficiencies
- Poorly developed muscles
- Oxygen-starved cells
- Partly responsible for baby's anemia that often occurs four to six weeks after premature birth
- Disorders of reproduction in research animals

VITAMIN K
(koagulations vitamin)

What it is
Vitamin K in foods includes the phylloquinone (K_1) of plants and several menaquinones (K_2) found in animals and synthesized by microorganisms. There are three K vitamins—the third (K_3) is a synthetic. The first two are formed by bacteria in the intestines. All are fat-soluble. Vitamin K is included in baby foods and formula as phytonadione. A Danish researcher found this vitamin while investigating hemorrhages among chickens. The Danish word for clotting of the blood is *koagulation,* and that's how the vitamin got its alphabetical identity.

Exercise and Nutrition 127

Where to find it

It is widely distributed in foods, usually at low concentrations. Aside from the intestinal flora, sources of the vitamin K group are green leafy vegetables (cabbage, kale, spinach), beef, pork, cauliflower, tomatoes, peas, carrots. It is present also in strawberries, potatoes, eggs, and bran. Yogurt quickly restores vitamin K if antibiotics have been administered for treatment of disease.

What it does for you

- Is necessary for clotting blood following a cut, injury, or surgery
- Helps to promote the health of red blood cells

Rx for daily supplemental doses

None (given to some people before surgery)

Results of deficiencies

- Hemorrhage
- Hypoprothrombinemia, a tendency toward bleeding, is a condition that results from deprivation.

VITAMIN P
(citrus bioflavonoids—rutin, narigin, hesperidin)

What it is

Vitamin P is water-soluble and required for the proper functioning and absorption of vitamin C. It contains citrin, rutin, and hesperidin, as well as flavones and flavonols. (Flavonoids are what make citrus fruits yellow.)

Where to find it

Citrus fruits are the chief source of vitamin P. The white substance under the rind, called albedo, is rich in bioflavonoids. It is also available in apricots, strawberries, buckwheat, cherries, and rose hips.

What it does for you

- Prevents bruising by strengthening capillary walls
- Promotes relief from feminine hot flashes when taken with C
- Builds resistance to infection

- Aids in preventing and healing bleeding gums
- Increases the effectiveness of vitamin C

Rx for daily supplemental doses

No daily minimum has been established. Nutritionists agree generally that for every 500 mg of vitamin C at least 100 mg of bioflavonoids is appropriate.

Results of deficiencies

- Loss of resistance to infection
- Bleeding gums
- Unnatural and painful bruising

INOSITOL (B COMPLEX)

What it is

This vitamin is not recognized by the Food and Nutrition Board as being essential to human health. Inositol can be partly manufactured in the body from other nutrients and also is quite widespread in foods. It is almost impossible to suffer a deficiency.

Where to find it

The best natural sources are brewer's yeast, beef brains and heart, liver, dried lima beans, wheat germ, peanuts, unrefined molasses, cantaloupe, grapefruit, raisins, and cabbage. Also a good source is pure soya lecithin granules. One tablespoon provides 250 mg of inositol.

What it does for you

- Essential for proper digestion of fats
- Essential for brain function
- Helps utilize vitamin E

Rx for daily supplemental doses

250–500 mg

Results of deficiencies

- Heavier deposits of cholesterol
- Sluggish metabolism of fat

Exercise and Nutrition

- Possible nerve damage
- Hardening of the arteries

PABA (B COMPLEX)
(para-aminobenzoic acid)

What it is
PABA acts as an essential coenzyme in the metabolism of proteins in the formation of red blood cells. PABA is an element in folic acid that assists in the production of folic acid by intestinal bacteria. PABA is a pantothenic acid synergist.

Where to find it
The vitamin occurs naturally in brewer's yeast, wheat germ, and yogurt. It is partially synthesized by intestinal flora.

What it does for you
- Affects glandular function
- Is thought to normalize function of pituitary gland

Rx for daily supplemental doses
30 mg

Results of deficiencies
- Digestive disorders
- Anxiety

Persons who give vitamins no thought could end up deficient in any number of nutrients. Such a situation may not be easily reversed. When it is so easy to eat right and feel great . . . to enjoy abundant energy . . . to allow your body to function at its maximum potential . . . and to ward off disease, why not get acquainted with all the vitamins God created and use them?

Test your moods and observe your reactions to foods. Eat as wisely as you can. Then give your body exercise so it can utilize the fuel you give it.

THE ROLE OF MINERALS

Minerals are the coenzymes with vitamins in numerous biochemical processes. Vitamins are delicate organic compounds; minerals are more hardy inorganic molecules. They can take a lot of physical and chemical abuse.

Although this is a section on vitamins, we shall list also the various minerals that the body needs (along with recommended supplemental doses when appropriate) because of the interdependence of the two.

Calcium

This important mineral can calm nerves and improve bone density. It's available in dairy products, greens, broccoli, and seafood. 250 mg

Chlorine

A trace (microelement) mineral, chlorine is available in table salt, meat, milk, and eggs.

Chromium

A trace mineral, chromium abounds in grains, fruits and vegetables, and brewer's yeast.

Cobalt

This trace mineral is found in liver, beef, kidney, milk, and seafoods. 1 mg

Copper

Liver, oysters, meat, fish, legumes, and whole grain foods offer copper. 2 mg

Fluorine

This mineral works with calcium to strengthen bones and teeth. Seafoods and gelatin are sources of fluorine.

Iodine

Most of the body's iodine is contained in the thyroid gland, which regulates the rate of energy exchange and controls weight. Onions, seafood, and vegetables are rich in iodine. 0.15 mg

Iron

This critical mineral is active in the production of hemoglobin (red blood corpuscles) and of myoglobin (red pigment in muscles), and is in certain enzymes. Red meat is a source, as are fruits. Heavy intake of coffee and tea interferes with the absorption of iron. The lack of adequate iron in women and children is one of the nation's most common defi-

Exercise and Nutrition 131

ciencies. 10 to 18 mg for adults and 30 to 60 mg for pregnant and lactating women.

Magnesium

A trace mineral, magnesium regulates the body's pH (a quantitative measure of acidity), and is quite active in the utilization of vitamins C, E, and the B-complex family. Figs, citrus fruits, milk, whole grains, and dark green vegetables are sources. 200 to 300 mg

Manganese

This trace mineral is an enzyme activator and important also for nerve and brain function. Deficiency is rare. 5 mg

Molybdenum

A trace mineral, molybdenum assists in the metabolism of carbohydrates and fat. It helps the body to use iron. Dark green vegetables and whole grains are rich sources. 0.1 mg

Nickel and Tin

These earthy minerals are isolated chiefly in experimental animals. Probably man does not need them.

Phosphorus

This trace mineral is present in every cell and needs vitamin D and calcium to operate properly. It helps to build bones and teeth and to buffer salts. Dairy products, fish, and legumes offer sources.

Potassium

A vital mineral, potassium operates with sodium to regulate heart rhythms and water balance. Beans, dark green vegetables, corn, wheat, oats, and bananas are sources.

Selenium

Helps to synergize vitamin E. Boys at puberty need more than girls. Improves use of oxygen. Tuna, onions, tomatoes, broccoli, and garlic are sources. 0.02 mg

Sodium

A common mineral, it keeps calcium and other minerals soluble in the blood. It regulates muscle contraction and nerve stimulation. Found in salt, shellfish, beets, grains, kidney, and kelp.

Sulphur

This mineral works with B-complex vitamins for basic body metabolism. Found in cabbage, onions, fish, eggs, and nuts.

Vanadium

The chief assignment for this trace mineral is to inhibit the formation of cholesterol in blood vessels. No known deficiencies.

Zinc

Many nutritionists believe that zinc is the most vital of the trace minerals. It is also a common deficiency. It directs the maintenance of enzyme systems and cells and helps the body to form insulin. Adequate zinc helps in eliminating prostate problems and is vital in fighting acne. Labeled commercially as the additive zinc oxide or zinc sulfate it is found in pork, wheat germ and bran, brewer's yeast, and eggs. 15 to 60 mg

Water

The most important nutrient of all is water. Nearly three-fourths of the body's weight is water. It regulates body temperature and carries varying quantities of minerals such as calcium and fluoride. These play a vital role in nutrition.

NATURAL VERSUS SYNTHETIC

A "natural" or "organic" vitamin comes from plants and animals. A "synthetic" vitamin comes from a laboratory.

Heated arguments center on which is better. Most scientists are agreed that the synthetic is just as good for the body as the natural; some health-food enthusiasts argue that the body uses more readily a vitamin that originates in plant and animal food.

Extracting organic vitamins requires high temperatures, harsh solvents, and pressure. The end result is a vitamin that is below essential strength. The required concentration must be boosted artificially; otherwise the pill would be too big to swallow.

Take vitamin C, for example, which is sold in health food stores as "Rose Hips C." It costs several times more than other C, but many people willingly buy it. Actually, the capsule is made up mostly of ascorbic acid. A small, unspecified amount of rose hips powder is added so that rose hips can appear on the label. The Food and Drug Administration does not require a manufacturer to state the source of vitamin C. As long as the capsule has ascorbic acid, the government is satisfied. Vitamin C is a definite chemical compound with a definite biochemical activity, whether it comes from oranges, rose hips, acerola berries, or pure ascorbic acid.

To manufacture a supplement of pure rose hips C, the capsule would be as big as a hen's egg. That's why the manufacturer includes 5 percent of the organic vitamin along with 95 percent of the so-called synthetic sources. The inflated price takes more money from consumers than they need to spend.

There are also hidden facts behind the multivitamin supplements that are labeled "natural." Most contain a small amount of liver or yeast, or both. To these are added synthetic vitamins; the supplements are then labeled organic and sold at inflated prices.

One gram (1,000 mg) of whole dried liver, says the National Formulary (an official compendium recognized by the United States government), contains 0.05 mg of vitamin B_2, 0.25 mg of niacin, 10 mg of choline, and lesser amounts of other B complex factors. The National Formulary also states that 1 gram (1,000 mg) of brewer's yeast contains 0.04 mg B_2, 0.30 mg niacin, 0.12 mg B_1, and lesser amounts of other B complex factors. Therefore, the average capsule, even if it were entirely composed of liver concentrate, or yeast, would fall far below the claim of the label on the average so-called "natural" vitamin supplement.

The manufacturers, therefore, add synthetic vitamins to bring the constituency up to the required strength. The customer, in turn, is asked to pay higher prices for synthetic vitamins sold as "natural" vitamins.

Robert Benowicz says in *Vitamins and You* "Synthetic vitamins are as poorly named as their 'natural' or 'organic' counterparts. Because most people associate the term with artificiality and inferiority, it is easy for hucksters to exploit your distaste for the 'synthetic.'"

MYTHS ABOUT VITAMINS

Myth 1: A Balanced Diet Provides All a Body Needs

In his eighties, while still cultivating the beautiful fruits and vegetables on his truck farm in Lancaster County, Pennsylvania, Pop Rohrer said, "Take care of the soil and the soil will take care of you."

This humble farmer who reads only the Bible, comics, and the newspaper, seems to know by instinct more than the learned scientists of the nation's finest schools. Pop knew when to fertilize, what cover crops to sow, how to rotate his crops, and how much manure to plow under. He took care of the soil, and as he predicted, the rich, nutritious food he harvested kept his body strong long beyond the biblical three score years and ten.

Since Pop began to farm, agriculture has become big business. America has become the world's largest exporter of wheat, soybeans, and even rice. Yankee know-how easily turned to agribusiness, using sophisticated fertilizers to produce record-breaking yields of grain, vegetables, fruit, and fiber. Agribusiness learned how to breed plants for better growth, how to breed fatter and healthier livestock, and how to increase the yields of all animal products.

Americans began to expect fresh produce all year long. Vegetables and fruits were harvested earlier and earlier, before they were fully ripe and before they achieved their full quota of vitamins and minerals. Some were artificially "ripened" by the use of ethylene gas. Some were waxed to make them appear inviting to shoppers and to avoid spoilage owing to water losses by evaporation. Lemons, oranges, apples, melons, cucumbers, new potatoes, and other produce are routinely ripened chemically today, then waxed for long life during shipping and shelf display.

In addition, vast cold-storage plants store food in controlled atmospheres manipulated by inert gases to retard spoilage. Antisprouting chemicals inhibit growth in fresh root vegetables such as potatoes. When extra color is needed to make a vegetable or fruit look appetizing, chemicals are found to do the job.

To say that a "balanced diet" gives a person all the vitamins and minerals necessary to sustain good health is to make many assumptions. One has to assume that the soil in which the food was grown had sufficient quantities of all the necessary minerals. One has to assume that the food was picked ripe at the peak of its maturity. One has to assume that harsh treatment by processors did not expose the food to air or through preservatives destroy or greatly reduce the vitamin content. One has to assume that the ground has been fertilized properly . . . that the iodine content of the plant is adequate . . . that there are essential trace elements in the soil such as zinc, cobalt, and selenium, to name a few.

The United States Food and Drug Administration has stated that about 70 percent of domestic corn and soybeans do not contain adequate amounts of selenium. Such a deficiency, the FDA said, can lead to decreased growth, disease, and death of animals feeding on such crops.

In Australia and New Zealand some years back, selenium and cobalt were absent in the soil, leading to nutritional problems among the populace. The absence of cobalt led to reduced vitamin B_{12} (which has cobalt in its molecule) in grazing animals. This led to diseased animals. In Australia and New Zealand the problem was eliminated when these essential micronutrients were added to fertilizers.

In special hearings in Washington, a representative of the United States Department of Agriculture declared: "The statement that the nutritional values of our crops are not significantly affected by either the soil or the kind of fertilizer used cannot be defended."

The myth of proper nutrition through a balanced diet alone is further exposed when you consider the decrease in food quality through time, exposure to light and heat, cooking, canning, and freezing.

Further misconceptions about balanced diet loom because food tables are rough averages at best. They do not show how much of the nutrient is available for absorption by the body.

The vitamin C content of potatoes, for example, fluctuates between 4 and 26 milligrams per 100 grams of potatoes. Nutritionists use the general figure of 15 milligrams per 100 grams, but that must be wrong half the time—even for the raw potato.

It is important to ask also how much of the nutrient is available for absorption by the body. The supposed vitamin C content of prepared cabbage is not available to the body since it is chemically bound up in the form of ascorbinogen.

Fresh food loses nutrients rapidly through enzymatic decomposition. Green vegetables lose nearly all their vitamin C in a few days when kept at room temperature. That is why produce purchased from a store where the turnover is slow might be nutritionally depleted.

The processing of TV dinners results in depleted food. Forty percent of the vitamin A, 100 percent of the vitamin C, 80 percent of the B complex and 55 percent of the vitamin E can be lost during the processing of TV dinners. (These figures were supplied by the United States Department of Agriculture.)

Although the nutritional sufficiency of a balanced diet is a debatable issue, it is obviously wise to eat a varied diet, ensuring that you will get a greater number of nutrients and reduce the concentration of any harmful substance (food coloring, preservatives, insecticides).

Try to eat from each of the four major food groups each day. Your daily menu should include the following:

1. green and yellow vegetables and fruits, 4 servings
2. milk and milk products, 2 to 4 servings
3. meat, poultry, fish, eggs, 2 servings
4. grains and cereals, 4 servings

These servings are recommended by the National Research Council and provide approximately 1200 calories per day. Adjustments can be made to provide for individual needs according to age, weight, calorie requirements, and for pregnant women.

Put on your table as much unprocessed, natural food as you can. Eating smaller meals five or six times a day is better than gorging three meals, or less, a day. Seek the advice of a nutritionist if you cannot eat right and are not feeling great. Supplements might be necessary for your diet.

Myth 2: Every Body Metabolizes in the Same Way

Each person is born with a chemistry personality. One body exudes energy, another is sluggish. Each type responds differently. The body may be efficient or it may lack the ability to respond to the nutrients that are fed to it. For this reason the nutritional requirements for different individuals are immensely varied.

Every body assimilates food differently, according to its biochemistry. As our family of four ate together recently we were reminded of this difference in metabolism. One son eats much more than the other and doesn't gain weight. He is like his father. However, the father doesn't have sensitive taste buds, so he doesn't enjoy his food as much as the son does. The other son eats but would rather talk about ideas and machines than concentrate on how delicious a salad is or how flavorful the vegetables are.

Pity the person in a nutritional rut. Favorite foods are consumed in large quantities while various other foods are ignored or shunned. The lack of variety in food intake can lead to serious deficiencies.

Be sensitive to your own special requirements.

Myth 3: You Can Take Vitamins or Leave Them

We have established in preceding pages the necessity for everyone to give their priceless bodies the maximum number of vitamins and minerals. This is not something you can ignore without paying a price.

You need about forty different nutrients to sustain good health. These include vitamins and minerals, as well as amino acids (from proteins), essential fatty acids (from vegetable oils and animal fats), and sources of energy (calories, carbohydrates, proteins, and fats).

Most foods contain more than one nutrient. Milk, for example, provides proteins, fats, sugars, riboflavin and other B vitamins, vitamin A, calcium, and phosphorus—among other nutrients. This single food has a marvelous variety of nutrients.

But no single food item supplies all the essential nutrients in the amounts that you need. Milk, for instance, contains very little iron or vitamin C. You should, therefore, eat a variety of foods to assure an adequate diet.

The official dietary guidelines prepared jointly by the United States Department of Agriculture and the United States Department of Health,

Exercise and Nutrition

Education and Welfare for distribution to the public are studiously inoffensive formulations. Here they are:

- Eat a variety of foods.
- Maintain ideal weight.
- Avoid too much fat, saturated fat, and cholesterol.
- Eat foods with adequate starch and fiber.
- Avoid too much sugar.
- Avoid too much sodium.
- If you drink alcohol, do so in moderation.

We find this list so innocuous that it must have been put together by politicians (and it was) so as not to offend. The greater offense is that the government apparently doesn't care if you operate to the maximum or enjoy tip-top health. They'll settle for a nation of averages in which people eat food that might or might not be grown in rich soil and thus have all their nutrients . . . food that might be violently shattered through processing and end up empty of important vitamins . . . food that might have death-dealing dye in it . . . food that is stale . . . or food that is picked green, waxed, gassed, and hauled from sea to shining sea.

You can take vitamins or leave them. But if you want to enjoy maximum health and protect your body against disease, then take vitamins, don't leave them.

Myth 4: Vitamins Are Drugs

"Don't forget to take your pills!"

This exhortation is so common in America today that we don't allow vitamin supplements in our house to be called "pills." Pills mean drugs. Vitamins are food, not drugs. We'll prove it.

Time and time again truthful physicians admit that they were given very little training in medical school concerning nutrition. Doctors who are honest say they learn more about the effect of vitamins from their patients than they do from their medical books.

The son of an eye, ear, nose, and throat specialist suffered chronic ear infections and was unable to resist infections after antibiotic treatments.

His father, the physician, had several patients who told him what vitamin and mineral supplements and the elimination of sugar had done to bring better health to their children.

The medical expert was open to the suggestions and tried them. His son was dramatically restored to health. As a result of this experience, the doctor left his traditional discipline and became an outstanding nutrition specialist in southern California. He has guided thousands to healing through food supplementation and the elimination of nonnutrient foodstuffs.

Noted nutrition columnist Jean Mayer, president of Tufts University and a professor at Harvard Medical School, is widely quoted as saying: "Our studies at Harvard among residents suggest that the average physician knows a little more about nutrition than the average secretary—unless the secretary has a weight problem, and then she probably knows more than the average physician."

This is the sad state of affairs because medical schools have accorded nutrition almost no place in the curriculum. "Clinical nutrition is not even taught in most medical schools, and not really adequately done in any of them," said Professor Nevin S. Scrimshaw of Massachusetts Institute of Technology.

Part of the reason that practitioners of the healing arts haven't paid much attention to nutrition and vitamins has been the rapid increase during the last three decades in the number and type of drugs now used by the medical profession.

Most drugs have narrow, specific effects; vitamins influence the entire body. A single vitamin may have a beneficial effect upon many tissues and body functions including skin, hair, mouth conditions, muscle spasms, cardiac stress, ulcers, mental state, vitality, and more.

Drugs work best alone; vitamins work best in consort with all the natural elements created to go with them. Drugs are like a pole vaulter—one man against the hurdle bar; vitamins are like a baseball team—each element plays a part toward victory for the whole.

Hundreds of children die each year from accidental aspirin poisoning. Antacids, which Americans swallow by the ton for upset stomachs, often give adverse effects. Fatalities are caused by antihistamines, also, along with nose drops and barbiturates. Many patients have suffered illness in hospitals due to wrong combinations of drugs. Many die every year due to side effects.

Vitamins are food. The human body loves them. They are natural to it. When they are consumed, the body uses them in the course of its regular processes.

Vitamins—except for excessive doses of A and D—are virtually harmless in any quantity to persons of average health. The water-soluble B vitamins and vitamin C, on rare occasions and with certain individuals, can produce slight distress if taken in very large quantities. Even this distress is merely stomach upset and laxative action. The A and D vitamins can harm the body, but only if taken in doses described as wildly excessive—such as one hundred times the amount proposed in a nutritional regimen. Nobody fears eating a medium serving of beef or calf liver, yet this por-

Exercise and Nutrition

tion contains more than twice as much vitamin A as a "high-level" supplemental vitamin regimen might prescribe. Excessive vitamins are gradually used up by the body or excreted.

Excessive use of drugs can be the forerunner of malnutrition. Drugs do this by depressing appetites, impairing the body's ability to absorb nutrients, causing a loss of minerals and vitamins, and interfering with the mechanisms for using vitamins.

When amphetamines are used as diet pills to control appetite and weight gain and to treat hyperactive youngsters, these foreign substances can take away appetites and run trace minerals dangerously low. Other drugs, used to treat psoriasis, high cholesterol levels, and blood disorders can interfere with the body's ability to absorb the fat-soluble vitamins A, D, and K. The popular birth control pill can cause deficiencies of vitamins D, C, and B_6.

The Food and Drug Administration requires that manufacturers of prescription drugs describe thoroughly all side effects. Just because a drug is sold over the counter (aspirin, antacids, cough medicines, and so forth) doesn't mean that it is without potential side effects that are frightening.

The unfortunate reality is that none of the drugs are sold with any indication to the consumer, patient, or even physician, that they can induce vitamin deficiencies.

Probably the best route to personal and national health is good maintenance over the long haul of that finely tuned instrument—our body. Well-nourished living cells respond to the demands of life and are a source of joy for the individual owning them. Take the long view. Avoid the quick fix in favor of the slow, healthful, more permanent cure.

Myth 5: Vitamin Supplements Are Only For the Sickly

Hippocrates, the father of modern medicine, observed that "extreme remedies are very appropriate for extreme disease."

A better plan would be to avoid extreme remedies by maintaining a consistent intake of vital nutrients. This is the sentiment in four lines in the *Epistle to John Dryden* of Chesterton:

> Better to hunt in the fields for health unbought,
> Than to fee the doctor for a nauseous draught.
> The wise for cure on exercise depend;
> God never made his work for man to mend.

Do you want to be well? Healthy? Vital? Bursting with energy? Don't expect to reach this state of being overnight. Your state of health is determined by what you do hour after hour, day after day, year after year.

This routine determines when or if you become ill and even perhaps when you die.

Proper vitamin and mineral intake day after day is something you can control completely. Most people mistakenly feel that illness is "something that can happen to anybody" and throw caution to the winds. To the contrary, illness is what can happen to people who consume too much fat (which can bring about cancer), too much sugar (which disrupts the pancreas and adrenal glands), too much caffeine (implicated as one of the causes of breast cancer and cancer of the bladder).

A recent two-year study commissioned by the National Cancer Institute turned up more evidence pointing to a link between most common cancers and diet. It has been determined by this group that 40 percent of cancer in men and 60 percent in women is related to diet.

"Habit, diet, and custom" were placed above genes as causes of cancer.

If you cannot determine whether or not you need vitamins, ask yourself how well you wish to be. If you want only to get by, proceed with what you're doing. If you'd like to prevent illness, to stay out of the doctor's office, and to enjoy freedom from fatigue, then adopt a program of vitamin supplementation coupled with proper exercise.

Women who expect to bear children should begin their regimen immediately, even though they are still youngsters dreaming of the day. When marriage occurs and a little one is expected, a pregnant mother should increase her intake of the necessary vitamins and minerals to nourish the little one growing inside. Pregnancy is *not* the time to go on a diet. Too little weight gain causes deficiencies for the baby; too much gain may make the birth difficult. Any weight loss should occur before the pregnancy starts. A woman who is overweight when she becomes pregnant faces the likelihood that medical problems such as high blood pressure, toxemia, and a difficult delivery may arise.

Good nutrition during a person's twenties and thirties pays the biggest dividends for life. Let meals consisting of a wide variety of food become a habit—meals drawing from whole grains and cereals, dairy products, both green and yellow vegetables, fresh fruits, fish, and poultry. Such a habit, once formed, will serve you well for the rest of your life.

Myth 6: Supermarket Food Is Adequately Fortified

A visitor to the United States was defensive during her tour of factories, construction sites, and other accoutrements of a modern American city. "We have the same in our country," she would declare. But when she stepped inside a supermarket, all she could do was stand and weep.

This eighth wonder of the world offers food once worth a king's ransom. Shelves are bulging with colorful, beautifully packaged, and tasty food in seemingly unlimited quantities. But when it comes to the nutritional value of the food, the visitor's farm market in the steppes of the Ukraine that offered unrefined food with almost no shelf life might have surpassed the quality of the supermarket's doctored fare.

Take wheat, for example—literally the world's largest and most widely cultivated food crop. The milling process in the United States separates wheat into two parts. Some people choose not to eat the most nutritious part consisting of the germ and bran. One part (from two-thirds to three-fourths) is used for human food; the remainder is fed to animals. What the animals eat is in most respects far more nutritious than that which is highly refined for human consumption.

In the developing countries, more of the nutritional quality of wheat is retained for human consumption. Even in most Western nations the food value of wheat is utilized better than it is in the United States.

Such inefficient use of wheat stems from a popular demand for white bread and bland-tasting wheat products. Widespread ignorance of white bread's bankrupt nutritional store is also to blame.

In 1941 the government began to require the enrichment of refined wheat products with four nutrients that were available and popular at that time. Not until 1974 did the Food and Nutrition Board of the National Academy of Sciences recommend fortification with six additional nutrients. Even so, the refined and milled white flour eaten by most Americans is nutritionally far below what it should be—and what it was in the original germ of wheat.

While minerals usually make it through the refining process, vitamins are more vulnerable. They are easily destroyed by heat, light, air, and chemical processing.

Although they are not changed at all, refined carbohydrates are not always welcomed by the body. Refined sugar contains none of the protein or vegetable oils that were in the original cane or beet. Only traces of copper and iron remain of all the wide range of minerals that were in the original food before processing. Therefore, refined sugar, flour, rice, and cereal grains are almost exclusively forms of carbohydrate. Processed vegetable oil is virtually all fat.

The process of refining food compromises the nutritional integrity of whole wheat, rice, cereal grains, vegetables, fruits, and vegetable oils. It does not destroy all food value, or Americans would be starving rather than getting fat. But enough nutrients are destroyed to cause marginal deficiencies that prevent the best of health.

Eat an abundance of "fast foods" and you will be getting a rich caloric store—lots of carbohydrates and fats, very little protein, minerals, and vitamins. Is it worth it?

Nutrients Lost When Wheat Is Refined

Thiamine	.86%
Riboflavin	.70%
Niacin	.86%
Iron	.84%
Vitamin B_6	.60%
Folic Acid	.70%
Pantothenic Acid	.54%
Biotin	.90%
Calcium	.50%
Phosphorus	.78%
Copper	.75%
Magnesium	.72%
Zinc	.71%
Chromium	.87%
Fiber	.68%

BY U.D. Register, Ph.D., Department of Nutrition, Loma Linda University.

Myth 7: Overeating Will Supply More of What's Needed

"Oh, what a tangled web we weave," cried the poet, "when first we practice to deceive!"

People who are overweight rarely eat to put more nutrition into their bodies. They eat compulsively, out of anger, frustration, stress, or defiance. Many are helpless about changing their habits. Overeating (usually the obese person selects refined sugars and other carbohydrates) does not mean eating better.

The problem of overeating usually runs in families. A child with one obese parent has a risk of about 40 percent of becoming an obese adult; if the child has two obese parents, the risk jumps to 70 percent. How much is genetic and how much grows out of poor family meal planning who can tell? But we do know wrong choices are made. Behavior modification is of utmost value.

The object of good nutrition is not to eat more but to eat better. Five or six smaller meals, for example, will accommodate the body's digestion and assimilation of food better than three heavy ones.

People who are overweight are not good eaters, just "eaters." Therefore, they should be encouraged to eat foods rich in the vitamin B complex group. They should vary the diet, increasing the intake of such foods as wheat germ, raw green and leafy vegetables, and liver (if pure), and drink more water. As a treat, popcorn is a good source of roughage and is

Exercise and Nutrition 143

low in calories. Try sprinkling popcorn with debittered yeast instead of salt.

People who crave sweets and alcohol are often deficient in the B vitamins. A vitamin supplement might include 10 to 50 mg of the entire vitamin B complex one to two times daily.

If your child is prone to obesity, don't encourage him to finish the last drop of formula, or eat that last spoonful in his dish, or keep him nursing when he's satisfied. This parental pressure day after day merely contributes to the wrong pattern of excessive eating.

Never refer to your child as "fat." Talk about how wonderful the body is and how it takes care of our needs if we don't abuse it with too much food.

It is best not to associate food with deportment, because food is necessary for life and must be considered a gift from God. Neither use food as a reward for good behavior nor withdraw it as punishment for poor behavior.

Include some form of exercise every day—if only brisk walking (which is best for many) or doing exercises on your living-room floor or running in place. Exercising can *decrease* the desire for food.

Sow a routine of relaxed, varied, and nutritious eating and reap glowing health for a lifetime.

HELPFUL USES OF VITAMIN SUPPLEMENTS

In Times of Stress

Stress is a part of life, but occasionally it disrupts the equilibrium. It can come from the inside through fear, worry, apprehension, or severe frustration; it can also come from the outside through hard work, burns, fractures, or the need to respond physically to danger.

Disease is also a stress on the body. A bacterial or viral infection is a stress. So are deficiencies of the metabolic requirements for certain cells. In other words, if your body doesn't have enough fuel for its functions, great stress is created. This section is concerned with ridding the body of this stress by fortifying it with sufficient nutrients.

Tranquilizers and depressant drugs cannot reduce stress. These types of medication are designed to lower the stress response but they do not remove the cause. Drugs can be administered to lower blood pressure, but they do not remove the problem. Taking drugs to decrease response to stress is like binding up an ugly wound. The bandage won't heal it, but it may hide the unsightly wound and prevent some new infection.

How do you know whether or not you need to supplement your diet with extra vitamins and minerals? Ask yourself: (1) Do I have adequate energy for my daily routine? (2) Is my body resistant to infection? (3) Do I have a cheerful mental outlook most of the time? (4) When I feel depressed, does it pass within a couple of days? (5) Do I feel like exercising enthusiastically (for my age)?

You may live in a community where a nutrition-oriented doctor or good nutritionist can map out a dietary program for you. If you do not, contact:

> Consumers for Nutrition Action, Inc.
> 3404 Saint Paul Street, Suite 1-B
> Baltimore, MD 21218
> Telephone (301) 235-9039

Referrals are made to nutritionally aware physicians as well as to organizations involved in food issues. Other sources of information include:

> International College of Applied Nutrition (ICAN)
> P.O. Box 386
> LaHabra, CA 90631
> Telephone (213) 697-4576 (Referrals are made)

> Society for the Protection of the Unborn Through
>   Nutrition (SPUN)
> 17 North Wabash Avenue, Suite 603
> Chicago, IL 60602
> Telephone (312) 332-2334 (Referrals are made)

Just beginning a program to supplement your diet—knowing that you have given your body what it needs—will in itself remove some stress in your life.

You can also experiment, if you don't do anything foolish. First, cut out stressors like coffee and tea with caffeine, and all other drugs, like nicotine, marijuana, and alcohol. Next, cut out refined sugar and see how you feel. Sugar lowers your resistance to infections and causes fatigue. It will be easier to get out of bed in the morning without it. It will not be without struggle, but just for the sake of the experiment, do it for thirty days. You will be amazed at the increase in energy.

Finally, note the good foods listed in the Vitamin Alphabet and eat those that are loaded with nutrients. Note how confident you feel as you face the day ... tackle new projects ... clean up old work you've been meaning to get to.

Avoid excessive doses of vitamins A and D. If you check with your doctor about other vitamin supplements, he or she will probably shrug and say, "It's your money. Certainly can't hurt you."

True. But it might help you.

Exercise and Nutrition

For People Who Smoke

Smoking speeds the aging process of the body. We need not argue against the habit; the habit argues well against itself through an abundance of statistics. Smoking leads to lung cancer, heart disease, and emphysema. An attractive face is changed into one with premature wrinkles, bags under the eyes, and dull eyes. Nicotine stains the teeth and fingers. In addition, smoking pollutes homes, restaurants, and airplanes while creating enemies among nonsmokers.

Smoking destroys vitamins. It puts carbon monoxide into the blood . . . constricts blood vessels . . . and thus reduces circulation. Smoking also lowers immunity to diseases and interferes with dozens of other body processes.

Smoking leads also to cancer of the mouth and bladder. Finally, smoking wastes your money.

A document called the Framingham Heart Study reveals that middle-aged men who smoke more than a pack of cigarettes a day are two to six times more likely to have strokes than nonsmoking middle-aged men. The hardest-hit smokers, as far as heart disease is concerned, are forty-five to fifty-four years of age.

Vitamin C does wonders for smokers. It can detoxify some of the poisons formed in the blood by smoke.

We probably will not know in our lifetime all that the scourge of chemicals is doing to our bodies. But we do know vividly and dramatically what smoking does. Pointing this out to a smoker will not cause him or her to quit. The habit is addictive and may stem from deep psychological need and that could be the subject of another book.

Women—especially teenagers—who smoke during pregnancy are particularly vulnerable to illness. Their infants face retarded growth and weakened respiratory systems. Smoking dulls the appetite of mothers so that they don't eat properly for themselves and for the baby they are carrying.

To sum up: Smokers need all the nutritional help they can get, especially from antioxidants such as vitamins A, C, E, and selenium. The rest is up to their willpower.

During Extensive Travel

Travel is hard work. (Don't tell that to people who are stuck at a menial task and who would like nothing better than to roam the world!)

People who have a private plane, and an unlimited budget, can schedule their own departures but not always their arrivals. Weather, strikes, and all kinds of interruptions throw a carefully prepared travel schedule out of kilter. The result is hours of inactivity, a body cramped in a seat, days of no exercise, strange meals that surprise the stomach, breathing of polluted air, and thinned oxygen in pressurized cabins. As a result a person's circadian (daily) body clock becomes so disoriented the body does not know when it's time to get up or go to sleep.

To minimize stress, make sure you supplement the body first with sufficient quantities of timed-release vitamin C. This will guard against colds and infection and help to keep the bowels regular. Large doses of C can act as a laxative. Second, take vitamins E and A along with selenium.

A handy guide for short-term use would be the following:

A high-potency multiple vitamin and mineral tablet
Vitamin C, 2,000 mg A.M. and P.M.
Vitamin E, 400 to 800 I.U. daily
Selenium, 50 mcg daily

To keep one's strength up during travel is to add much to the trip. Avoiding stimulants such as coffee and wake-up pills means that you will be able to sleep at night. Eliminating rich desserts will help the body to resist infections since sugar weakens the immune system. For extra protection, a gamma globulin shot will build antibodies against hepatitis.

Presurgery and Recuperation

"I treated him, God cured him," said Ambroise Paré four centuries ago.

In the hospitals and clinics of America, the dedication and skills of doctors, nurses, and medical technicians is superb. Impressive gains have been made in wiping out disease, in improving surgical procedures, and in making patients comfortable.

Most of these same skilled practitioners of the healing arts are either ignorant of, or indifferent to, the basic nutritional needs of recuperating patients under their care.

Dr. Charles E. Butterworth, an official of the American Medical Society, wrote in *Nutrition Today* that the lack of therapy through nutrition is a scandal of national scope, which he branded "inexcusable" and "tragic."

"It is well-known," Dr. Butterworth said, "that malnutrition interferes with wound healing and increases susceptibility to infection. It thus becomes imperative to ensure that preventable malnutrition does not contribute to the mortality, morbidity, and prolonged bed-occupancy rates of our hospital population. So it's time to swing open the door and have a look at this skeleton in the hospital closet."

A twenty-four-month study in the mid-1970s by United States surgeons on the quality of their own work revealed that approximately half

Exercise and Nutrition 147

of surgical complications were preventable. So were 85 of the 245 surgical deaths investigated.

The Study of Surgical Services for the United States, an undertaking sponsored by the American College of Surgeons and the American Surgical Association, investigated the details of 1,696 deaths or complications associated with surgical procedures on 1,493 patients in 95 hospitals of 7 states. An impressive 796 (47 percent) of the 1,696 incidents were assessed as preventable and 900 as nonpreventable by the cooperating hospitals.

You might not be able to control the surgical knife, but you can increase your chances of recovery from disease by preventing it in the first place by keeping yourself fit, or by fortifying your body so that recuperation is as swift and complete as possible.

If you face surgery, get started now to strengthen your body for the ordeal. Select protein-rich foods so that each organ of your body has material with which to build.

A friend of ours who broke his nose in an automobile accident arranged for rhinoplasty (corrective nasal surgery) to remedy the injuries. Before the surgery he fortified himself with a high-protein diet and vitamin/mineral supplements.

Following the operation our friend was rewarded by the exclamations of surprise when the surgeon removed the bandages and made his first inspection. Far less bruising had occurred than normal. Not one nosebleed occurred in the following days. The surgeon declared it was one of the cleanest cases he had ever seen—all attributable, we are convinced, to the preoperative nutrition carried out by the patient.

Troops of the United States armed forces were studied by the National Academy of Sciences, National Research Council. Therapeutic nutrition, the council found, dramatically increased the number of soldiers who survived battle injuries.

If you face surgery, prepare a "hospital survival kit" to hasten your exit from the bed of pain:

1. Pack a supply of multiple vitamin-mineral tablets in your personal belongings. If your physician has not prescribed a supplement, tell him or her that you wish to continue your daily habit of diet supplementation during your hospital stay.
2. Select the following menu choices:

- Fresh green salads as much as possible (unless restricted by your doctor), and fresh fruits
- Turkey, chicken, fish, lean beef, cheese, eggs, or soybean products (at least one of those protein foods at each meal)
- Baked potatoes instead of mashed or fried (most cooked vegetables

are waterlogged and a nutritional fiasco). Ask if you can order cottage cheese, sliced tomatoes, or another salad in place of the cooked vegetable.
- Sugar-free yogurt for dessert (especially important if you have been taking an antibiotic)
- Whole wheat bread

3. Add protein powder to the milk or juices if permitted. Your doctor should be informed of any extra intake of nutrients in case they affect laboratory tests.
4. Avoid all sugar and chocolate served from the hospital kitchen or given as gifts from well-meaning but thoughtless visitors. Sugar weakens the body by affecting the white blood cells that fight infection.
5. Avoid caffeine drinks including coffee, tea, chocolate, and colas. Request juice or milk. Have your family bring you herbal tea bags and blackstrap molasses to add to your milk.
6. Fill your mind with the comfort available from the Holy Scriptures.
7. Maintain an optimistic outlook. Inner peace and serenity contribute to the healing process.

Who knows? With daily fare like that you might never have to go to the hospital in the first place!

BIBLIOGRAPHY
Airola, Paavo. *How to Get Well.* Phoenix: Health Plus Pubs., 1974.
Benowicz, Robert J. *Vitamins and You.* New York: Grosset & Dunlap, Inc., 1978.
Blaine, Tom R. *Mental Health Through Nutrition.* Secaucus, N.J.: The Citadel Press, 1974.
Cousins, Norman. *Anatomy of an Illness.* New York: W.W. Norton & Co., 1979.
Passwater, Richard A. *Supernutrition: Megavitamin Revolution.* New York: The Dial Press, 1975.
Pauling, Linus and Cameron, Ewan. *Cancer and Vitamin C.* Los Angeles: Cancer Book House, 1979.
Price, Weston A. *Nutrition and Physical Degeneration.* La Mesa, Calif.: Price-Pottenger Nutrition Foundation, 1977.
Rohrer, Virginia, and Rohrer, Norman. *How to Eat Right and Feel Great.* Wheaton, Ill.: Tyndale House Publishers, 1977.
Rohrer, Virginia Page. *Total Health Cookbook.* Wheaton, Ill.: Tyndale House Publishers, 1980.
Williams, Roger J. *Nutrition in a Nutshell.* New York: Doubleday & Company, Inc., 1962.
Williams, Roger J. *Nutrition Against Disease.* New York: Bantam Books, 1973.
Williams, Roger J. *The Wonderful World Within You.* New York: Bantam Books, 1977.
American Journal of Clinical Nutrition. Bethesda, Md.: March, 1981.
American Journal of Clinical Nutrition. Bethesda, Md.: November, 1981.
Canadian Medical Association Journal. Ottawa, Canada: September, 1981.
Canadian Medical Association Journal. Ottawa, Canada: February, 1982.
Clinical Science, #62, 1982.
Food Science & Nutrition, 1980.
New York Academy of Science, 1980.
Prevention Magazine. Emmaus, Pa.: Rodale Press.

Part II

Self-destructive Habits

Up-to-date information and statistics are quoted by the authors on each of these topics. In particular, the harmful effects of marijuana, formerly thought erroneously to be relatively innocuous, are freshly presented, with a summary of the mechanisms of action of its active ingredient (THC). Young adults and adolescents should be persuaded by all means to read this section.

The physically harmful effects of alcohol, and tar and nicotine, especially in cigarettes, is well-documented in these sections. Some very sobering facts are given in an interesting and easy-to-read way. All who indulge in these self-destructive habits should be strongly urged to think through the information presented and to evaluate the implications for the health and well-being of their internal organs, especially the brain, the liver, the heart, and the lungs.

5
Marijuana
O. Quentin Hyder, M.D.

Many young people today are experience seekers, and taking drugs with others (peer identification) provides them with a community experience. Some are looking for a personality change; feeling inadequate and dissatisfied, they hope drugs will give them more self-confidence and status. Others use drugs to escape emotional pain by "dropping out" or entering temporary, blissful oblivion. For example: The psychotic may use drugs to escape depression and suppress painful symptoms such as delusions, hallucinations, and other nonreality thoughts or feelings; the neurotic indulges in order to relieve tension, stress, or anxiety, or to elevate low mood; and the psychopath (personality disorder) craves the thrill of the euphoria he gets when he "turns on," or seeks to alleviate social or sexual problems.

Why do young people take drugs? Here are some possible answers:

1. They see their parents smoking and drinking and grow up with the attitude that drug use is socially acceptable behavior.
2. Peer-group pressure is a major factor. A young person with even slight feelings of inferiority or insecurity finds greater acceptance in his group if he joins them in a pot party.
3. Simple curiosity can lead to the desire to try it "just once," but the pleasure derived from the relaxation, seemingly heightened sensibility, uninhibited emotional (and sexual) expression, and group acceptance can lead to frequency of practice.
4. The risk of being caught and the fear of coming to any physical harm seem less when involved with a group of friends.

Self-destructive Habits

5. Drug use is often seen by youth as a symbol of independence from adult authority figures. Precisely because it is illegal, smoking pot gives expression to the normal adolescent rebellious phase. Even though he knows deep down that he still needs support, guidance, and instruction from parents and teachers, the impatient adolescent finds in this form of self-assertion a boost to his desired sense of maturity and independence.
6. Escape from an unhappy home situation, peer-group rejection, loss of a friend, parent, or sibling, financial difficulties, boyfriend or girl friend conflicts or misunderstandings, broken love affairs, or social or academic failure can sometimes be temporarily alleviated by withdrawal into drug use. Unhappily, the reality situation, however, remains unchanged and has to be faced eventually.
7. Internal problems are the most tragic causes of drug use. Low self-esteem and feelings of worthlessness, hopelessness, guilt, anxiety, or depression from whatever cause can all be temporarily escaped by taking drugs. Permanent solutions, however, remain elusive, and the dejection continues to hang like a black cloud over the sufferer, unless and until time eventually heals the wounds.

Marijuana

Let us now consider marijuana specifically. It is obtained from the flowers and leaves of Indian hemp, a plant with the botanical name of *Cannabis sativa,* which grows naturally in temperate climates. Its products have been used since ancient times for intoxication or stimulation. Its only possible medical uses, which are still very experimental, are the prescription of its active ingredient (Delta-9-THC) in the reduction of nausea in terminal cancer patients being treated with chemotherapy or in the reduction of high pressure in the eye in the condition of glaucoma. Other medications, however, without mind-altering side effects, are equally effective in these conditions. Marijuana is usually called pot, grass, hash, bhang, reefers, tea, or sinsemilla, and is usually ingested by inhalation, like smoking a regular cigarette.

Let us not kid ourselves that pot smoking is confined to youth. Many in their thirties, forties, and even fifties are experimenting with it. Some use it to help themselves cut down on alcohol, some to revive failing sexual powers, some use it as a tranquilizer, others to keep up with the younger generation. All these can indeed be achieved temporarily, but the key to recently published findings, which should cause serious concern, is the discovery of long-range effects of use over an extended period of time.

Now, how can you recognize someone on pot? Consider these physical, emotional, and behavioral changes. A person in the early stages of use will appear from time to time to be "stoned." He may have a glazed appearance in his eyes, which may also be slightly red. He will be animated, talkative, giggly, have uncontrollable hilarity and be apparently very happy. He tries to dominate any conversation and seems unable to listen or to remain quiet. He may well say things out of character for him: He may use words of profanity, or express opinions which are silly, unkind, untrue, hurtful, meaningless, or hostile. He may possibly complain of thirst, hunger, craving for sweet foods, dizziness, nausea, drowsiness, or abdominal pain. He may well seem very confused, apprehensive, or depressed, be inarticulate or mentally dull. He is usually quite restless or agitated, and manifests loss of reality contact by saying or doing foolish or inappropriate things. You might think he is drunk, but his breath does not stink of alcohol.

When not high on a recent dose, because so much marijuana is retained in the body, other signs are manifested between trips, especially after protracted use. Experienced pot smokers suffer from distorted emotional responses, dullness and disorder of thought processes, impairment of judgment, slothfulness, lethargy, difficulty with verbalization, and a slowing down of a sense of passage of time. They manifest poor motivation, proneness to error, reduced capacity to take responsibility, memory loss, especially for important details, carelessness, and lack of attention or ability to concentrate. They usually tell lies to parents or friends to avoid admitting to their habit. This deception can only lead eventually to alienation. Those with higher intelligence or education show the greatest deterioration, usually leading to job or school failure. The user's proficiency at driving a car is impaired, even when he has not smoked pot recently, by reduced ability to gauge distance, speed, or road conditions.

The impaired judgment tragically leads to loss of control and inhibitions. This can lead to the use of more dangerous drugs, mixing the pot with alcohol, which potentiates the symptoms, or acting sexually in a manner often later regretted. Intoxication with marijuana specifically lowers sexual inhibitions and exposes the user to unhealthy sexual temptations. Interpersonal relationships invariably suffer because of easy irritability, hostility, impatience, and even the delusional thought processes of paranoia. People with poor ego strength or a borderline (potential) schizoid personality can easily be pushed over into a psychosis (serious mental disorder) by the use of marijuana. Adolescents or young adults who have not yet developed a strong sense of personal identity are especially vulnerable to drug-induced mental or emotional breakdowns.

If you are in discussion with a teenager be prepared to give him or her this summary of adverse effects of heavy marijuana use (heavy use is five or more "joints" per week):

Physical Effects: Lung damage leading to breathing impairment and possibly cancer; destruction of brain cells leading to abnormal or reduced intellectual functioning or capacity; lowered immunity to infectious diseases; slowed down visual and muscular reflex actions and changes in perception of time and space, leading to impaired driving ability; increased heart rate, leading to decreased efficiency and chest pain; risk of a variety of unexpected effects when a fresh supply of marijuana is much more potent than that previously used.

Psychological Effects: Slowing of thought processes and speech; impairment of memory, concentration, logical thinking, and ability to abstract and synthesize concepts; reduction of self-control by the will in any behavior or relationships involving moral choice; anxiety or depression after the high, panic attacks, or even schizophrenic disorientation in those vulnerable or predisposed to it; loss of ambition and motivational drive—the "drop-out syndrome."

Sexual Effects: Lowered testosterone (male hormone) levels in adolescent boys and men, affecting growth and sexual maturation; lowered sperm count and motility and, most sinister, increased *abnormal* sperm; damage to chromosomes, which can cause procreation of deformed offspring, altered menstrual cycles in women with reduced fertility; toxic effect on fetus in pregnant women and on babies being breast-fed, enlarged breasts in adolescent boys, and facial hairs in girls passing through puberty.

Cocaine

Because of the alarming rise in its use recently, parents and other loved ones need to know the following basic facts also about cocaine: Cocaine's legitimate medical use is as a local anaesthetic, but it is also a stimulant with definite psychological dependence potential and possible physical dependence as well. Commonly called coke, flake, snow, or dust, it is a white powder derived from coca leaves. It is usually sniffed through the nose and, within a few minutes, leads to a feeling of excitement, euphoria and increased alertness, but also to an increase in pulse rate and blood pressure, loss of appetite, and insomnia. Overdose can lead to acute agitation, hallucinations, tremors, convulsions, coma and death. Long-term effects include infections of the nasal passages, apathy, and irritability, and when supplies run out, to acute withdrawal symptoms including depression leading sometimes to suicide.

Remember that our bodies and minds are the temples of God's Holy

Spirit. Paul warns the Corinthians, "If any man defile the temple of God, him shall God destroy; for the temple of God is holy, which temple ye are" (1 Corinthians 3:17). In addition to incurring the wrath of God by defiling the body, there are several reasons why Christians should not partake of marijuana or cocaine.

First, remember that our bodies are intended by God to be used for His purposes, and that we are to live by faith. To be fully yielded to this is impossible while under the influence of intoxicants. Our bodies cannot be effective vehicles for expressing the Spirit within if we fool around with them as if they were experimental laboratories. It is not possible to "glorify God in your body" if that body is not physically and mentally in first-class working order, and if you are not living by faith. Remember that "... whatsoever is not of faith is sin" (Romans 14:23).

Second, since God Himself is the ultimate reality, the Christian's personal relationship with God is his ultimate source of joy. The pot smoker is trying to escape from reality by obtaining his artificial "high." The Christian, by contrast, finds his high by relating to reality and doing God's will in the real world. Jesus is the best high. The joy of relating to Him cannot remotely be duplicated by temporary trips into euphoria, illusion, excitement, exaggerated sensations, erotic stimulation, or altered perceptions.

The oft-heard claims that marijuana heightens one's sense of reality and deepens insights are purely subjective experiences. The high mood and insights cannot be shared with others, and objective creative ability is not, in fact, increased. The experience does not lead to anything of value beyond itself. It is narcissistic pleasure for its own sake, unable to lead to any lasting measurable achievements.

On the other hand, as the Reverend Peter Moore has written,

> Hobbies, sports, good music, and exciting conversation, spirit-filled worship of God, the expression of some creative gift, the reading of a good book, the discovery of new places, the making of new friends all have value at many levels [and] they continue to have a positive effect on the individual. Sobriety is not the grim quenching of joy, but the positive engagement of one's mind [and body] for all that leads to personal wholeness.

Listen also to the apostle Peter: "Wherefore gird up the loins of your mind, be sober.... As obedient children, not fashioning yourselves according to the former lusts in your ignorance.... be ye holy in all manner of conversation" (1 Peter 1:13-15).

Third, the Christian is not at liberty to disobey the laws of the society in which he lives, even if he thinks that some of them are overly strict or that their penalties are too severe. The only possible exception to this would be situations in which civil laws are actually morally unjust or contrary to the revealed Word of God, such as the civil rights problems in this country or as in the cruel laws of totalitarian regimes. Drug-abuse laws, however, are hardly in this category and, like it or not, the facts are the sale of marijuana is illegal, and God's Word clearly teaches that we are to submit to civil authority. "Let every soul be subject unto the higher powers. For there is no power but of God: the powers that be are ordained by God.... For rulers are not a terror to good works, but to the evil.... Wherefore ye must needs be subject, not only for wrath, but also for conscience sake" (Romans 13:1, 3, 5).

Finally, the Christian should heed his calling as the "salt of the earth" and the "light of the world." Rather than being led astray by others, he should seek to lead others to experience the new life in Christ he has himself found. Smoking marijuana is learned behavior, an acquired taste. Pot smokers are lured into the habit by the enthusiasm of others. They are led astray, as Peter Laurie writes in a book on drugs "... by an active society of smokers who will welcome the novice and persuade him that the unpleasant sensations he first gets from the drug are in fact delightful and worth repeating." The victorious Christian, by contrast, resists such seductions and heeds the words of Paul: "And be not conformed to this world: but be ye transformed by the renewing of your mind, that ye may prove what is that good, and acceptable, and perfect, will of God" (Romans 12:2).

Note: For information on the *Mechanism of Action of Marijuana,* see page 182 at end of section.

6
Alcohol
O. Quentin Hyder, M.D.

Almost 10 million Americans are either outright alcoholics or "problem drinkers" whose consumption is enough to cause serious problems both to themselves and others. This still leaves 70 to 80 million men and women in this country, many of them Christians, who drink in moderation, and are rather proud of the fact that they never get drunk. Whereas I do not share the view that if someone partakes of alcohol, he cannot be a Christian, I nevertheless am committed to the belief that temperance is a personal quality to be aimed at by all who profess Christ as Lord in their lives.

One doesn't have to get drunk or become an addict for alcohol to cause serious problems in one's own life or the lives of others. *Alcoholism* is the term used to describe any condition in which the influence of alcohol is disruptive to functioning or relationships.

Alcoholism is an illness, and is America's third most prevalent disease, behind heart disease and cancer. But this only numbers the patients themselves. Add to this alcoholism's other victims: family, loved ones, friends, business associates, other users of the highways, and so on, who are adversely affected by it. Now we see that, in addition, about another 50 million people (almost a quarter of our national population) have a drinking problem, their own or someone else's.

Alcoholism is now recognized by both the medical and legal professions as being a chronic, progressive, and eventually fatal illness. There is no known cure. This means that there is no known way in which someone can indulge in the relaxing and other pleasurable effects of alcohol with-

Self-destructive Habits 157

out also experiencing the adverse bad effects, both immediate and long-term.

Although Christians differ in their opinions as to whether or not drinking alcohol is a sin, most would agree that the Christian virtue of self-control is required of all of us. Although total abstention is the perfect standard, Christians who do drink are obligated to be strict with their own self-discipline. We are in danger of losing the protective and guiding influence of the Holy Spirit when alcohol, in clouding intellectual functioning and loosening emotional restraint, usurps the control the Spirit should have over us, thereby forming a barrier between us and God.

There is no guaranteed "safe" level of drinking because individuals differ widely in their vulnerability. Alcohol, being extremely water soluble, is rapidly absorbed through the stomach, enters the bloodstream in seconds, and immediately is carried to the brain, a few heartbeats later. There it interferes with the release of oxygen to the brain cells, many of which die as a result. Alcohol, even in very small doses, causes blood cells to clump together, or sludge, and these can block minute capillaries, depriving local areas of the brain of vital nutrients. For reasons not yet clearly understood, some people are apparently much more sensitive than others to this highly destructive mechanism.

Remember that relaxed, woozy sensation you experience when the alcohol gets to the brain? Remember that pleasant feeling you get when it first hits you? Well, that's several hundred brain cells dying. They are permanently lost; brain cells cannot regenerate.

Even though our brains contain between 15 and 20 billion individual cells, the loss of thousands of them, with each drink, over a period of several years, eventually leads to atrophy, or actual loss of substance. This causes an undeniable loss of intellectual ability, which compounds the inevitable changes of senility in one's declining years, the very time of life when one is concerned to stay "with it" for as long as possible. Cassio said to Iago: "O God, that men should put an enemy in their mouths to steal away their brains! That we should with joy, pleasance, revel, and applause transform ourselves into beasts!" (Shakespeare's *Othello:* Act II, Scene 3.)

Alcohol is broken down in the liver to sugars which are then stored as fat, leading to undesirable weight gain, unless adequate exercise prompts further breakdown to waste products. Taken daily, even in small doses, it eventually begins to damage the liver, especially if taken on an empty stomach. Fortunately, unlike the brain, liver cells can regenerate, but only during periods of abstinence, when they are not being overwhelmed with yet more alcohol. These periods of relief are essential to recovery. It is less harmful to the liver to have a binge on a Saturday night and then abstain totally for the rest of the week, than to inflict it daily with no letup. This doesn't mean that the binge is okay. It still kills brain cells, but daily, small amounts of alcohol can cause the liver to become fatty, and, after about fifteen years of continuous abuse, it may become the victim of cirrhosis, an irreversible and potentially fatal degenerative condition.

How can you tell if a family member or friend is in danger of progressing from social drinker to a problem drinker? When should such a one either quit completely or at the least seek professional help? Here's what to look for:

1. He/she makes stronger drinks for himself than for his guests.
2. He seems to be able to enjoy drinking alone, as much or more than if in the company of family or friends.
3. He craves his first drink of the day, and may even have it before noon. Morning drinking is an especially sinister symptom.
4. He tends to be evasive about his habit and usually divides his admitted number of drinks by two or three when stating his consumption.
5. He may slip alcohol into his orange juice or coffee or otherwise try to disguise his intake.
6. He may have had an alcohol-related traffic violation.
7. He may be unable to sleep without a stiff drink.

Two of more of these signs are strong indications that something firm must be done at once to halt an otherwise irreversible downward spiral.

Whereas I am personally convinced that alcohol is harmful, I recognize that some Christians are less concerned. I have, therefore, a few words of caution for Christians who do not feel convinced that they ought or need to be total abstainers. By these comments I am in no way condoning the use of alcohol in any form, but rather advising of some vital principles to be remembered by those Christians who do choose to drink.

Morris Chafetz, M.D., former director of the National Institute on Alcohol Abuse and Alcoholism, has stated that one and a half ounces of pure alcohol per twenty-four hours must be regarded as the upper limit of "safe" drinking. (This is, of course, only a statistical average. For thousands of alcoholics now in Alcoholics Anonymous, and many other people, even one drop is too much.) This one and a half ounces is contained in three one-ounce shots of 100-proof liquor (which is 50 percent alcohol), or in twelve ounces of wine, or in thirty-two ounces of any light beer. More than this consumption will increase the concentration of alcohol in the blood to above 0.05 percent, at which point many brain functions begin to be adversely affected. It would take the liver at least two hours to fully metabolize the one and a half ounces, if taken all at once.

What about the types of alcohol? Within the limits of the amounts just recommended, remember one or two other relevant points. Beer, lager, ale, and stout are all very fattening, have a high calorie/low nutritional quotient, give a gassy, bloated feeling, and have the danger that, though low in alcohol percentage, they are usually drunk in large volumes. Frequently, therefore, at the end of an evening, the drinker has taken in a total of more ounces (and therefore calories) of alcohol than the slow martini sippers. Beers are *very* effective in producing weight gain, especially around the belly and hips!

Hard liquor such as whiskey, gin, vodka, rum, and liqueurs such as brandy and sweet cordials are very high in both expense and alcohol percentage.

The high alcohol content of hard liquors relatively quickly produces in the body a biochemical imbalance. This leads to certain internal adjustment mechanisms which the system adopts in anticipation of continued supply. The victim then experiences craving, a condition in which he can only be comfortable if he indeed keeps the supply coming. This is habituation. As he persists with his habit, he needs increasing doses to produce his required level of comfort. His biochemical systems have by now progressed beyond the stage of mere adaptation. They now have to have alcohol to avoid the acute pain of withdrawal symptoms. This is addiction.

Wines, also, though containing good nutrients from grapes, are just as much of a problem as hard liquors, because of the large quantities usually consumed. Almost all of them contain as much as three times the volume of alcohol as beers, and their high sugar content significantly contributes to fat deposition.

The alcoholic (an addicted person incapable of disciplined restricted "social drinking") can never drink in moderation. He is *unable* to control him/herself. (That is why alcoholism is an illness.) He *is* able however to choose not to drink at all and can learn to live a happy, productive life without alcohol. Recovery begins with admission of one's incapability of self-control and is accomplished successfully by making and acting upon the life-changing decision to quit completely and permanently.

Paul also wrote to the church at Ephesus, "And be not drunk with wine, wherein is excess; but be filled with the Spirit" (Ephesians 5:18). To the Galatians he said: ". . . temperance: against such there is no law. And they that are Christ's have crucified the flesh with the affections and lusts. If we live in the Spirit, let us also walk in the Spirit" (Galatians 5:23–25).

7
Smoking

S. I. McMillen, M.D.,
with David E. Stern, M.D.

The manager of a grocery store phoned me one day. "Doctor," he said, "Mrs. Henderson secretly slipped me a note when I delivered groceries to her house this morning. She says that her husband is very sick—so sick that he is almost out of his head. He won't allow her to leave the house for fear she will never come back. She is afraid he may kill her. She wants you to go to her house to examine her husband."

Mr. Henderson stood over six feet tall. He had been a burly muscular man; but now, his flesh wasted away from his bones and his eyes sunk deep in their sockets, he appeared more like a skeleton than a man. Coughing up masses of blood, he had not slept well for months. His suffering had been long and horrible.

After I questioned and examined him, a diagnosis of cancer of the lung seemed highly probable. By phone I arranged to admit him to the hospital, and it was a big relief to all concerned when the day of his admission arrived. During his first night in the hospital, however, he hemorrhaged severely and drowned, gurgling in his own blood. An autopsy revealed widespread cancer of both lungs.

How often does this sanguinary horror occur in the lives of men and women? In 1983, over 100,000 Americans were strangled to death by lung cancer. The following graph shows that no cancer statistic has ever skyrocketed as high or as rapidly as deaths from lung cancer.

Despite exposure to many new industrial chemicals, Western man has suffered a devastating increase in only one type of cancer—cancer of the

Self-Destructive Habits

AGE-ADJUSTED CANCER DEATH RATES* FOR SELECTED SITES
MALES, UNITED STATES, 1930–1978

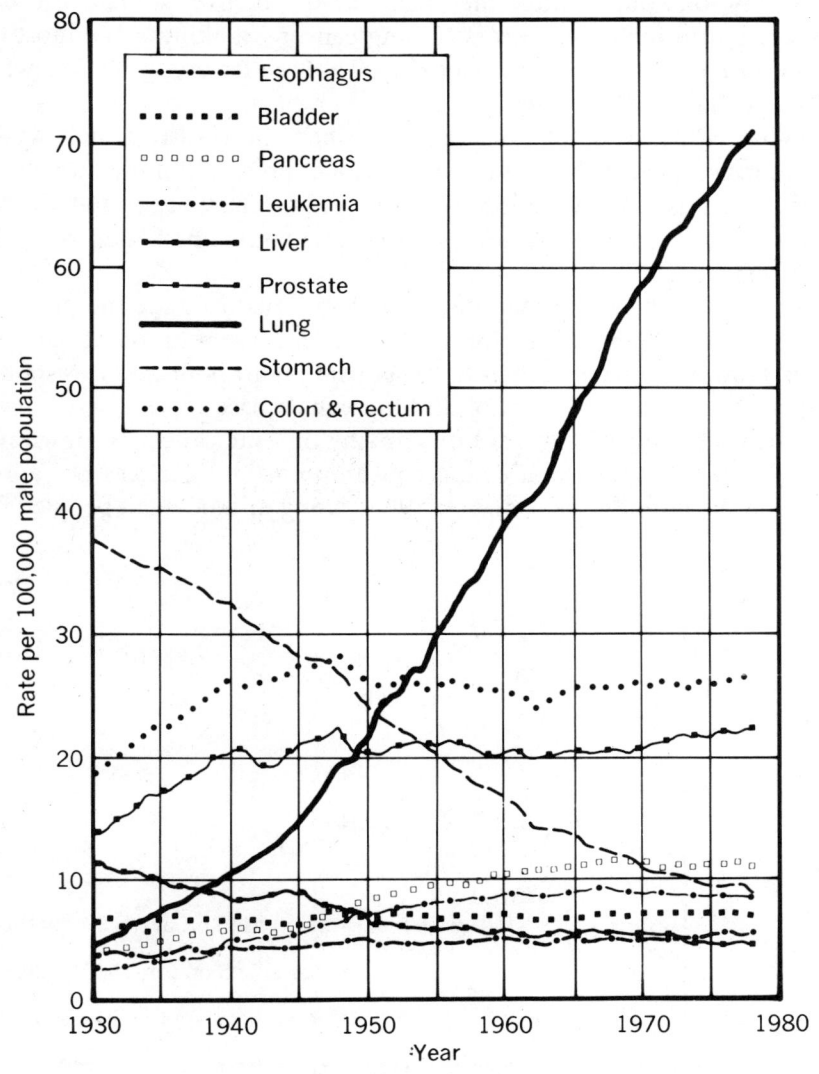

[Graph showing age-adjusted cancer death rates per 100,000 male population from 1930 to 1980 for the following sites: Esophagus, Bladder, Pancreas, Leukemia, Liver, Prostate, Lung, Stomach, Colon & Rectum]

Sources of Data: U.S. National Center for Health Statistics and U.S. Bureau of the Census.
* Adjusted to the age distribution of the 1970 U.S. Census Population.

FIGURE 1: Age-adjusted death rates from the most common cancers in American males since 1930.[1]

lung. The reason for the decrease in stomach cancer is unknown; however, it has nothing to do with smoking.

Back in 1912, lung cancer was called "the rarest of diseases."[2] Then, in the 1920s, it began to increase. In the 1940s and 1950s, the mortality figures zoomed upward at an unbelievable rate.

Today, one out of three men and one out of five women who die of cancer go through the horrors of lung cancer—making it the most common form of cancer in America today. That is a far cry from 1912 when it was the "rarest of diseases."

What is the cause of lung cancer? When the statistics shot skyward, surgeons suspected the cause, but statistical proof did not come until the middle of this century. In 1950 Wynder and Graham reported 605 proven cases of lung cancer. Among these 605 men, only 8 had been non-smokers.[3]

In the past, cigarette manufacturers have tried to dupe the public into believing that these increases in lung cancer have been due to air pollution. However, recent studies have shown that air pollution is responsible for no more than 5 percent of all lung-cancer cases.[4]

The international influence of smoking on lung cancer is shown in figure 2. This graph compares the consumption of cigarettes per adult in 1950 to the rate of lung cancer in 1970 among middle-aged people. Those

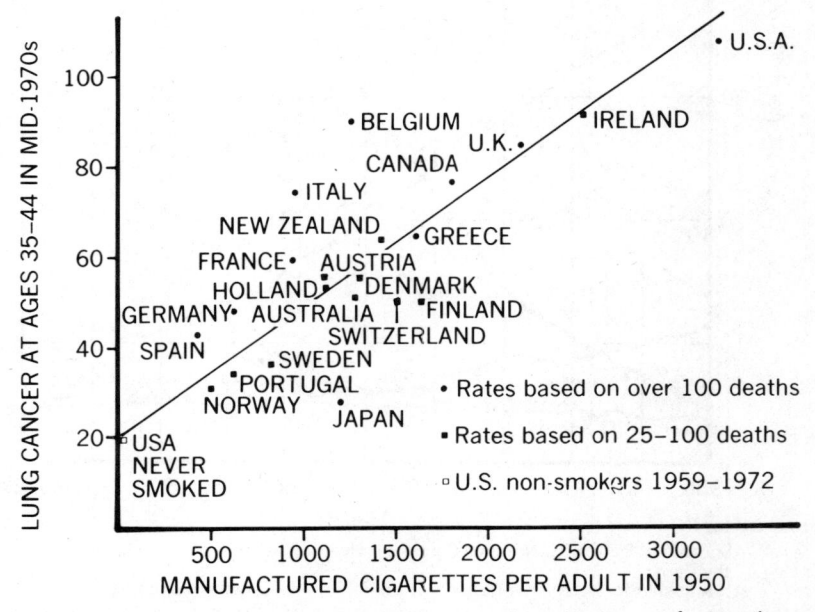

FIGURE 2: International correlation between cigarettes manufactured per adult in 1950 and lung cancer rates in 1970.[5]

countries in which cigarette consumption was high when a certain generation was entering adulthood had much higher lung-cancer rates when that generation reached middle age. Those countries that had lower cigarette consumption subsequently had much lower rates of lung cancer.

In 1979, the Surgeon General released a vast summary of all the research to date on the effects of smoking on health.[6] In this immense volume, hundreds of studies of literally hundreds of thousands of people were cited. The results of these studies not only proved that smoking is the major cause of lung cancer, but they also demonstrated that smoking is responsible for many deaths from other cancers and other diseases. The Surgeon General reports that smokers are particularly susceptible to:

1. **Cancers:** including cancers of the lung, larynx, mouth, esophagus, bladder, and pancreas
2. **Cardiovascular Disease:** including coronary heart disease, hypertension, and aortic aneurysms
3. **Lung Diseases:** including emphysema, chronic bronchitis, influenza and pneumonia
4. **Gastrointestinal Diseases:** including ulcers of the stomach and duodenum.

Figures 3 and 4 illustrate how the number of cigarettes smoked influences the risk for dying from various diseases. People who smoke more than two packs per day have a rate of lung cancer that is seventy-two times greater than that of the nonsmokers! Heavy smokers contract cancer of the larynx (voice box) over thirty-four times more often than nonsmokers.

In addition to the 100,000 Americans who die yearly from lung cancer, tobacco habits slaughter thousands of men and women from cancer of many other organs. The surest way to die a painful and premature death is to buy cancer by the carton.

One wonders how smoking can produce cancer in organs such as the urinary bladder, which is far removed from cigarette smoke. Scientists have now identified in tobacco smoke over forty-two different chemicals that can cause cancer when injected into animals. These products, when inhaled into the lungs, dissolve in the blood, spread throughout the body, and are excreted in the urine. Thus, the chemicals in cigarette smoke contact every organ in the body. The carcinogens and toxins in cigarette smoke include carbon monoxide, ammonia, cyanide, acetone, benzene, phenol, DDT, methyl alcohol, arsenic, formaldehyde, nitrobenzene, and a radioactive element Polonium-210. From this partial list, you can see

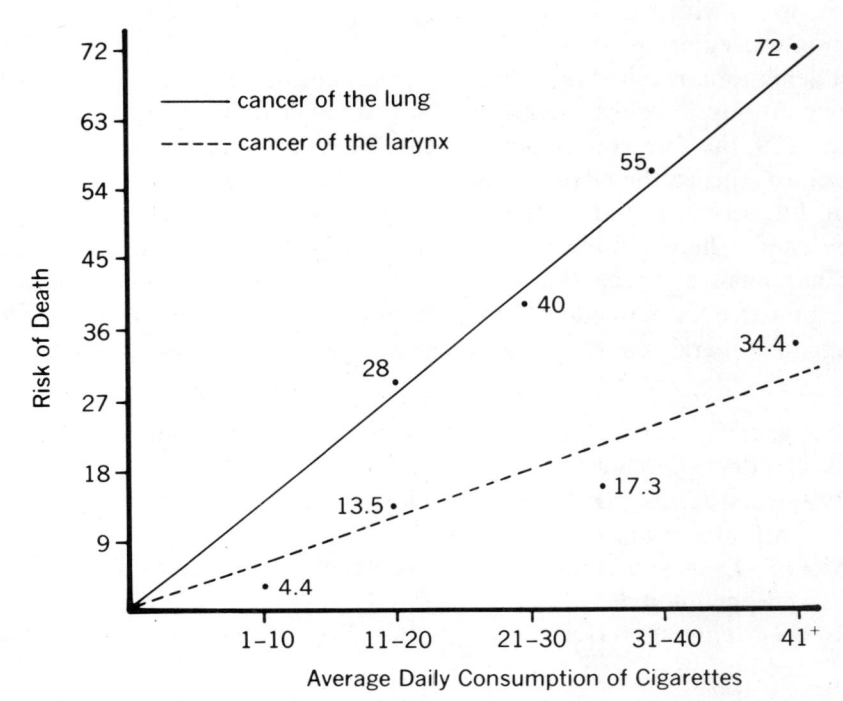

FIGURE 3: Risk for lung and laryngeal cancer death related to amount smoked.[7]

that a smoker uses his lungs and body as a veritable toxic-waste dump, rivaling anything created by pesticide companies.

A few years ago I was called out of bed to treat a man who was experiencing severe, crushing chest pain. When I arrived, the man lay on the floor. His face was ashen gray. His eyes stared motionless at the ceiling. He was not breathing; his heart was not beating. He was dead. A clot in his coronary artery had shut off the supply of blood to his heart and had changed his muscular blood pump into a lifeless bag of tissue. The blocked coronary is the master of executioners, killing over 700,000 men and women in America every year.

In my patient's shirt pocket was a partly empty pack of cigarettes. Can smoking cause heart disease? Yes! Looking at figure 4, you can see that the more a man smokes, the more likely he is to die of heart disease. The American Heart Association studied over 7,000 men and found that smoking was indeed associated with death from coronary-artery disease. Those who smoked more than one pack a day were three times more likely to die from a heart attack than were their nonsmoking counterparts.[8] About one-third of the 700,000 Americans who die from coronary artery disease are killed by the fire in their mouths. Thus, in addition to

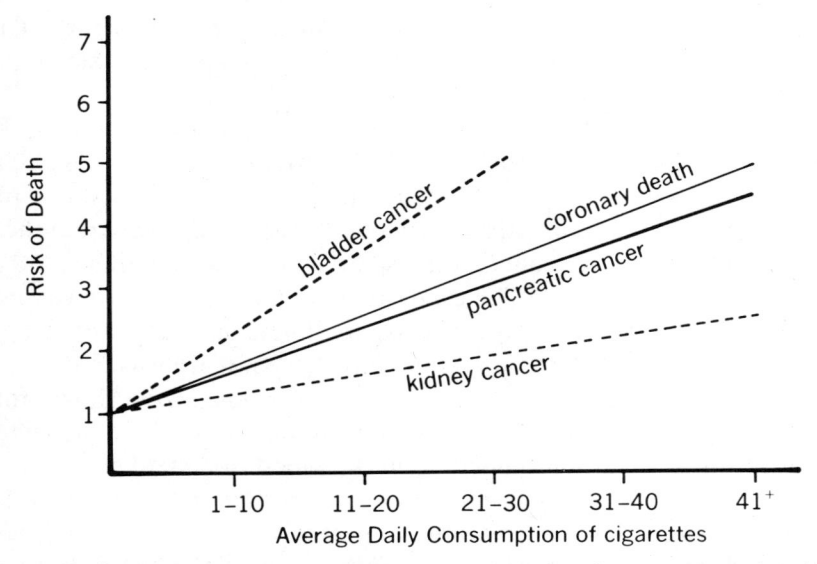

FIGURE 4: Risk for death due to heart attacks and various cancers related to amount smoked.[9]

the 100,000 Americans who yearly succumb to lung cancer, cigarettes kill about 230,000 more with heart disease.

Not only is smoking the major cause of lung cancer, it is also the most important preventable cause of fatal heart attacks. Comparing a cigarette to a coffin nail is far more than a figure of speech.

Cigarettes use several mechanisms to bring about coronary death. The chemicals in cigarette smoke promote the formation of atherosclerotic plaques in coronary arteries. Researchers autopsied over 1,000 veterans and found that heavy smokers were more than four times as likely to suffer from advanced coronary-artery atherosclerosis.[10] Smoking also increases the stickiness of certain blood cells; thus, a smoker's blood is more likely to clot within the already-narrowed coronary arteries.

When the vessel is finally clogged up, the smoker is at a distinct disadvantage. The nicotine in his blood stimulates his heart to work harder than normal, so his heart needs more oxygen to support its higher work load. However, carbon monoxide from cigarette smoke binds very tightly to hemoglobin—the oxygen-carrying molecule—thereby lowering its capacity to transport oxygen. Thus, blood that gets through or around a clogged artery carries less oxygen to a heart that requires more oxygen due to its increased work load.

Reduction of blood flow and damage to the arteries can cause serious trouble in other organs. In the brain, the damaged arteries are prone to induce clots, thereby causing strokes. The Surgeon General reports that the death rate from strokes is about 70 percent higher in smokers.[11] This percentage is truly startling, since strokes annually strike dead about 120,000 Americans.

Tobacco companies have responded to this vast amount of evidence by producing and heavily advertising "safer" cigarettes. In 1968 these cigarettes made up 2 percent of the United States market; but today, one out of three cigarettes sold is a "safer" cigarette. However, tobacco from these "low nicotine" cigarettes contains the same amount of nicotine as other cigarettes! How can this be? The cigarette manufacturers have developed ventilated filters and porous cigarette papers. These modifications change the way that cigarettes burn, so that the nicotine content measured by the government's machines are falsely low. In fact, studies have shown that the labeled "tar and nicotine" content of cigarettes does not influence the level of nicotine or carbon monoxide in the blood of a smoker.[12]

One study even showed that the risk for heart attacks was the same for those who smoked "low tar" cigarettes and those who smoked "high tar" cigarettes. A person's risk for heart attack was determined by the number, not the type, of cigarettes smoked.[13] Thus, there is no such thing as a "low risk" cigarette.

Emphysema is another common and serious condition caused by smoking. New evidence indicates that emphysema results from several enzyme changes. One enzyme, named *elastase,* circulates in the blood. Elastase breaks down the stretchy lung protein, elastin, that expands all of the tiny air sacs and the air tubules in the lung. Fortunately, however, the body makes another molecule, *antitrypsin,* that blocks the breakdown of elastin in the lung. Cigarette smoke destroys the function of antitrypsin; so, the unblocked elastase is free to break down lung tissue. Not only does smoking destroy lung tissue, it also retards repair of the damaged elastin. Cigarette smoke blocks the formation of another enzyme, *lysl oxidase.* Without this enzyme, the body is unable to replace the smoke-damaged elastin. Therefore, cigarette smoke not only causes the body to "digest" its own lungs, but also blocks repair of this damage. Unsupported by elastin, all of the tiny air passages in the lungs collapse; and the smoker slowly suffocates.

The Surgeon General reports that the average sixty-three-year-old female smoker has destroyed her lungs to such an extent that they function as poorly as the lungs of the average eighty-year-old non-smoking woman.[14]

One of David's patients had such severe emphysema that he could not even dress himself without becoming breathless. Through a hole in his windpipe, he was connected to a continuous supply of oxygen. Unable to

Self-destructive Habits

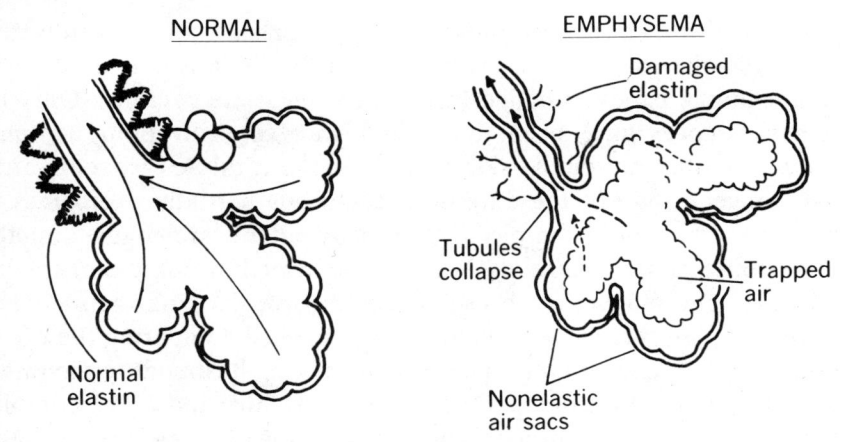

NORMAL   **EMPHYSEMA**

(Diagram labels: Normal elastin; Damaged elastin; Tubules collapse; Trapped air; Nonelastic air sacs)

FIGURE 5: Mechanism of suffocation in emphysema.

completely exhale through his collapsed airways, his lungs trapped air and blew up like balloons until his chest assumed the shape of a pickle barrel. For the past seven years, he had limited his activity to rolling over in bed, changing the channels on his TV, and smoking his demon cigarettes.

Another effect of smoking is wrinkled skin. One study showed that "crow's feet" were much more common in smokers.[15] One has to question the sanity of a society that spends billions of dollars to get and preserve better looks, yet smokes billions of cigarettes, which irreparably destroy those looks.

Smoking not only decreases sexual appeal, but also decreases sexual fertility. Male smokers are more likely to be infertile. They have decreased sperm count in their semen, and the sperm tend to be abnormal in motility and shape.[16]

Tobacco smoke even affects others in the room. How many times have we all seen a mother cuddle her child while exhaling a cloud of smoke into his face. I have treated many such a child for frequently recurring runny noses, raspy coughs, and sore throats. I have told these parents that their children are so susceptible to these viral infections because their mucous membranes are constantly being irritated by the "second hand" smoke from their parents' cigarettes. Even after my careful explanations, most of them inquired if it would help to try a new medicine for colds, massive doses of some vitamin, or nighttime humidification of bedroom air; yet they seldom asked me how to quit the habit that had caused these colds.

One study showed that after a little over an hour in a smoke-filled room people had inhaled the amount of carbon monoxide equivalent to smoking one cigarette.[17] In addition, at least thirty-nine cancer causing or toxic chemicals have been found in higher concentrations in sidestream smoke (smoke wisping into room air from the lit end) that in the mainstream smoke (smoke inhaled through the cigarette column). Only four such substances have been found in higher concentrations in "mainstream" smoke. Although "sidestream" smoke is diluted by room air, its high concentration of these harmful chemicals partially overcomes this dilutional effect. For example, an extremely potent carcinogen, dimethylnitrosamine, is up to 830 times more concentrated in sidestream smoke.[18]

Has anyone shown that this so-called "passive smoking" actually leads to cancer? Yes, three studies have been published comparing the rates of lung cancer in nonsmoking wives of nonsmoking husbands to the rates of lung cancer in nonsmoking wives of smoking husbands. The combined data from these three studies suggests that nonsmoking women have a rate of lung cancer about 50 percent higher if they are married to men who smoke.[19]

Although tobacco products are heavily taxed at several levels of government, the economic burden of smokers on society is astounding. The following table itemizes the economic costs of smoking in the United States.

Total Economic Costs of Smoking in 1975[20]	
Cancers	$ 4.4 billion
Cardiovascular diseases	12.7 billion
Lung diseases	8.4 billion
Fires	0.4 billion
Cost of tobacco (retail)	15.7 billion
Total cost	$41.6 billion

Although smokers paid $5.6 billion in tobacco taxes, their habit cost themselves and society $41.6 billion—an average of $692 per smoker per year. Their excess health costs made up over half of the costs for all lung diseases, about one-third of the costs for all cardiovascular disease, and about one-quarter of the costs for all cancers. Tell that to a smoker the next time that you hear one claim that his habit supports the economy!

Mention should be made of the effect of smoking on women. The only reason that fewer women are suffering medical tragedies today is that they have not been smoking for as many years as men. In fact, the main reason that women live an average of seven years longer than men is that

AGE-ADJUSTED CANCER DEATH RATES* FOR SELECTED SITES
FEMALES, UNITED STATES, 1930-1978

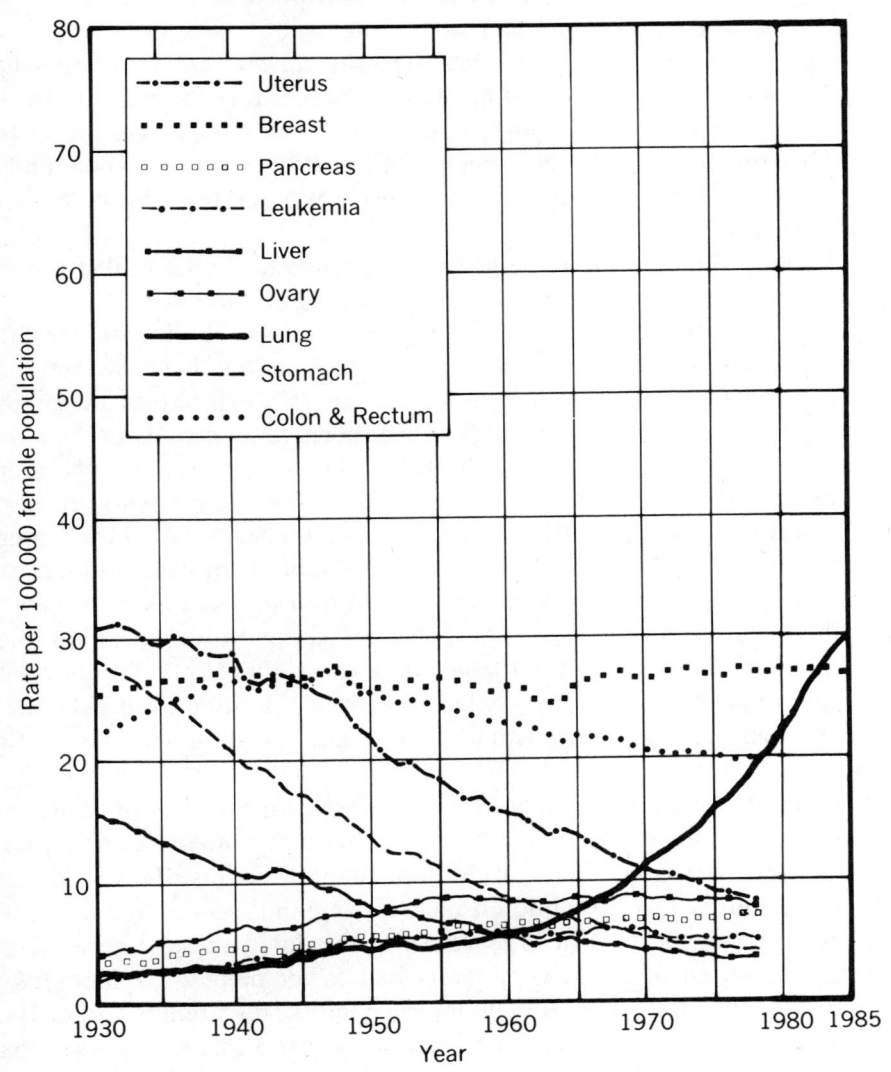

- —·—·— Uterus
- ▪ ▪ ▪ ▪ ▪ ▪ Breast
- ▫ ▫ ▫ ▫ ▫ ▫ Pancreas
- —·—·— Leukemia
- ●——●——● Liver
- ●——●——● Ovary
- ▬▬▬▬ Lung
- — — — — Stomach
- ● ● ● ● ● ● Colon & Rectum

Sources of Data: U.S. National Center for Health Statistics and U.S. Bureau of the Census.
* Adjusted to the age distribution of the 1970 U.S. Census Population.
Based on projected statistics *Beyond* 1978.

FIGURE 6: Age-adjusted death rate for the most common cancers in females since 1930.[21]

fewer women than men have smoked over the last several decades. In 1924 only 6 percent of women smoked, but by 1944 about 36 percent of women were smokers. In the 1980s, more teenage girls smoked than teenage boys; thus, in future years, we can expect the life expectancy of women to begin to drop to near that of men.

Figure 6 shows that since 1965 the lung-cancer rate of women has begun to skyrocket just as fast as the lung cancer rate for men did in the 1940s (figure 1). In 1985, lung cancer will surpass breast cancer as the number-one cancer killer of women. In the last twenty years women have more than tripled their rate of lung cancer. Women truly have "come a long way, baby."

Women who take the pill and smoke are five times more likely to die from fatal heart attacks than their nonsmoking counterparts.[22]

Even more frightening is the effect of a mother's smoking on her children. Women who smoke more than one pack per day have two times as many premature babies as nonsmoking mothers. Their babies are, on the average, 6.4 ounces lighter than babies born to nonsmokers.[23] A few ounces may not seem like much, but these lighter babies are much more likely to suffer complications of all types. Thus, infants who are born alive have an increased death rate if their mothers smoked during pregnancy. Smoking mothers, also, more than double their chances of delivering a stillborn child. They are also almost four times as likely to have a stillborn due to abruption of the placenta—a condition where the placenta prematurely tears away from the mother's uterus.[24] Abruption of the placenta often results not only in death of the infant; but also often leads to serious, sometimes lethal, clotting and bleeding disorders in the mother.[25]

Smoking during pregnancy also has long-lasting effects on children. Researchers studied the children of mothers who smoked during pregnancy and compared them to children of nonsmokers. This study included almost all 17,000 children born in England, Scotland, and Wales during a six-day period in 1958. Eleven years later, these children were tested. Children of smoking mothers had lower mental abilities. Even after adjusting for social and biological factors, researchers found that children of smoking mothers had mathematical and reading ages that were an average of about six months behind. These children also had stunted physical growth in that they were an average of 1.5 centimeters shorter.[26]

If one were to tally the excess deaths due to tobacco habits—including those from cancers, strokes, pneumonia, influenza, tuberculosis, emphysema, asthma, ulcers, stillbirths, and coronary heart trouble—the annual total would be about 400,000 Americans.

Self-destructive Habits

What should be done about this proven killer? In the early seventeenth century, Turks who were caught smoking were beheaded, hung, and quartered. In Russia under the first czar, smokers had their noses slit, their testicles castrated, their backs flogged, and their bodies exiled to Siberia. Few would endorse such severe methods today, but there are many ways by which our country could reduce tobacco consumption.

Since almost all smokers start before the age of twenty, much effort has been directed at deterring teenagers from beginning this lethal habit. Education and fear, however, have proven to be insufficient motivators; for one study found that even three out of four teen smokers believe that smoking is a bad habit and that it can harm their health.[27]

Why has the widespread knowledge of the dangers of smoking not led to decreased smoking by teenagers? The major obstacle to discouraging smoking is the association of smoking with adulthood and independence. Researchers asked teens to describe two almost identical pictures: one depicted a man with a cigarette in his hand, and the other had the cigarette removed. Teens were more likely to describe the man with the cigarette as adventurous, rugged, daring, energetic, and individualistic. Without the cigarette, the man was more often described as shy, gentle, timid, and awkward.[28] From these studies, we can see that cigarette ads—by associating smoking with rugged, individualistic men and beautiful, sophisticated women—have exerted a tremendous deleterious influence on the impressionable minds of teenagers. Although almost all teens consciously realize that smoking is extremely harmful to their health, cigarette advertisements have successfully sabotaged the onslaught of scientific evidence by attacking at the point where teens are most vulnerable—their subconscious desire to appear grown-up.

Any government that continues to allow smoking advertisement is irresponsible. A survey of Americans found that 62 percent of nonsmokers and 43 percent of smokers felt that cigarette advertising should be banned.[29] The reason that tobacco companies agreed to discontinue television advertisement was a law called the "Fairness Doctrine," which had stated that for every dollar spent on cigarette advertisement, the tobacco companies had to give another dollar to antismoking campaigns. Although prosmoking TV ads resulted in an average yearly increase of 75 cigarettes per person, the antismoking ads resulted in a yearly reduction of over 500 cigarettes per person.[30] In order to get this "Fairness Doctrine" repealed, the tobacco companies were even willing to give up television advertising. Thus, because it resulted in a decrease in antismoking commercials, the net effect of the ban on TV advertisement was an increase in cigarette sales. Many people thought that this ban was a victory

a) Reading Comprehension

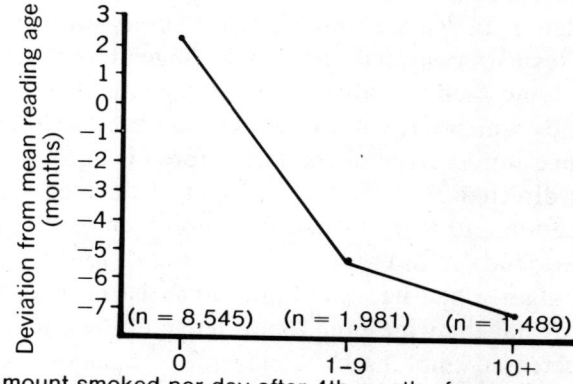

[Graph: Deviation from mean reading age (months) vs Amount smoked per day after 4th month of pregnancy. Points at 0 (n = 8,545), 1-9 (n = 1,981), 10+ (n = 1,489).]

b) Mathematics Ability

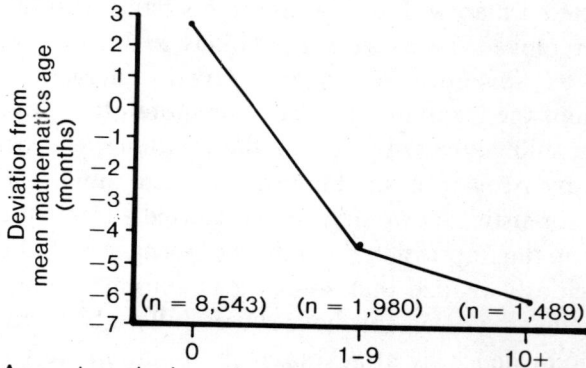

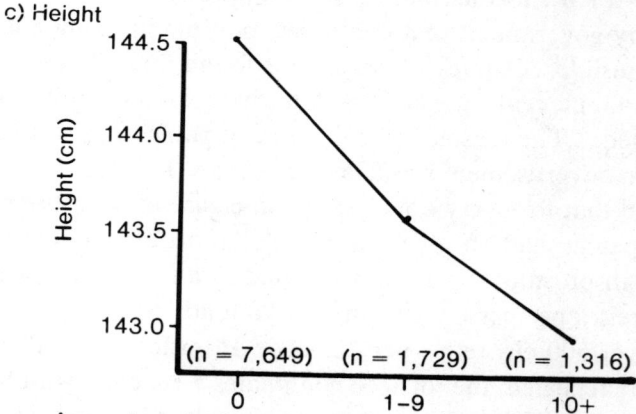

[Graph: Deviation from mean mathematics age (months) vs Amount smoked per day after 4th month of pregnancy. Points at 0 (n = 8,543), 1-9 (n = 1,980), 10+ (n = 1,489).]

c) Height

[Graph: Height (cm) vs Amount smoked per day after 4th month of pregnancy. Points at 0 (n = 7,649), 1-9 (n = 1,729), 10+ (n = 1,316).]

FIGURE 7: Intelligence and height of eleven-year-old children related to the smoking habits of their mothers after the fourth month of pregnancy.[31]

Self-destructive Habits

for public health, but it turns out that it was just another demonstration of the evil cunning and manipulative power of the giant tobacco industry.

Tobacco is a proven killer of hundreds of thousands of Americans each year, yet the government seems to close its eyes to the evidence. Let us face squarely the reason behind this paradox. Any political party that attacked the $15 billion tobacco industry would be committing political suicide. Although this country counts its tobacco killings by the hundreds of thousands, its politicians count their profits from political contributions by the millions of dollars. Congressmen and senators from tobacco states (even those men who claim to espouse Christian principles) staunchly defend the nicotine giants with the rhetoric of "free trade." Our senators and congressmen seem as devoid of conscience as home computers. As Nero kept aloof and fiddled while Rome burned, so our government appears to be detached while the nicotine giants annually incinerate over 400,000 Americans.

We should demand immediate government action before tobacco habits claim more multitudes of American lives. All tobacco advertisement should be banned. Tobacco products should be taxed to pay for a deluge of antismoking advertisements. Increased production of cigarettes should be halted, and slow but significant reductions should begin at once.

Reducing cigarette consumption would soon result in improved health for many Americans and reduced health-care costs for all Americans. As the government's health representative, the Surgeon General, states, "The highest priority in the field of public health is that individuals who have not started smoking should not begin and that those who currently smoke should quit."[32] We should demand that our government act toward this end.

If you have been trapped by nicotine, you may wonder how you can best keep your children from starting the habit. Statistics show that one of the most important factors in determining whether children smoke is whether their parents smoke. If both parents smoke, over 20 percent of their children will smoke; but if neither parent smokes, less than 10 percent of their children will become trapped in this filthy habit.[33] Quitting smoking will do more to influence your children's smoking status than anything else you can do. In fact, several studies have shown that parents' *attitudes* toward their children's smoking have no influence on whether their children take up the habit.[34]

Why do people stick their heads into the noose of the smoking habit? A person enjoys the first encounter with smoking in spite (not because) of nicotine, for this drug usually induces nausea and dizziness at the first encounter. Why do they begin? I recall our arrival in Philadephia from one of our African missionary terms. While we were shopping in the large stores, our three-year-old daughter kept putting little pieces of paper between her lips, and I kept pulling them out. Finally I said, "Linda, why are you putting these pieces of paper between your lips?"

"Daddy, everybody in America has fire in their mouths. This is my fire."

Why do they continue? To many preteenagers and teenagers, smoking is the hallmark of maturity. It is a status symbol to show the world that they have arrived. Smoking soon becomes a "useful accomplishment" to adolescents who are struggling for acceptance and peer status. In difficult situations, instead of fidgeting, they have something to do with their hands. Sharing cigarettes with others gives them a feeling of belonging to a group of friends.

The most important reason, however, that people continue smoking is that they become addicted to nicotine. Nicotine, whether inhaled or injected with a needle, is a habit-producing drug that calls for more and more. Ninety percent of the nicotine in smoke is absorbed into the blood. Within seven seconds it reaches the brain where it is rapidly concentrated. In the brain, nicotine mimics a chemical messenger. First, nicotine stimulates certain neurons by activating nicotine receptors; later, it inhibits these neurons by sticking to their surfaces. Since these neurons are important in portions of the brain responsible for physical and mental arousal, learning, memory, and emotions—it is little wonder that stimulating and inhibiting these centers has a tremendous effect on the nicotine addict. In fact, nicotine is so potent and these neurons are so essential that one drop of pure nicotine placed on the tongue of a dog results in rapid and agonizing death.[35] Serious and sometimes lethal nicotine poisoning occurs when a small child accidentally eats a pack of cigarettes.

The importance of nicotine addiction has been dramatically demonstrated by Dr. M. E. Jarvick. Dr. Jarvick found that monkeys normally preferred to breathe pure air rather than air polluted with cigarette smoke. He forced his monkeys to puff on cigarette smoke, and they soon preferred to breathe air polluted with cigarette smoke. However, when Dr. Jarvick administered a drug that blocked their brain receptors for nicotine, these monkeys again preferred to breathe clean air.[36]

Smokers also continue to require nicotine "fixes" to relieve their anxiety. One researcher found that smokers were able to tolerate high levels of electric shock when they smoked nicotine-enriched cigarettes. Their tolerance to shock, however, decreased when they smoked extremely low nicotine cigarettes.[37] Because of their increased anxiety these nicotine-deprived smokers become unable to tolerate as much aggravation from electric shocks.

Self-destructive Habits

The reason that smokers require such frequent "shots" of nicotine is that nicotine is so rapidly broken down and excreted in the urine. In fact, smokers smoke more cigarettes when they are nervous because stress acidifies their urine. Acid urine causes the nicotine to be excreted at a faster rate. Thus, smokers undergoing stress must smoke more cigarettes in order to maintain the same nicotine blood levels.

Another reason that people smoke is simply that it becomes a habit. We are creatures of habit; anything that we repeat daily, hourly, or by the minute—we soon do without thinking. Habits may include tying shoelaces, kissing a spouse, biting nails, or shaking hands. Marcel Proust observed that the strength of a habit is generally in proportion to its absurdity; the absurd habit of inhaling harsh tobacco smoke into delicate lung tissues certainly follows this rule.

I remember a young woman who attended a nearby college where smoking was forbidden. She thought it was sophisticated and smart to sneak a cigarette when no one was looking. She considered the anti-smoking college standards fanatical and foolish. Because her style was cramped, she finally went elsewhere.

Many years later she called me to see if there was anything that she could possibly do to stop smoking. Something had come up, and she wanted to get rid of her habit. Was there any drug I could send her to deliver her from her bondage. Now she recognized that the maturity she was proud of a few years ago was actually a most disappointing immaturity. The freedom she had sought had slowly enslaved and now constantly tortured her.

Sigmund Freud was a classic example of a slave to nicotine. Smoking twenty cigars a day, he suffered forty years of heart disease and endured thirty-three operations for mouth cancer, from which he eventually died. His doctors strongly warned him that his smoking was probably the cause of his afflictions, yet he found it impossible to quit. On the few occasions that he tried to quit, he suffered the classic symptoms of nicotine withdrawal. Because his brain missed the nicotine-induced amphetaminelike high, he became depressed and soon returned to his lethal habit. Once, when confronted by a physician, he replied, "I am not following your interdict from smoking; do you think then it is so very lucky to have a long miserable life?"[38]

The benefits of quitting smoking, however, are immense. After only three weeks of abstinence, young adults have decreased heart rates, more efficient breathing, more elastic lungs, and increased exercise tolerance.[39]

Smokers usually find it much easier to quit when they finally get lung cancer or heart disease, but it makes a lot more sense to quit before one gets a fatal disease. Ex-smokers decrease their risks for heart attacks, strokes, and lung cancer. After quitting for five years, smokers more than halve their risk for lung cancer; and after fifteen smokeless years their lung-cancer rate approaches that of nonsmokers.[40]

Although gradual withdrawal has been successful for many drug addicts, this technique does not work well for nicotine addicts. People who try to cut down slowly or even just to low-nicotine cigarettes experience all of the symptoms of the smoker who goes "cold turkey," but their discomfort is more severe and more protracted. Dr. Saul Schiffman found that those who quit "cold turkey" had a very rapid decrease in their craving for a cigarette and that their physical symptoms practically disappeared by eight days after quitting. However, those who tried to quit slowly had physical symptoms of discomfort and severe cravings for cigarettes that lasted for the entire two-week study.[41]

I once asked one of my medical colleagues—who, after smoking for most of his life, had quit—if he had found it difficult to stop. "No," he said, "not after I really made up my mind. When I quit, I got rid of the biggest nuisance in my life."

"What do you mean?" I asked. "I thought people smoked because they enjoyed it."

"It's not like that at all," he replied. "I got rid of a grand nuisance. I was always looking for cigarettes, for matches, for ashtrays. I burned holes in my suits and the furniture. When I quit, I got rid of the biggest annoyance anybody can ever have."

He is only one of many thousands of physicians who decided they were fools to continue smoking. Among physicans, a surprising change of attitude has occurred during the past thirty years. Years ago at meetings I had to struggle to see the speaker through a smoky haze. For a day or two afterward I smelled like something smoked. Even the *Journal of the American Medical Association* carried ads for various brands of cigarettes. Today, however, the rare physician who smokes at a medical meeting is considered to be something like a stock market analyst who advises his clients to buy bullish stock but himself buys stock that he knows is going to crash. In David's medical-school class, there were very few students who smoked. Most of those who did smoke tried to hide their habit because their fellow students regarded them with disdain for their lack of self-control. In 1949, about 60 percent of physicians smoked cigarettes. In 1975, a survey of physicians found that only 21 percent of physicians still smoked and 37 percent had quit.[42]

These changes in attitudes and habits have occurred because medical science has discovered and proved that smoking is the greatest single preventable cause of:

Public Killer No. 1—Heart disease
Pubic Killer No. 2—Cancer

Self-destructive Habits

Everybody should be thankful that medical science has opened its eyes to the dangers of smoking. How much more thankful we should be to the Lord because He warned many of His people about and saved countless thousands of His followers from a variety of horrible deaths many years before any scientific studies were done.

I recall the testimony of a man who had been converted in an environment where there was no preaching against smoking. The Spirit of God told him to stop smoking. He thought it very strange for God to make such an odd request of him, but he obeyed. Sometime later he came across passages in the Bible that confirmed the course he had taken.

Tobacco was not used in the Middle East when the Bible was written. It is, therefore, not mentioned specifically in the Bible. The impact of many Bible passages, however, gave sufficient warning to keep millions of Christians from using tobacco in any form even before medical science had proven the dangers of these habits. These admonitions—coupled with observation of tobacco users with their spittoons, smells, smokes, and sicknesses—deterred many believers from indulging.

As early as 1604, King James I of England attacked smoking as, "lothesome to the eye, hatefull to the Nose, harmfull to the braine, dangerous to the Lungs, and in the blacke stinking fume thereof, neerest resembling the horrible Stigian smoke of the pit that is bottomles."[43]

In 1653, Jacob Bald, a Jesuit priest, asked, "What difference is there between a smoker and a suicide; except that the one takes longer to kill himself than the other?"[44]

To a Christian, indulgence would be inconsistent with obedience to such Scriptures as:

> Do you not know that your body is a temple of the Holy Spirit, who is in you.... You are not your own; you were bought at a price. Therefore honor God with your body.
> 1 Corinthians 6:19, 20 NIV

> If anyone destroys God's temple, God will destroy him; for God's temple is sacred, and you are that temple.
> 1 Corinthians 3:17 NIV

> So whether you eat or drink or whatever you do, do it all for the glory of God.
> 1 Corinthians 10:31 NIV

Guidance by the Holy Spirit and obedience to the Holy Bible have allowed many Christians to suffer from "none of these diseases"—these diseases caused by tobacco and nicotine.

HOW TO QUIT
O. Quentin Hyder, M.D.

How to quit? It takes motivation and courage. Here are some hopefully helpful suggestions.

There are several systems that use conditioning therapy, with self-imposed rewards for success and penalties for failure. These take several weeks, but work well if you stick with it. The Schick Stop-Smoking Clinics use aversion therapy in which taking certain controlled substances so alters the taste of cigarettes that one quickly loses all desire to smoke again. This is thoroughly unpleasant, but quick and effective.

Hypnosis can sometimes be effective, though I have some reservations. Occasionally, after treatment, an alternative habit may develop, such as nail biting, gum chewing, excessive coffee drinking, or taking tranquilizers, if any underlying problems are not dealt with. Also, Christians generally are resistant to the prospect of submitting control of their minds to another person. For these reasons, although I don't recommend a trial of hypnotherapy, I strongly urge anyone intent on giving it a try to go to a well-qualified person, preferably a psychiatrist or other medical doctor.

The department of psychiatry of your local county or city hospital should be able to advise you what number to call to obtain one of these therapies.

"Cold turkey," or ending smoking abruptly by yourself, is the quickest, but the most painful. If you choose this method, pick a definite date: the first of next month, a birthday, an anniversary. It helps the significance of the commitment. Withdrawal symptoms, such as craving, last from two to three weeks, and you may experience temporary nervousness, sleep disturbance, fatigue, slight weight gain, and inability to concentrate. But stick with it. The long-term benefits of quitting far outweigh the brief discomfort period.

Cutting down gradually is less painful, but may take several weeks. In my view this is the best method, if you can be both patient and determined. Use of the four-stage filter system which progressively reduces the tar and nicotine inhaled has helped some to quit over a period of a few weeks. Try also these tested and effective methods which have worked for many who have attended Smoke Enders classes.

1. Realize that smoking is a learned habit and, therefore, through the behavior modification of constant practice, you can relearn the habit of nonsmoking.
2. Motivation is essential. Establish your incentive to quit. Write down a list of reasons: health needs, economics, self-concept, aesthetics,

effect on others, example to your children, self-mastery, and so forth. Be positive. Have the attitude that you are achieving something, not that you are denying yourself something.

3. Keep a cigarette count sheet and carefully record every one you use, at what time, under what circumstances, and how you are feeling. Keep the sheet wrapped round your pack and don't light up until you've noted it down.
4. Start breaking the habit by carrying your pack in a different place. At home or in the office store them out of easy reach. Start smoking without inhaling. Hold the ciragette in the hand you don't usually use. Do not carry matches or lighters. Take fewer puffs and use only half the cigarette, or even less. Mix a variety of different brands of cigarettes in your pack. This will begin to make smoking unpleasant.
5. Pick substitute habits to meet needs formerly met by smoking. (This does not include pot, alcohol, or eating!) When you desire a smoke, wait at least five minutes before giving in. Try these distractions first; the desire might go away: Find something small you can play with with your fingers. Take a short but brisk walk, if you can get out. In the office do some isometrics or knee bends. Half a dozen slow, very deep breaths held for a few seconds both at the full and empty points are very therapeutic.
6. Agree with yourself that you will smoke at least one less cigarette tomorrow than today. Again, don't regard this as a sacrifice or feel sorry for yourself. Be glad you're actually succeeding in quitting. The end is in sight. Drink plenty of water to wash the nicotine out of your body.
7. Set a definite date in the near future for your absolute last cigarette. Tell many close friends of your resolve. Such public commitment will bolster your determination. Find a friend who has also successfully quit smoking and encourage each other to stick with it.
8. Committed Christian believers have one additional resource: the power of the indwelling Holy Spirit. "Praise the Lord and Pass the Ammunition" we used to sing in World War II. Any battle in this life needs a combination of personal courage, effort, and determination, with God's invoked strength and help. "God helps those who help themselves" is a well-known, though nonbiblical, truism commonly used in our culture. "Fortune favors the brave" is a similar secular motto of a prep school I attended in England.

As Christians, we don't believe in luck, but God so often does seem to bless those who strive to serve Him. In my life's experience I have found that once I have made my own utmost human effort, somehow things work out for the best eventually. God seems to come through with the answers, and the help. Smoking (like drinking, overeating, and drug dependence) is a form of lust which can be conquered with a combination of guts and God.

My discipline, motivation and commitment, plus God's support, wisdom, and strength, is an unconquerable team. My part is to "... make not provision for the flesh, to fulfil the lusts thereof" (Romans 13:14). God's part is committed in His promise of Spiritual power: "... Walk in the Spirit, and ye *shall not* fulfil the lust of the flesh" (Galatians 5:16, italics added).

A final sobering thought. The graph of cigarette consumption by women has climbed dramatically in the last twenty years, and the graph of their mortality rates from lung cancer and cardiovascular disease has almost exactly paralleled it. It is rapidly approaching the male graph, a doubtful achievement in equality of the sexes. Truly we can say with Virginia Slims, "You've come a long way, baby!"

Source Notes

1. E. Silverberg and J.A. Lubera, "A Review of American Cancer Society Estimates of Cancer Cases and Deaths," *Ca—A Cancer Journal for Clinicians* 33 (1983):15. © 1983 American Cancer Society, Inc.
2. Alton Ochsner, *Smoking and Cancer* (New York: Julian Messner, Inc, 1954), p. 12.
3. *Ibid.,* p. 4.
4. G. Hammond and L. Garfinkel, "General Air Pollution and Cancer in the United States," *Preventive Medicine* 9 (1980):206.
5. Surgeon General, *The Health Consequences of Smoking: Cancer* (Washington, D.C.: Government Printing Office, 1981).
6. Surgeon General, *Smoking and Health* (Washington, D.C.: Government Printing Office, 1979).
7. Surgeon General, *Health Consequences of Smoking: Cancer,* pp. 41, 69.
8. O. Auerbach et al., "Cigarette Smoking and Coronary Artery Disease," *Chest* 70 (1976):699.
9. *Ibid.,* pp. 111, 129; Surgeon General, *Smoking and Health,* chap. 4, p. 30; chap 4, p. 49.
10. Surgeon General, *Smoking and Health,* chap 4, p. 51.
11. The Pooling Research Group, *Journal of Chronic Diseases* 31 (1978):201.
12. N.L. Benowitz et al., "Smokers of Low-Yield Cigarettes Do Not Consume Less Nicotine," *New England Journal of Medicine* 309 (1983):139; J.H. Jaffe et al., "Carbon Monoxide and Thiocyanate Levels in Low Tar/Nicotine Smokers," *Addictive Behaviors* 6 (1981):337
13. D.W. Kaufman et al., "Nicotine and Carbon Monoxide Content of Cigarette Smoke and the Risk of Myocardial Infarction in Young Men," *New England Journal of Medicine* 308 (1983):409.
14. Surgeon General, *The Health Consequences of Smoking for Women* (Washington, D.C.: Government Printing Office, 1980), p. 162.
15. H. W. Daniell, "Smokers Wrinkles: A Study in the Epidemiology of 'Crow's Feet,'" *Annals of Internal Medicine* 75 (1971):873.

16. C. Schirren, *Geburtshilfe und Frauenheilkunde* 35 (1975):334.
17. M. A. Russel, P. V. Cole and E. Brown, "Absorption by Non-smokers of Carbon Monoxide from Room Air Polluted by Tobacco Smoke," *Lancet* 1 (1973):576.
18. Surgeon General, *Health Consequences of Smoking: Cancer,* p. 214.
19. T. Hirayama, *British Medical Journal* 283 (October 3, 1983):916.
20. B. R. Luce and S. O. Schweitzer, "The Economic Costs of Smoking Induced Illness," in *Research in Smoking Behavior,* ed. M. E. Jarvick et al. (Washington, D.C.: Government Printing Office, 1977), pp. 221–229.
21. Adapted from Silverberg and Lubera, "A Review of American Cancer Society Estimates of Cancer Cases and Deaths," p. 14. © 1983 American Cancer Society, Inc.
22. Surgeon General, *Smoking and Health,* p. 60.
23. Surgeon General, *Health Consequences of Smoking for Women,* p. 192.
24. J. Goujard, C. Rumeau and D. Schwartz, "Smoking During Pregnancy: Stillbirth and Abruptio Placentae," *Biomedicine* 23 (1975):20–22.
25. J. Andrews and J. M. McGarry, "A Community Study of Smoking in Pregnancy," *Journal of Obstetrics and Gynecology of the British Commonwealth* 79 (1972):1057.
26. N. R. Butler and H. Goldstein, "Smoking in Pregnancy and Subsequent Child Development," *British Medical Journal* 4 (1973):573.
27. R. I. Evans and A. Henderson, "Smoking in Children and Adolescents: Psychosocial Determinants and Prevention Strategies," in *The Behavioral Aspects of Smoking,* ed. N. A. Krasnegor (Washington, D.C.: Government Printing Office, 1979), pp. 69–96.
28. B. Mausner and E. S. Platt, *Smoking: A Behavioral Analysis* (New York: Pergamon Press, 1971).
29. *Report of the Task Force on Tobacco and Cancer, Target 5* (New York: American Cancer Society, Inc., 1976).
30. J. L. Hamilton, *Review of Economics and Statistics* 54 (1972):401.
31. Butler and Goldstein, "Smoking in Pregnancy and Subsequent Child Development," p. 201.
32. Surgeon General, *The Health Consequences of Smoking; The Changing Cigarette* (Washington, D.C.: Government Printing Office, 1981), p. 99.
33. The Pooling Project Research Group, *Journal of Chronic Diseases* 31 (1978):201.
34. H. M. Annis, "Patterns of Intra-familial Drug Use," *British Journal of Addiction* 69 (1974):361.
35. P. S. Larson, H. B. Haig and Silvette, *Tobacco: Experimental and Clinical Studies* (Baltimore: Williams and Wilkins, 1961).
36. M. E. Jarvick, "Tobacco Smoking in Monkeys," *Annals of the New York Academy of Science* 142 (1967):280.
37. B. Silverstein, *An Addiction Explanation of Cigarette-Induced Relaxation* (Ph.D. dissertation: Columbia University, 1976). pp. 1–68.
38. E. Jones, *Sigmund Freud: Life and Work,* 3 vols. (London: Hogarth Press, 1953), p. 339.
39. R. A. Krumholz, R. B. Chevalier and J. C. Ross, "Changes in Cardiopulmonary Functions Related to Abstinence from Smoking," *Annals of Internal Medicine* 62 (1965):197–207.
40. Surgeon General, *Smoking and Health,* chap. 5, p. 25.
41. Saul M. Schiffman, "The Tobacco Withdrawal Syndrome," in *Cigarette Smoking as a Dependence Process,* ed. N. A. Krasnegor (Washington, D.C.: Government Printing Office, 1979), pp. 158–184.
42. Surgeon General, *Smoking and Health,* chap. 22, p. 10.
43. James I, *A Counterblaste to Tobacco* (London: 1604).
44. Count E. C. Corti, *A History of Smoking* (London: Harrap, 1931), p. 119.

Mechanism of Action of Marijuana

Most drugs taken repeatedly lead to three related and progressive states within the user.

1. *Psychological dependence,* in which pleasurable or calming effects on the nervous system, produced by the drug, become necessary to maintain an optimal state of well-being
2. *Tolerance,* which is the need for increasing dosage to produce the required effect
3. *Physical dependence,* in which, because of an altered biochemical state, repeated doses have become necessary to prevent the discomfort of withdrawal symptoms

Located deep in the cerebrum (forebrain) are reflex centers recently discovered to be associated with the subjective sensations of pleasure. Stimulation of these pleasure centers by sensual drugs produces a psychological response in the brain, below a conscious level. This, in turn, adjusts the brain's internal controls so that discomfort results if the chemical is not supplied. The problem is that such unnatural, artificial stimulation of the pleasure centers eventually impairs their normal operation. A state of sensory deprivation then results, in which pleasurable responses actually become suppressed. Hence the tendency to take higher doses, leading to addiction.

Some have argued that a drug such as marijuana, which is not chemically addictive, but only psychologically addictive, is for that reason less dangerous, because it is considered to be more susceptible to rational control. In fact, however, because of the above-described mechanism of action, the two forms of addiction are so closely related as to make the argument false, because control or abstention becomes more than simply an act of the will. The late Dr. Hardin B. Jones of the University of California stated, "There is an inseparable relationship between chemical and psychological addiction, and the two forms coincide when the addictive substance is a pleasure-giving drug."

The problem with marijuana specifically is that its active ingredient, tetrahydrocannabinol (THC), is fat soluble and is, therefore, retained in the body for long periods (unlike water-soluble alcohol, which, if not stored as sugars or fat, is relatively quickly metabolized and excreted as carbon dioxide and water). Molecule for molecule, THC is ten thousand times more potent than alcohol in its ability to produce intoxication. Once dissolved, the THC is deposited in the fatty outer membranes of cells, including those in the brain, liver, and lungs, and on both red and white blood cells and sperm.

Postmortem specimens of brains of heavy users of marijuana reveal cerebral atrophy (shrinkage), the degree of which can be correlated with duration of use. This brain damage undoubtedly accounts for well-recognized behavioral changes in long-term pot smokers.

Genetic and embryologic damage has been shown in malformations in offspring of either male or female monkeys exposed to marijuana. In humans in the U.S.A. since the mid-1960s, when the use of pot increased greatly, there has been a parallel increase in birth defects in children of users, such as malformations of the hip joint and cardiovascular system. In the lungs, Swiss research has shown that marijuana smoke causes a greater degree of damage than tobacco smoke to lung cells, which eventually turn permanently from pink to black.

Physical effects of longtime use of marijuana include weight loss, wasting of muscles, loss of ability to enjoy any sensual pleasures, insomnia, irreversible brain damage, lowered resistance to infections, chromosome breakdown, genetic damage, emphysema and other related lung diseases, and sexual impotence and infertility. Recovery after cessation of longtime use takes months, or even years, and sometimes some of the damage done, such as in the brain or lungs, is permanent.

One frequently hears it said from the ignorant or wishful thinkers that marijuana is safer than alcohol. This is *not* true. Whereas an ounce of alcohol is completely metabolized from the body in a few hours, the THC in one joint of marijuana takes up to seven days to be half eliminated and thirty days to be totally eliminated. The cumulative effect therefore from frequent weekly or daily use saturates those parts of the body that are high in fat content, especially the brain and the reproductive organs.

Part III

Common Medical Problems

Next to the common cold the flesh is most commonly heir to stress, leading to various forms of pain, which, if heeded as a warning, can prevent more serious problems developing. Headaches in particular are a valuable indication that stressors in one's life need to be reduced. Pain and headaches can be a friend if they effect the red-light warning of impending harm.

The relationship between a stressful life-style and heart attacks also is well-presented here. To read these chapters could be the most important step to be taken in the cause of preventive medicine by a middle-aged man or woman who is overextended and in danger of potentially life-threatening consequences.

8
Stress
Dr. Angharad Young

WHAT IS IT?

One of the most misunderstood words in our language today is *stress*. What is stress? Do you have stress? How much is too much? As a counselor I find that it is a major concern for most of my patients. It is also a major concern for me. There are times when I have to determine what I can do to cope with my own stress.

What is the meaning of this term that is used daily. I believe that stress is the wear and tear of life. There is virtually no way to escape stress in this sense. To be alive is to be stressed.

The psychological usage of the term stress was made famous by Dr. Hans Selye in his book *The Stress of Life*. Dr. Selye defined stress as the "nonspecific response of the body to any demand made upon it." His research findings note three stages following an intense or threatening demand.

The first is the *alarm stage* in which adrenaline and other hormones are released to increase your heart rate, elevate your blood pressure, put sugar into your blood stream, and strengthen your muscles. Your body mobilizes and you are prepared to "fight or flight." (Here I might add that if the odds are heavily against you, I would suggest you opt for flight.)

As soon as the threat is over, you enter the *resistance stage* in which your bodily functions return to normal. Your entire system breathes a sigh of relief and slows down. However, if you should perceive that the danger is continuing over a prolonged time, your body will go into the *exhaustion stage* where the continued wear and tear can begin to do some

Common Medical Problems

damage to your system. You cannot function well on red alert all the time.

Stress can be helpful or harmful. It can be friend or foe; yet I believe that if stress is not dealt with it is more often than not foe instead of friend.

Stress does come with the general wear and tear of life. The pressure that we feel is not going to go away. Instead we are going to have to determine some ways of coping with our stress and not let it erode our relationships. There are various ways of coping and that is what we are going to consider.

WHAT CAUSES STRESS?

Do you look at your calendar and wish that you could add another day to your week? Is that what you really need or do you need a better way to handle the stress of your life? The amount of stress varies, but sometimes it can be extremely great, applying pressure to you physically, mentally, emotionally, and spiritually.

Intense stress can be compared to the shock measurement of an earthquake on the Richter Scale. The stronger the amount of stress the stronger will be the stress reaction and the ripple effects.

If you are under a large amount of stress, you will have physical signals to warn you such as indigestion, headaches, high blood pressure, fatigue, nausea, muscle spasms or aches, perspiration, or heart flutters. My own physical signal for too much stress is a stiff neck and tight back muscles. Whenever I feel such tightness I know that I'd better slow down or get some relief from the wear and tear. Mental and emotional reactions can include feelings such as anger, frustration, anxiety, or depression. Such reactions usually manifest themselves in relationships. Some of the problems that appear to warn you of too much stress are impatience with others, irritation with their requests, resentment toward those you love, desire to be away from family and friends, anger toward everyone, and arguments with anyone. I have a friend who is an accountant, and during tax season she asks her family to please go the extra mile in tolerance as she is so stressed that she is very irritable and will snap at almost anyone. Even your relationship with God can be affected.

Evaluate yourself in these areas by answering the following general questions.

1. What is my physical condition?
2. How am I responding to daily wear and tear mentally and emotionally?
3. What is my evaluation of my spiritual and personal relationships?

Stress comes from every direction. It can come from financial problems and work situations, or it can be generated by everyday occurrences such as driving in heavy traffic or standing in the slowest checkout line at the store.

If you want to know where your stress originates, you need to contemplate your own life situation and expectations. You can obtain some insight into this area by considering these questions.

1. What situations or people cause me stress?
2. Are there any of these that I can reduce or avoid?
3. Are there any of these that can be changed in the future?
4. What are the ones with which I must cope immediately?

Earlier I mentioned that some stress is more intense than other stress. Certainly a serious illness is far worse than a traffic jam or the loss of a job is worse than a missed appointment. Prolonged and intense stress can be damaging to your health and is of more danger than brief annoyances.

A useful tool in measuring the intensity or amount of serious stress has been the Social Readjustment Rating Scale, which was developed by Dr. Thomas Holmes and Dr. Richard Rahe at the School of Medicine of the University of Washington. Their research spanned twenty years and included over 5,000 interviews. From these interviews they sought to determine the relationship of illness and injury to the major happenings of life.

Some of these events were regarded as positive, such as marriages, trips, or promotions; some were classified as negative, such as the death of a loved one, divorce, or financial loss. The situations were listed according to the frequency and importance that those interviewed accorded them. Following the listing the doctors asked other people from varying backgrounds and experiences to rank these events. After many interviews and rankings, they found that the values were very similar for people among all social levels.

Study Dr. Holmes and Dr. Rahe's chart. It can give you an idea of how intense your stress may be. Add the points for the events that have occurred within the last twelve months of your life. Record the total at the base of the chart.

The Social Readjustment Rating Scale

Life Event	Mean Value
1. Death of spouse	100
2. Divorce	73
3. Marital separation	65

4.	Jail term	63
5.	Death of close family member	63
6.	Personal injury or illness	53
7.	Marriage	50
8.	Fired at work	47
9.	Marital reconciliation	45
10.	Retirement	45
11.	Change in health of family member	44
12.	Pregnancy	40
13.	Sex difficulties	39
14.	Gain of new family member	39
15.	Business readjustment	39
16.	Change in financial state	38
17.	Death of close friend	37
18.	Change to different line of work	36
19.	Change in number of arguments with spouse	35
20.	Mortgage or loan for major purchase (home, etc.)	31
21.	Foreclosure of mortgage or loan	30
22.	Change in responsibilities at work	29
23.	Son or daughter leaving home	29
24.	Trouble with in-laws	29
25.	Outstanding personal achievement	28
26.	Wife begins or stops work	26
27.	Begin or end school	26
28.	Change in living conditions	25
29.	Revision of personal habits	24
30.	Trouble with boss	23
31.	Change in work hours or conditions	20
32.	Change in residence	20
33.	Change in schools	20
34.	Change in recreation	19
35.	Change in church activities	19
36.	Change in social activities	18
37.	Mortgage or loan for lesser purchase (car, TV, etc.)	17
38.	Change in sleeping habits	16
39.	Change in number of family get-togethers	15
40.	Change in eating habits	15
41.	Vacation	13
42.	Christmas	12
43.	Minor violations of the law	11
	Total	—

Reprinted with permission from *The Journal of Psychosomatic Research*, vol. 11: T. H. Holmes and R. H. Rahe, Social Readjustment Rating Scale. Copyright 1967 by Pergamon Press, Ltd.

If your total was 300 or more, you are under an intense amount of stress, which means that you might want to postpone changes or delay any major decisions that would add more stress. For instance, a young man I'll call Joe is working through the grief experience of his father's death six months earlier. Since it takes about a year to recover enough from a loved one's death to rejoice in the times you had together and not feel intense pain with memory, Joe will wait to make any major changes in his plans, such as changing his job, since his stress points already total more than 300.

This underscores our belief that stress is wear and tear. And Dr. Richard Lazarus, another eminent stress researcher, has developed the Hassle Scale, which measures stress caused by minor irritants, instead of major ones. He believes that these little things "are psychodynamically more important. They often suggest inner agendas that keep troubling a person, such as an ineptitude in handling a particular person."

You may have found that your life experiences—major or minor—are not causing a great deal of stress; however there is another condition that can produce stress.

ARE YOU TYPE A OR TYPE B?

It is possible for your behavior to add stress to your life. In a book entitled *Type A Behavior and Your Heart* Dr. Meyer Friedman and Dr. Ray Rosenman, who are heart specialists in San Francisco, reported on a ten-year study in which they had discovered a personality type that was prone to heart attacks.

They noted that people fall into two categories—Type A or Type B. Type A personalities are much more likely to suffer from stress and have a high risk factor for heart attacks. They feel compelled to achieve and are always in a hurry. Because of their impatience and obsession with time, they hate to be caught in traffic, to wait for appointments, or to stand in line. Often Type A people are workaholics and are the first to arrive at the office and the last ones to leave. Most of their activities or projects require deadlines and add pressure to their crowded schedule. Since it is very difficult for them to say no, they often have multiple projects to oversee or meetings to attend.

In order to meet this increased load they simply speed up all activities, so they will speed through traffic or become upset with family or co-workers if they do not move fast enough. Sometimes they will take up sports to allow for some relaxation; however, these sports are usually fast-paced and very competitive. Type A personalities feel that they are the only ones with the responsibility and ability to get a job done. Often their speech is short and abrupt, and in a conversation they will be tapping a pencil, clenching their fists, or making some type of extra body movement. The Type A wants to prove something and is in a hurry to do so, so he or she may finish sentences for the speaker or interrupt the speaker.

In contrast Type B people are more flexible concerning life circumstances, and when they participate in sports, they play for fun as well as competition. Many Bs are also ambitious, but they have learned a different or less stressful approach, and Type B people have often learned how to be successful and happy and satisfied too.

Type B people will usually handle only one or two projects at a time for they have learned to pace their time so that they do not feel the pressure that all must be done immediately. These personalities can also work with a team concept and delegate responsibility, and they do not feel that all the work has to be done by them or that they alone are responsible for progress.

Usually Type B personalities can listen to another's point of view or enjoy a slow-paced conversation. Often they are more patient in traffic or with minor delays. Sometimes the fast-paced Type A man or woman may accomplish more in a short term, but usually the Type B lives longer, so he or she may accomplish more in the long run. The comparison of the two personality types brings to mind the old story of the tortoise and the hare.

It is possible to be a combination of the two types, and Type B personalities can also learn to be Type A personalities or vice versa. You may find that you are a combination of the two. Many of us are, but it is important to be sure that the Type A part of us does not always have control. In myself I see Type A tendencies in traffic, standing in line, or waiting for appointments. To alleviate my frustration I try to have something with me to read. It is relaxing but it also solves my problem of feeling that time is being wasted.

Think about your behavior and assess your personality type by answering the following questions:

1. Am I always in a hurry?
2. Do I worry at night?
3. Do I feel compelled to try to win all the time?
4. Am I impatient with slow people?
5. Do I explode in speech or action?
6. Do I find it difficult to sit still and relax?
7. Do I eat my meals as quickly as possible?

If you answered yes to most of these questions, you may be a Type A personality. If so, you are adding stress to your life and your heart.

It is also possible for some occupations to cause Type A tendencies. In my counseling experience, I have found, for example, that people who constantly face deadlines are stressed. Editors, students, orderlies, seamstresses, or truck drivers represent some of the occupations that require the constant awareness of time and sometimes a race with time.

Don't despair if you have found that you are Type A or that your life or work situation is causing Type A behavior. There are ways to cope with stress and we will discuss them later.

AREAS OF STRESS

Family

The family is often a source of stress for an individual. Also, family structure itself is under much stress in today's society and the breakup of marriages is tragically increasing.

As Dr. Gary Collins points out in his book *You Can Profit from Stress,* there have been some definite changes in family structure. He notes that family size is smaller, which should make for a calmer home; however, there are fewer older children to help with the younger ones. Family members are educated and entertained away from home. In addition family members often live far away from one another as our society is very mobile. Family styles are less traditional, and there are many single parents who are playing two roles. Intense stress is a given in some of these situations. Your family relationships can be stressful just because of the close proximity of family members. Dr. Virginia Satir, who has worked extensively in family therapy, has noted that "when one person in a family has pain which shows up in symptoms, all family members are feeling this pain in some way."

There have been many studies which indicate that the family operates as a unit. The family is intricately linked, and seeks to maintain a comfortable and familiar balance within relationships. Dr. Don D. Jackson, director of the Mental Research Institute in Palo Alto, has done much study on family life and has described this unit behavior as "family homeostasis." Thus, any time the family has stress every member of that family will try to react in some way that will return the unit to its accustomed balance.

Many statements are made about the outside forces or society's changes that create stress for the family. For instance Dr. Keith Sehnert in his book *Stress/Unstress* reports that certain trends are placing stress on families of today. For example:

1. Nearly half of all marriages end in divorce.
2. Forty percent of all children born in this decade will spend part of their youth in homes with only one parent.
3. Households headed by women have doubled in the last 20 years.
4. Only sixteen percent of today's families fit the traditional concept of mother, father, and children—with Dad the breadwinner and Mom staying home to care for the family.
5. The number of unmarried couples living together has more than doubled since 1960.
6. The average homeowner stays in a single home for about seven years.
7. Twenty percent of all families in America move each year.

However, it is my observation and opinion that more stress is placed upon the family from within. Each family member is experiencing stress and if one family member begins to experience really intense stress, he or she will bring that stress into the family unit. If individual members can cope and can help one another in coping with stress, they can in turn aid and strengthen their own family units.

Job

As I have noted, it is possible for some jobs to cause Type A behavior. I have heard people relate intense stress feelings to deadlines or too many projects. For instance Ted, who is a truck driver under constant pressure from the moment he accepts a job, reported, "I begin to race against the deadline and try to deliver the material sooner than the contract requires." Ted is not really a Type A personality but is behaving like one and is adding a great deal of stress to his life.

Deadlines are not the only cause of stress in job areas. The National Institute for Occupational Safety and Health did a study on occupational stress. In their study they found that waiters, waitresses, practical nurses, dishwashers, and laboratory technicians are under a great deal of occupational stress.

What causes job stress in such areas? Often you think of high-level executives being under pressure and stress. Many times they are, as Scott, a financial analyst and president of his consulting firm, exemplifies. He states, "A heavy sense of responsibility seems to hang over my head all the time. I feel responsible for my family, my employees, and clients' investments."

However, the occupations that were listed above don't seem to carry the responsibility that Scott's does. These jobs exhibit lack of control in the work situation. For instance at one of my favorite restaurants there is a waitress named Cathy. She is excellent in that she is friendly and you sense she is happy to be helping you. Yet, as I've watched Cathy I notice that she is constantly busy and does not have too much control over what is happening. The cook determines the quality of the meal; however, if it is not good, Cathy takes the blame. The busboy cleans the tables, but if he does not do his job quickly customers may be seated in another waitress's area. The customers decide when they will enter the restaurant and how agreeable or disagreeable they may be.

In other words Cathy does not have control in her work situation; she cannot decide to sit down for a coffee break when customers are waiting nor can she do anything about the food preparation. Another stressful factor in Cathy's job is that often it is feast or famine. If her customers tip well, then she has more than her low salary; however, if the customers do not tip well, she has even less money and that can cause some family stress and financial stress.

Cathy's situation points up that it is often low-paying job positions that have the most stress. An interesting study by E. I. du Pont de Nemours and Company indicated that initial heart attacks among male employees over forty-five years old most often occurred in the lowest salaried positions. Those in the highest paying positions had the fewest heart attacks. The researchers surmised that the executives received more satisfaction from their jobs and had more assistance from secretaries and executive aides. They had more control of their work than employees in low positions so they felt much less stress.

Now let me add that every situation is different and the general economic climate varies. No matter what your position in a business or company, if it is a difficult time for your industry, stress is produced at all levels.

Finances

Of course one of the primary purposes behind work is to provide income for your necessities, your wants, and your dreams. However, this same income is sometimes the cause of much stress. If there is too little income or it is mismanaged you will feel the stress of trying to pay bills and buy necessities without enough money. The control of money within the family can cause distress among its members.

Also what is your viewpoint on money? A study was done at Johns Hopkins University by Harvey Brenner concerning psychiatric admissions in New York State over the past 127 years. He found that whenever economic conditions were going down or were bad, admissions to psychiatric hospitals increased. His study also revealed that alcoholism increased among the working class and suicides increased among the higher economic levels. Another factor that came to light in his study was that among males in the 45- to 60-year age group the number admitted for emergency treatment of emotional distress increased.

Dr. Louis Kopolow, staff psychiatrist with the National Institute of Mental Health, noted that "the change in the economy has created a feeling of insecurity, financial strain, and fear of the future. For the first time in their lives, millions of Americans are losing confidence in their ability to achieve a more prosperous future or even to maintain their present economic condition."

Inflation continues to shrink the amount of money that families have to take care of their needs. Living expenses continue to escalate, forcing most of the money to be used for necessities, leaving little or none to be used for dreams or entertainment. Sometimes monetary stress can come from an unexpected illness.

It is possible to estimate your financial stress on a comparison with the Richter Scale, too. If you are experiencing extreme stress because of an insufficient amount of money, there will be shock waves or ripple effects sent out to other areas of your life. For instance if you had hoped that this year would be the time to take that dream vacation, but the air conditioning system is going to have to be replaced or there are some major plumbing repairs to be completed and the vacation money has to be used for repair, what happens to the stress level of the family? If the vacation was being happily anticipated by all, you can understand what moods might follow.

Financial stress usually is experienced by every one of us. You can probably think of a time (or it may even be now) when money was very tight and you could only dream about what you would like to do. Sometimes there can be another aspect to such a situation. Overindebtedness is certainly a stressful situation.

On the other hand there are people who have so much money that they fear losing it. The *Peoples Almanac II* made up a chart which indicated that a large income produced stressful "high living." Harry Levinson in his book *Executive Stress* also alluded to such a dilemma. (I realize many of us are thinking—Oh, for such a dilemma.) My hunch is, though, that sometimes the credit-card craze and even the high living can be a result of others' expectations.

Appearances

What about others' expectations? I think that whomever your thoughts turn to when you think of success, or dream of what you would like to be, has a big impact on what you say and do—and your stress.

Dr. Gary Collins writes in his book *You Can Profit from Stress* that "in Western society, money means power, it brings status, and it is a mark of success. The person who drives an expensive car or lives in a big house is saying to the world, 'I'm a successful person in a world which values success.'"

There are other kinds of appearances besides financial success that you might try to project. In an interview for *Guideposts* magazine J. B. Phillips noted that as the success of his New Testament translation began to grow, he succumbed to "an image of 'J. B. Phillips' that was not Jack Phillips at all. I was no longer an ordinary human being; I was in danger of becoming the super-Christian! Everything I wrote or said had to be better than the last. The image grew and grew until it was so unlike me that I could no longer live with it. And yet the thought of destroying it was terrifying too. It was on this dilemma that I hung."

He found that he was afraid to be himself. Ministers, professors, doctors, teachers, counselors, principals, and policemen are some examples of those who can be caught in the "I-must-look-better-than-I-am" appearance game. You can be caught in such a bind and find that a fear of being found to be something you are not places stress upon your actions.

What about the ads that pay homage to our youth-oriented culture? As Dr. Collins noted, "Old age doesn't have a very good image in our society." So many times the physical-aging signs such as growing waistlines, energy loss, and grown children are very stressful. Thus many people spend large sums of money trying to appear or stay young. It can be stressful to try to be much younger than you are. The term midlife crisis is a well-known phrase in our society.

Sometimes appearances take other forms. I have a friend who is very self-conscious about not finishing college, so she often leaves the impression that she did. If someone specifically asks about her degree, you can almost see the stress she begins to feel. Others are sometimes guilty of pretending to have a fine family background or to know important people as close friends. All of these attempts to "keep up appearances" can add stress to life.

WRONG METHODS OF COPING WITH STRESS

Some people appear to be in control when they really are not. I have talked with people who believe that they can ignore the stress and hurt they feel and all will be all right.

Obviously ignoring stress or pretending that you have no stress is not a way to handle it. I believe that there are some other methods that do not really teach a person to cope with stress. Some of these techniques simply

Common Medical Problems

ignore the problem temporarily. The pressure is still there and is still causing some type of reaction. Also, some of these methods can not only add to stress but also cause other problems.

One of the popular ways to unwind is to consume alcohol. It is estimated that there are 9 million alcoholics in America. Dr. Clarence Row believes that alcoholism results from psychological needs. The alcohol "is used to deal with insecurity, anxiety, depression, or stress." Often the drinking begins in a social way and on a limited scale; however it can become much like a runaway train and be used as an escape. It does not take too much imagination to see how heavy drinking can add more stress to life instead of relieving it. Ask someone who has had his or her driver's license suspended if it is stressful to have to be driven everywhere or to have one's insurance revoked.

In her book *The Booze Battle: A Common Sense Approach That Works* Ruth Maxwell states that approximately 36 million people in the United States are affected by drinking relatives or friends. The scenario can include car wrecks, drunken behavior, brutality, arguments, broken promises, and attempts by the family to keep the problem hidden. The family is much more likely to try to hide the problem if Mom is the one who is the alcoholic.

The problem drinker may begin with one or two drinks each evening in order to relax or bolster self-confidence. Soon though it may be three, four, or more, and the process of going to sleep each evening is simply a matter of passing out. The pattern soon becomes one where the person drinks alone and has to begin the day with a drink. Even with such a pattern an alcoholic will often still deny that there is a problem.

Yet it's a problem that affects the person and his or her family or friends. There are some actions or treatments that can be of help in such a situation. Usually there is need for direction or guidance from someone outside the family or inner circle of friends. I believe that the most successful helps for alcoholics (with the help of God) is Alcoholics Anonymous and its support groups of Al-Anon for wives or husbands of alcoholics and Alateen for teenage relatives of alcoholics. Alcohol is not any kind of answer for stress.

Another way that is equally as destructive in trying to face stress is drugs. Unfortunately many people seem to think that getting high on drugs is a way to conquer the pressures of life. When drugs are used correctly to ease pain, to prevent infection, or to cure diseases, they are marvelous. Unfortunately drug use has been much abused, and for some people drugs are not helping but harming. Many people carry Valium just as you would aspirin. A few years ago a very popular movie had a rather sad-comic scene in which a man needed to be calmed and his brother asked if anyone had any Valium. At that instant everyone in the crowd began searching pockets and purses. The comic exaggeration had a large amount of truth.

Sleeping pills have also become a popular medication. In his book *Executive Health* Philip Goldberg reports that more than $100 million a year is spent on sleeping pills. Dr. Anthony Kales who is a sleep researcher believes that "over the counter sleep drugs should not be sold. The use and availability of these drugs are not to the advantage of the average patient." Again you must realize that taking such a pill does not really do anything about the source of the problem. Dr. Peter Hauri, the director of the sleep clinic at Dartmouth, notes that "the individual may, because he believes the drug is putting him to sleep, actually be able to relax enough so that he can doze off. But the pill isn't doing a thing. On the contrary, the pills are most probably going to disturb the pattern of his sleep."

Tranquilizers and sleeping pills are considered socially acceptable. However, these medications can cause problems and become addictive. I can think of a lady named Doris whose husband had died a few months earlier. During her initial stages of grief she began to take Valium. Then she was able to stop the tranquilizer, but she felt she still needed something to help her sleep. So she bought a well-advertised brand of sleeping pill. Yet, even though she slept at night, she would awaken tired and feeling as if her nerves were frayed. They were, and she had to give up her dependence on sleeping pills before she could really begin to rest.

Sleep researchers tell us that sleeping pills do not really cause restful or natural sleep. Instead they depress the central nervous system by blocking impulses to the brain. Sleep comes because the nerve cells are paralyzed. However, the sleep is a tiring process instead of a recuperative process.

The researchers have also found that the pills interfere with the REM (Rapid Eye Movement) stage of sleep where dreaming takes place. REM sleep is considered a must for physical and mental balance. Thus it is important to limit sleeping pills or try to avoid them. Dr. Ernest Hartmann, who has written a book entitled *The Functions of Sleep,* has said, "I think of insomnia as a symptom, not as a disease. It is not an illness for which the sleeping pill is a cure." So if you are not sleeping well because of your negative stress, sleeping pills are not your answer.

Neither is compulsive eating the answer to stress. Many people overeat and use favorite foods (or even unfavorite ones) as tranquilizers. Food can be instant gratification; however it is obvious that overeating can cause obesity, which is usually stressful to the individual and is also bad for physical health. Health problems which occur from being overweight have been highlighted in many studies. One such study by the Methodist

Common Medical Problems

Hospital in Indianapolis found that overweight has a measurable influence in many diseases, especially heart trouble.

However, you may not find that compulsive overeating results from stress. Stress may sometimes cause so much tension that a person is unable to eat. I recall a college student who was painfully thin. After some discussion she noted that she was so uptight about problems at home and her courses at school that she was unable to eat. Obviously the problems associated with a lack of sound nutrition are many. The human body requires essential nutrients for maintenance, energy, and rebuilding.

Now I want you to consider a happening that sounds so innocent, yet, it adds negative stress. What am I talking about? I am referring to the "coffee break." Wherever you work, even if your work setting is your home, you probably take a break. The problem, of course, is not the break. The problem is what you do during the break.

Perhaps the first thing you seek on your break is a cup of coffee. If so, consider this. Caffeine is a stimulant. In moderate amounts it can increase your alertness and give you some added energy. However, in large amounts is can cause nervousness and anxiety. Caffeine also causes an increase in stomach acids and can cause headaches, heartburn, and ulcers.

Coffee seems to be the most popular source of caffeine, but it is also consumed in soft drinks, chocolate, and tea. Dr. J. F. Greeden in an article for the *American Journal of Psychiatry* has noted that caffeine intake of more than 250 mg per day is considered excessive.

The *Journal of the American Dietetic Association* lists the following amounts of caffeine in various items: A cup of coffee (5 ounces) contains 66–146 mg; tea (5 ounces) has 20–46 mg; cola drinks (12 ounces) have 32–65 mg.

Another popular item for relaxing at coffee break is the cigarette. Studies show, however, that nicotine causes a release of adrenaline, a rise in blood pressure, and an increase in the heart rate. Dr. Robert Anderson has noted in his book *Stress Power* that people who smoke more than a package of cigarettes a day shorten their life span by about seven and one-half years. There are also a number of respiratory diseases such as pneumonia and bronchitis caused by smoking. Perhaps the biggest reason to stay away from cigarettes is the possibility of lung cancer. In his book *Executive Health* Philip Goldberg reports that "moderate smokers have eight times the amount of lung cancer as nonsmokers, and heavy smokers have twenty times the risk."

In spite of the fact that smokers look to the cigarette for relaxation, I have observed that smokers are usually nervous, show tension, and have a habit that controls them. Usually heavy smokers have a chronic cough. All of these factors seem a high price to pay for a cigarette.

Rounding out the "menu" at coffee break is often a sweet roll loaded with sugar. It has been reported that the average individual consumption of sugar in the United States is 125 pounds a year, with children eating approximately 140 pounds a year. Partly to blame is food processing. Sugar is used in almost every commercially prepared food. Also there are many delicious sugary enticements such as pies, ice cream, cake, candy, and syrups. Even cereals are a problem. The *Journal of Dentistry for Children* reported on a study of seventy-eight brands of cereal. Shredded wheat had the low with only 1 percent sucrose; but with some of the others the percentage rose to a high of 68.

So what of the sweet roll at coffee break? It doesn't really help as the lift in energy does not last long. Also, the consumption of refined sugar has been linked to tooth problems, blood-pressure changes, insulin imbalance, and other related health problems.

Alcohol, drugs and caffeine, tobacco, sweets—these are some of the ways *not* to cope with stress.

STRESS AND ILLNESS

You may be thinking that you do not use any of those methods that really take away from life. However, there are consequences that people do not realize they inadvertently cause. Scientists, psychiatrists, psychologists, and physicians are beginning to monitor the relationship of illness and life change. Allen Wyler, Minoru Masuda, and Thomas Holmes published a paper, "Magnitude of Life Events and Seriousness of Illness." They had ranked 126 illnesses, based on the opinions of physicians and laymen as to the seriousness of the illness.

All 126 were rated accordingly by considering such factors as duration, threat to life, amount of disability, and amount of discomfort, and each was assigned a "Seriousness of Illness Unit" value. They ranged from dandruff at 21 units to leukemia at 1080 units.

Later they conducted a most fascinating study in which they randomly selected 252 patients for study. These people as a group had 42 of the 126 diseases. The study noted some interesting findings. There was a correlation between the numerical value of life change (*see* the Social Readjustment Rating Scale in the first section) and the seriousness of illness. Thus the greater the amount of life change the more serious was the illness that was manifested. A selection of their findings is listed on the next page.

All of this data should give us cause to carefully consider coping skills when we experience dramatic life changes or even in dealing with routine stress. Obviously illness would add even more stress; so you really do not

Common Medical Problems

Illness	Seriousness of illness units	Number of patients	Mean average life change units in the 2 years preceding the illness
Headache	(88)	5	209
Acne	(103)	6	311
Psoriasis	(174)	6	317
Eczema	(204)	7	231
Bronchitis	(210)	8	322
Hernia	(244)	9	457
Anemia	(312)	7	325
Anxiety reaction	(315)	4	482
Gallstones	(454)	6	563
Peptic ulcer	(500)	17	603
High blood pressure	(520)	4	405
Chest pain	(609)	7	638
Diabetes	(621)	6	599
Alcoholism	(688)	3	688
Manic-depressive psychosis	(766)	4	753
Schizophrenia	(785)	12	609
Heart failure	(824)	9	772
Cancer	(1020)	15	777

Reprinted by permission of Elsevier Science Publishing Co., Inc., from "Magnitude of Life Events and Seriousness of Illness" by Allen Wyler, Minoru Masuda, and Thomas Holmes; PSYCHOSOMATIC MEDICINE 33:115–22, copyright © 1971 by The American Psychosomatic Society, Inc.

want to use wrong methods such as the ones in the previous section in coping with your stress.

POSITIVE METHODS OF COPING

There are some positive ways to handle stress so that it does not diminish the joy in our lives, ruin our health, damage our relationships, or cause us to mismanage our money.

We know that if our stress is too heavy or out of control there is little else that we can think about. As a matter of fact sometimes there is little we do except think of our stress load.

Dr. Donald Dudley and Elton Welke in their book *How to Survive Being Alive* note that "survival in the real world depends upon your ability to cope. Coping depends on what you learned about the factors that contributed to success before you and/or successes around you."

One of the best ways to cope with stress is to be a good friend to yourself. Praise and affirm yourself for the good things you do and for your past accomplishments. Do not speak negatively to yourself. Give yourself the same respect that you would give a very special person, for you are special.

Share your thoughts, hopes, and dreams with someone you trust. Many times the stress you feel can be eased just by talking. It is comparable to a steam valve. It releases a lot of pressure just to be able to talk safely and express yourself.

Another way to help yourself is to be sure that you allow yourself to rest. If your thoughts come crashing in on you and panic descends when you lie down, then keep reminding yourself that you must rest in order to do anything about your problems or the stress you feel.

Anticipation can be another factor in coping. Usually no situation is permanent. Life and events are always being altered. Perhaps it would help to plan a vacation or visit that you would enjoy. Circumstances might not permit the happening in the present or near future, but it could be anticipated for some point in time. You cannot live in the future, but many times the hopes for the future can be the stimulus for the now.

Also remind yourself of the good aspects of your life. List these aspects and then name some things you would like to do for yourself.

Often your feelings toward yourself may not be good because your actions toward yourself are not good. As Dr. Frank Minirth and Dr. Paul Meier point out in their book *Happiness Is a Choice*, "Therapists have often tended to go to one extreme or the other in dealing with people's feelings versus their behavior. Some therapists (such as psychoanalysts) emphasize feelings, whereas others (such as therapists from the school of behavior modification or reality therapy) emphasize behavior. We believe both should be dealt with."

Dr. David Viscott in his book *The Language of Feelings* notes that "the language of feelings is the means by which we relate with ourselves, and if we cannot communicate with ourselves we simply cannot communicate with others. When a person assumes responsibility for his feelings, he assumes responsibility for his world."

I would concur with those opinions. It is your feelings that tell you if something is wrong or how much a happening may have affected your life.

Coping Through Relationships

Some of the most satisfying successes in life come from good relationships. You may not have had the best of training or family patterning in this area, but that does not mean that you cannot change. Suggestions for improving your family relationships can be applied to other relationships also.

Check yourself on your attitude and actions toward family, friends, and co-workers. You may be more charming to a total stranger than you are to the people who share life with you and make memories with you.

Your family members need to be a high priority and they need to know it. Let them hear you say that you love them and believe the best of them. Hugs and kisses should be given also. Good family relationships relieve a great deal of stress. Even when there are disagreements, if family members are sure of one another's love and support, stress can be positive.

You and your family should be able to truly relax and know that you can be your own true self, with your ups and downs. Such a climate does not come automatically. Love and acceptance must be cultivated. Both attributes must be learned and practiced.

One good way to cultivate acceptance is to really listen to one another. All behavior is purposeful, says Dr. Ben Patrick, who is a Christian counselor. Many times if you learn why a person has done, said, or thought something, your reaction will be different. Do not judge them by your own thoughts and actions.

Do not get caught up in the Madison Avenue picture of relationships. In the ads the families look perfect, neat, and loving. That is merely a pretend situation, yet somehow we would like our family to be or appear perfect. It is often hard to admit that just a few minutes before arriving at church the family was arguing.

Accept the uncomfortable times along with the wonderful times. Sometimes a family may be wrestling with a problem that cannot be solved or changed, as with a death in a familly. Yet, pieces of the problem can be solved or members can give love and support as they grieve together and go on with life.

It is also important for you and each member of your family to have some personal freedom. In other words, give family members and yourself life space. Each one needs an opportunity to grow and use innate talents. This process is lifelong. Many people learn new jobs or new hobbies later in life. People are not rigid static beings.

One other must for good family relationships is the willingness to compromise or apologize. Sometimes things cannot simply be one way or another. Compromise can be a solution. Many people are reluctant to apologize; yet an apology notes that you value another person's feelings and that you want the relationship restored. Such an action can often strengthen bonds and encourage open honest relationships. In his book *The Friendship Factor* Alan McGinnis says that "a true apology is more than acknowledging a mistake. It is recognition that something you have said, or done, has damaged a relationship—and you are concerned enough about that relationship to want it repaired and restored."

Not long ago a man confided to me that he often had dreams of apologizing to his father. The last memory he had of his father was an argument where neither would give in to the other. His sad words were, "If only I could see him for five minutes to say I'm sorry."

Some of these same considerations should be given to friends. Your social relationships can be a source of great pleasure and satisfaction. Much stress can also be relieved by spending enjoyable times with good friends. Laughter and good family and friend relationships reduce stress.

Coping at Work

In their book *Stressmap—Finding Your Pressure Points* Dr. Michele Haney and Edmond Boenisch report that "the 'average' worker spends eight hours a day, five days a week, fifty weeks a year on the job. This is an investment (or loss, depending on how you look at it!) of approximately 2,000 hours every year. Since a career is so time-consuming, it may be impossible for some to separate the career from the rest of living. Job literally becomes life, twelve hours a day, evenings and weekends."

Stress can be a part of work that adds just the right amount of tension and excitement to keep things moving. If in surveying your job status, however, you find that there are far more negative aspects than you want, then you might consider a change. Now you may be saying that you cannot change jobs or that you are not trained for anything else. You do not have to change jobs immediately. If the stress of your job is too much, you can begin to cope by reading ads or beginning to train for something else.

Sometimes you may be weighed down by assuming that you will never be out of a situation; however there may be other avenues or possibilities if you look for them and are open to them. For example, many people have become successful by creating a business from a hobby or sideline. Plans for taking control of the situation are very helpful to you in coping with stress. For what you are doing is changing your attitude. When you do that, the problems do not seem so overwhelming, and you can better cope with them.

Now if the negative aspects are not so many that you believe you must leave, then take a sheet of paper and rewrite your list of negative aspects. Then to the side of each write a possible solution or a possible way for you to think differently about it. For instance if one of the negative aspects is a specific person, then there are some ideas for you to consider: Can you avoid that person in a natural way? There is nothing wrong with putting some distance between you and a personality with whom you clash. You do not have to feel guilty about having a problem with someone. Do you expect your best friend to get along well with everyone? Your problem may lie in the fact that you think that everyone can be a good friend. That is not possible with different interests and perspectives. You can, though, have a productive working relationship with someone who has a totally opposite view of your work, especially if the two of you are willing to discuss perspectives and arrive at a compromise. In fact there is great strength in compromise in business as no one has a corner on all wisdom or knowledge.

It is also possible for your work to be stressful simply because it occupies all of your attention. Dr. Keith Sehnert has a definition of workaholics. "These individuals are the people who pride themselves at being the first at the office in the morning, and the last out at night. They have no time for recreation, exercise, family, or friends,"

If you think that some of your stress could be related to such an attitude then perhaps you should consider the following questions:

1. Do I exist solely for my job?
2. Is my work the only worthwhile aspect of my life?
3. Am I slave to my work?
4. Does my work dictate my life and activities?

Even if you should lose your job, you are still you with all your talents. Is not work merely one aspect of life? Yes, an important aspect and probably a satisfying one, but it is not all there is to you. You can increase your horizon by socializing with people in other walks of life through church, neighborhood, sports, or organizations. If you see only the people with whom you work, you have a tendency to discuss only work. Tension can build at work and an outlet is needed.

There are even some minor changes that you can make to cope with your stress at work. Here are a few suggestions that you might try:

1. Rearrange your office.
2. Get a new picture.
3. Bring a favorite magazine for your break.
4. Don't talk "shop" on your break.

Finances

There are general concepts to be considered for coping with your financial situation. Finances can get out of hand without business setbacks. Sometimes you may find yourself struggling with wants instead of needs.

It can be most helpful to make a list of financial goals. What do you plan to accomplish and hope to do?

It might be necessary to obtain some objective advice on a budget or ways to better manage your money. In most cities there are free money management counseling services. If not, talk to your banker and ask for some advice. Another possibility would be an older friend or acquaintance who seems to have sound money management skills. Information about budgets can be found in books at your library.

Meanwhile, ask yourself the following questions:

Do I have a will?
Are my birth certificate, marriage certificate, etc. accessible?
Do I have hospital, medical, and accident insurance?
Do I have automobile insurance?
Do I have home and fire insurance?
Do I have a record of valuables and personal property?
Do I have a savings account?
Do I keep personal records of payments, debts, and taxes?
Do I have a budget?
Do I have a list of financial goals?

If you could not answer yes to all of the items, then you can see some areas that you need to get in order. Even though you may have a number of debts to pay, you will remove or lower some of your stress by knowing that your personal business is in order.

Perhaps you may be thinking, "How can I make more money?" Certainly increasing your income is a way to turn off a certain amount of stress. You can be watching classified ads or talking with people you know to hear of other possibilities or suggestions. Sometimes a hobby or sideline can become not only a way to relax but may also make some money for you. Woodcarvers, artists, and many others have found ways to make some extra income.

Another general suggestion in the area of money management is comparative shopping. In our competitive system it is helpful to watch the ads and clip coupons. Many times you can save yourself some money by being alert. Some of the stores will give double value to the coupons which can make them even more worthwhile to save.

If you are a home owner, you might consider an energy audit from your utility company. It may be that your costs for heat and electricity can be reduced. Along this same line, be sure that lights or appliances are not left on unnecessarily. There are other things that you might do in order to help your financial situation. The following list can give you some ideas or spur you to think of others.

Car servicing and repair
Car pooling
Babysitting cooperatives
Quantity buying with neighbors
Food cooperatives
Making gift items
Having a garage sale

Money is a necessity and an asset; however, you need to control it and use it to your advantage. With sound planning your financial stress can be relieved.

Time Management

Obviously, there are other areas in life that bring stress besides family, job, or finances. Watching or racing the clock can be a source of stress.

Barry found that he was becoming extremely uncomfortable each day as he had to drive through heavy traffic to and from work. Often he had to wait in long lines. However, he turned his feelings around when he began to see this time as a time of opportunity. Barry began to keep books and tapes in his car with material that he needed to review. Thus, his time of waiting became an opportunity instead of a burden as material that would previously have been read or heard at home was covered on his way to and from work.

Barry's situation is one example of the ways in which time can be a friend instead of a foe. The initial step in making that adjustment is a conscious change of attitude. In order to do that you need to view time as a gift or an opportunity to accomplish your hopes and to solve your problems. Have you seen the bumper sticker, "Today is the first day of the rest of my life"? Such a statement has a positive outlook on time and opportunity. Another point it makes is concerning the past—don't look back. It will do you no good to keep dragging up past failures or wasted opportunities. In fact such perspective will keep you from taking advantage of current and future opportunities.

Many times in working with people who are under a great deal of stress, I find that they are not resting. They feel pressure to continue with a project or a job even when it means they must give up their necessary rest. The ramifications from such action are obvious. As sleep is lost exhaustion sets in (and sometimes poor sleep patterns) which keeps one from doing well.

R. S. Schuler noted in an article for *Personnel Journal* that the real importance of time management lies in the fact that many people have too many tasks to perform and not enough time for what they really want to do. The relationship between stress and time management then starts to surface. If individuals are not able to attain or fulfill a need or desire, then according to definition they are in stress. Time management is a process by which they are more likely to be able to attain or fulfill a desire or need.

There are many ways to manage or control your time. One of the best is to maintain a monthly calendar by your telephone where you can see at a glance which days or weeks are the heaviest. Of course you can carry a small pocket calendar that also shows your weekly schedule.

It is also helpful to make a list the night before or early in the morning of things that you need to do during the day. Prioritize them by A, B, C or 1, 2, 3. The As and the 1s are things that must be done. The others can be put off another day or longer if necessary.

You can be more specific by making your own schedule, listing the days of the week with a space for each hour. You probably would not want to do that each day but it might be helpful for you to get an overall view of the way you spend your time.

By analyzing your time expenditures you may find that you are using up your time in ways that are not what you want nor are they to your advantage.

Thus you have to learn to say no to nonproductive activities. Expend your energy on activities and projects that will have the best long-term benefits. You may have to say no at times to some good friends, in order to be free to spend your time on your interests. A time trap often exists when you cannot say no.

If you are involved in community activities and are reluctant to state a flat no, then limit yourself to a certain number of major projects per year. When you are at your limit, simply explain that you already have allocated your time and commitment.

Obviously if you are overcommitted because of your work you have another problem. Discuss your schedule with your boss and show him or her what is happening to your time. If you are your own boss, then go back to the time schedule you made and talk things over with yourself. What good will it do to have such a high level of stress that you cannot be as effective as you would like. Remember, too, when the negative stress level is too high, you run the risk of illness or injury.

A way to relieve stress and save time is to delegate whenever you can.

You do not have to be responsible for every detail. In fact you decrease stress all around when you can trust others and share responsibilities. It is a heavy and lonely load if you believe that you must do everything and are the only capable person you know.

The telephone is also a terrific time saver when it comes to running errands. Never just start off looking for something unless you have a lot of time that you can waste (money, too, on gasoline). Telephone stores or offices to be sure they have what you need.

Another time-saver is organization. Have a place for everything, as much time can be lost in looking for something that you have misplaced. The classic example is car keys: A drawer or hook especially for the keys can often save people much time and aggravation. Along the same vein, you would be wise to carry an extra set of car keys as it often happens that people lock their keys in the car. It can also be helpful to choose your outfit for the next day before you go to bed. Thus, if something needs pressing or a spot removed, it will not be a crisis in the morning.

Whatever your situation, use your creativity or seek advice on ways to organize your time and your work. Remember to think about the positive possibilities of time and all that they offer.

Gaining time will help your stress, but after it does help, there is another aspect of life that goes hand in hand with it. It involves planning or goal setting. Goal setting provides direction and keeps you from drifting. There is also a sense of accomplishment in reaching goals.

Goals

Eugene Walker in his book *Learn to Relax: Thirteen Ways to Reduce Tension* suggests that you make long-range and short-range goals. Most of our long-range goals are general, such as wanting to be a good spouse and parent or wanting to be good in our work. The short-range goals deal with specifics and usually are set within a certain time frame. An example might be to have lunch with a son or daughter during the week or to have a certain amount of money in savings in six months. In other words what are your plans for your work, your family, your life? While it's true that you should not live always in the future, it is equally true that you need a destination or direction. Such things are goals that aid in turning negative stress to positive and providing purpose for our actions.

It is my belief that within each of us are some positive hopes that are often suppressed and maybe even abandoned. Yet, if they are, then negative stress begins to build. A favorite saying of mine is that "A bird dog doesn't know he's a bird dog. He only knows he likes to chase birds."

What do you *really* like to do? What would you *really* hope to do? If you have a strong interest or wish to do something (positive of course) you probably have some aptitude for that endeavor that training or preparation could develop.

You probably have some hopes and dreams concerning family and friends. That sometimes is an area a little more difficult to plan because you have to take into consideration others' wills, hopes, and dreams.

A good way to put family and social relationships into a more objective view is to ask what kind of memories you are making with them. In this imperfect world you are very vulnerable. If you should not live to ninety-two, how will they remember you? Will happy memories give them strength or will memories bring sadness and regret? How close are you to the people you care about and how much support do they give to you and you to them? Ask yourself the following questions in order to further examine your goals:

1. What two or four things do I really want?
2. Will they make me happy if I receive them?
3. Will they be good for me and the people I care about?

In light of these thoughts it may be that one of your goals for your family is to spend more time with them. Perhaps you will want to plan a vacation that can be relived in conversation and pictures; maybe take the time to spend an evening with friends whom you have not seen in awhile.

Your physical, mental, and spiritual condition may lead you to make new commitments to exercise or learning. In today's society there are many possibilities to continue learning in every area. Never before have so many options for hobbies or avocations existed. It may be that you even want to learn an entirely new skill or occupation. The possibilities are endless with community programs, church programs, and local colleges offering a variety of courses.

These plans for continued learning may be linked to your financial occupational goals. If you are not planning to change occupations, then you may want to try for a certain position or open your own business.

Determining your needs and goals can relieve stress. You will enjoy a sense of purpose and direction. Obviously just setting goals does not always mean that you will accomplish them. But how much will be accomplished if you never set any?

Exercise

As you set goals in the area of physical conditioning you should consider a medical checkup, diet improvement, and an exercise plan. Currently there are many popular plans for exercising and health spas seem to be springing up everywhere.

There are some very strong positive results from exercise. As Dr. Anderson in the School of Medicine at the University of Washington has noted, physical exercise provides three advantages: "(1) the maintenance of a good muscular tone to provide a reserve for activities we do not commonly engage in; (2) the maintenance of a healthy cardiovascular system through challenge to near-capacity on a regular basis; and (3) the sense of well-being which is due to the escape of excessive tensions through this means."

As you can see, not only is exercise being recommended as a must for our physical condition, it is also advocated for its effects on your mental condition. Dr. Keith Sehnert reports that in 1976 Dr. John Greist, a psychiatrist, did a study with eight clinically depressed patients. These patients were involved in a ten-week running program. Of these, six were cured of their depression. Dr. Greist expanded the sample size to twenty-eight in 1978 and again found jogging to be effective psychotherapy.

There are many other studies being done in this area. Even though the evidence is not all in, the indications seem to be that jogging or active exercise can affect mental outlook and relieve stress. You should, of course, see a physician before you begin an exercise program.

Hal was a young executive who had much to do and aspired to do even more. However, he began to feel fatigued and depressed and lost some of his concentration. In examining his schedule, I could see that he had cut out almost everything except work. He began to build an exercise program and found that even though he still had many responsibilities, his energy level began to return and his depression lifted.

There are many avenues for exercise. You are free to explore various possibilities for your life-style and ability. An average of three twenty-minute sessions per week can be considered a minimum. Also it is better if you spread your exercising throughout the week instead of on three consecutive days. Some of the activities that are best for physical fitness are jogging, swimming, bicycling, aerobics, or skating.

However, you might prefer setting up a tennis match with a friend or taking part in a team sport. Exercise does not have to be drudgery. Find an activity that you enjoy. With some creative thought it can relieve your stress and provide some added enjoyment to your schedule.

Epilogue

We have given you some suggestions on these pages for relieving stress. One certainty is that you will have stress in your life and in this imperfect society. Yet, stress will give you a measurement of your strength and provide insight into your satisfaction with your life and work.

Hopefully your attitude toward stress will be positive and optimistic. Such an attitude can be a powerful agent for turning negative to positive. Also, as you handle each stressful event you build strength and confidence for the next one.

It may be that as you consider your life situation and your work, you will realize that you need to make some changes not just in attitude but also in actions. Lists are great aids; make a list of the possibilities in every area. Don't be afraid to take some risks and branch out in challenging new areas.

Here are some more possibilities that might work for you. Some have been suggested earlier but bear repeating. The more you understand and know about yourself the freer you are to respond to life and to change. Be flexible and see opportunity in every problem. There are many avenues open to you to find out about yourself. Listen to your feelings and your body. Your hurts can often tell you what is really important to you.

Use the helping professions. You might go to a counselor and take an interest inventory or a temperament analysis. If you do, be honest and kind to yourself. You do not expect your friends to be perfect in every area. Why do you expect it of yourself? Life is a growing and learning process. Throughout history kings and heads of state have known the value of objective counsel. There is much logic in seeking advice on life situations.

Continue to read self-help books; go to the library and look up topics of interest. Use some of your waiting time to read them. Enroll in a course or attend classes to learn a new hobby. Many classes are available and often free. Your mind will be challenged and you will enjoy the fun.

A journal will also help you to know yourself. It is also a way to record and enjoy again small fun happenings that you sometimes forget. Remind yourself of the nice people you know and see, and relive happy memories when you relax or take a break.

Continue with your own list and don't accept more stress by feeling overwhelmed. See the possibilities of using stress for opportunities. Nothing has to be done at once. You have a lifetime, and you never really finish some things.

Permit yourself to grow and develop just as you would a good friend. Take one thing at a time and work at your own pace. Fast changes are not always lasting or meaningful.

In our world change is inevitable, so be flexible. From time to time consider whether or not you are being true to yourself and those who mean the most to you. Reexamine your possibilities and goals. Your challenge is to creatively use and enjoy your life and talents.

9
Heart Attacks
Section I. What They Are and How to Avoid Them

Daniel MacNeil, M.D.

As a physician, cardiologist, and medical educator, much of my energy is devoted to the evaluation and treatment of patients with established heart disease. The majority of the problems deal with coronary artery disease, which is an acquired illness. Although the list of diagnostic and therapeutic achievements over the past one and one-half decades is impressive, the fact remains that we are dealing with the symptoms and consequences of a problem that has already occurred. Once a heart attack has taken place, the damage is permanent. It is the proverbial situation of attempting to close the barn door after the horse is out.

It was refreshing for me to be asked to write about *preventing* a heart attack. I believe that prevention of disease is the ultimate goal of medicine. All the answers are not in yet; but we certainly know much about the events that lead up to a heart attack as well as ways to minimize our risk. In my portion of this work, I would like to share with you the miracle of the design and function of the heart, the catastrophe of its disorder, and some of the ways in which we can engage in preventive maintenance. In the physical as well as the spiritual realm, a healthy heart is essential to the wellness of the individual. "A good man brings good out of the treasure of good things in his heart; a bad man brings bad out of his treasure of bad things" (*see* Luke 6:45).

THE MARVELOUS MACHINE—GUARANTEED FOR A LIFETIME

Not long ago many newspapers carried a picture of Henry Kissinger waving as he left a hospital. He had just undergone coronary artery bypass surgery. His medical problem is one that affects millions of people in the United States. It is so common that almost all of us have a family member or personally know someone who has heart disease.

A review of the facts about heart disease helps us to understand how serious the problem is and why it is important for us to attempt to reduce our chances of having a heart attack. According to the most recent United States statistics, an estimated 975,550 persons per year die from disease of the heart and blood vessels. This makes heart disease the leading cause of death in our country. Twice as many people die of heart problems as die of cancer, which is the second leading cause of death. The facts reveal that more people die from heart disease than all other causes combined.

LEADING CAUSES OF DEATH IN UNITED STATES*

Cause	Number
Heart and blood vessel disease	975,550
Cancer	403,780
Accident	105,420
Chronic obstructive lung disease	49,980
Pneumonia and influenza	44,110
All other causes	327,160

* As projected for 1979. Source: National Center for Health Statistics, U. S. Public Health Service.

Additional figures about heart attack also are alarming. The American Heart Association estimated that 1,500,000 Americans would have a heart attack in 1982. Of these people, 550,000 would die. More than half of the deaths would occur outside the hospital. It is no wonder that many people are concerned about heart disease and how to prevent it!

An unusual experience that points out the prevalence of coronary disease occurred while I was in practice in California. One afternoon I admitted a young man in his thirties to the coronary care unit for evaluation of chest pain, which proved to be caused by a heart attack. He had no prior history of heart trouble although he was a heavy smoker. He began to develop his chest symptoms while digging a grave for a member of his family, also in his thirties, who had died from a heart attack!

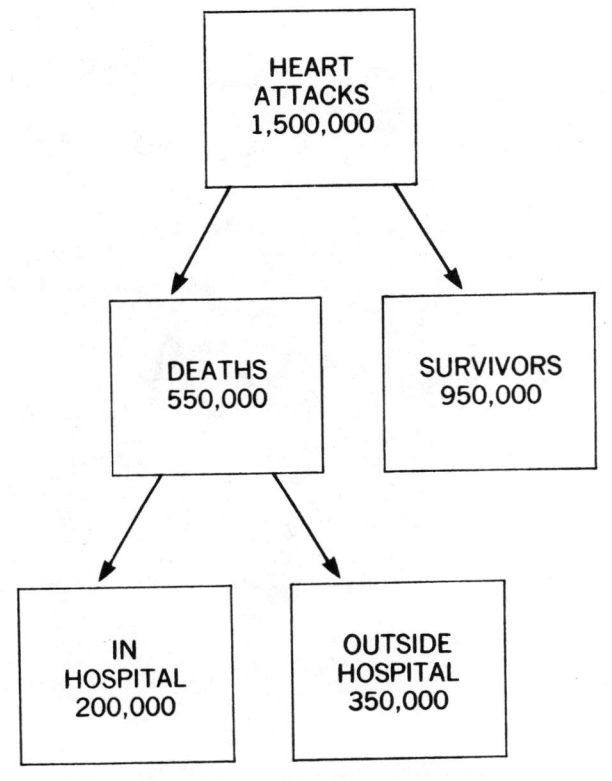

```
                    ┌─────────────┐
                    │   HEART     │
                    │  ATTACKS    │
                    │ 1,500,000   │
                    └─────────────┘
                      ↙         ↘
            ┌─────────────┐   ┌─────────────┐
            │   DEATHS    │   │  SURVIVORS  │
            │   550,000   │   │   950,000   │
            └─────────────┘   └─────────────┘
              ↙         ↘
    ┌─────────────┐   ┌─────────────┐
    │     IN      │   │   OUTSIDE   │
    │  HOSPITAL   │   │  HOSPITAL   │
    │   200,000   │   │   350,000   │
    └─────────────┘   └─────────────┘
```

Projected Figures for 1982.
Source: American Heart Association

Structure of the Heart

Knowing how the heart is put together is the best way to understand what can go wrong and how to prevent it. After a cardiac catheterization, I frequently draw illustrations of the normal heart in order to help patients understand why their heart may be functioning abnormally. The heart is a muscle that constantly squeezes, or contracts, and then relaxes.

The heart is divided into a right and left side (*see* figure 1) with each side having an upper and lower chamber. The upper chambers are called *atria* after the Latin word for room. The lower compartments are called *ventricles.* The right side of the heart receives blood from the body and pumps it to the lungs. The left side of the heart receives blood from the lungs and pumps it to the body. The blood travels in pipes called *arteries* and *veins.* These blood vessels can branch like a tree, getting so small that you need a microscope to see them. Some are as large as a half-dollar.

The heart itself is the size of your fist. It is located in the chest behind

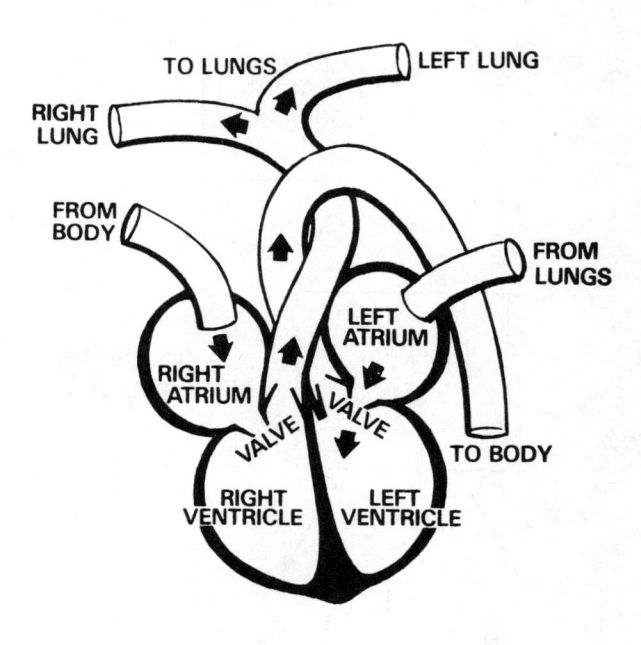

Figure 1

and slightly to the left of your breastbone (*see* figure 2). The majority of the pumping work is done by the ventricles, so these chambers have thicker muscles than the atria. The thickest muscle is found in the left ventricle since this chamber must pump blood to the entire body at about four times the pressure of the right ventricle.

Inside the heart there are delicate doors called valves, which are found on each side of the heart (*see* figure 3). These doors can open only in one direction, allowing the blood to flow in only one direction through the heart. The valves on the right side are called the *tricuspid valve* and the *pulmonic valve*. On the left side the valves are called the *mitral valve* and the *aortic valve*. When one valve on a side is open, the other is closed and vice versa.

Since the heart is constantly at work pumping blood, it has to receive oxygen and nutrients continually to maintain its energy. The pipes that supply blood to the heart run over the surface of the heart in a crownlike fashion and are thus called coronary arteries. There are three major pipelines that supply the energy needs of the heart (*see* figure 4). When any of these coronary arteries develop significant blockage, a heart attack can occur. Names of the major branches of these vessels are *left anterior descending, circumflex,* and *posterior descending arteries.*

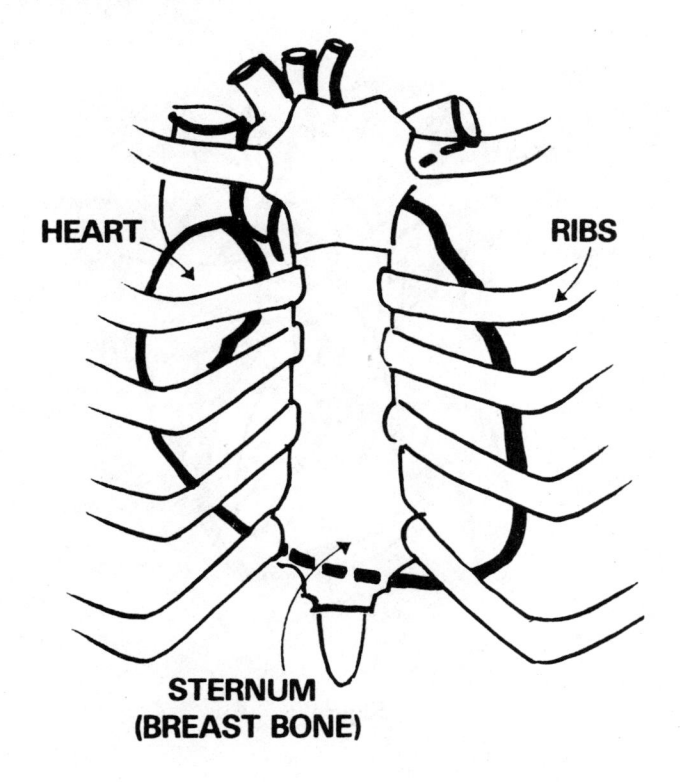

Figure 2

How It All Works

Given all of these parts, how do they work together? Inside the heart there is a little electric regulator called a *pacemaker*. Normally, sixty to one hundred impulses are sent out every minute from the pacemaker. Each electrical impulse causes first the atria to contract and then the ventricles. When these muscles contract, they squeeze all of the blood out of the heart chambers. The atria squeeze the blood into the ventricles and then the ventricles squeeze the blood into the lungs and body. Normally, about five quarts of blood are pumped every minute. That amount can be increased several times if necessary. Exercise is one of the things that requires the heart to pump more blood.

You might wonder why blood has to be pumped to both the lungs and the body. The reason is that all of the blood pumped by the heart to the body is rich in oxygen. The body then uses the oxygen and puts waste gases into the blood. When blood is pumped to the lungs, the waste gases can be eliminated and oxygen from the air can be put back into the

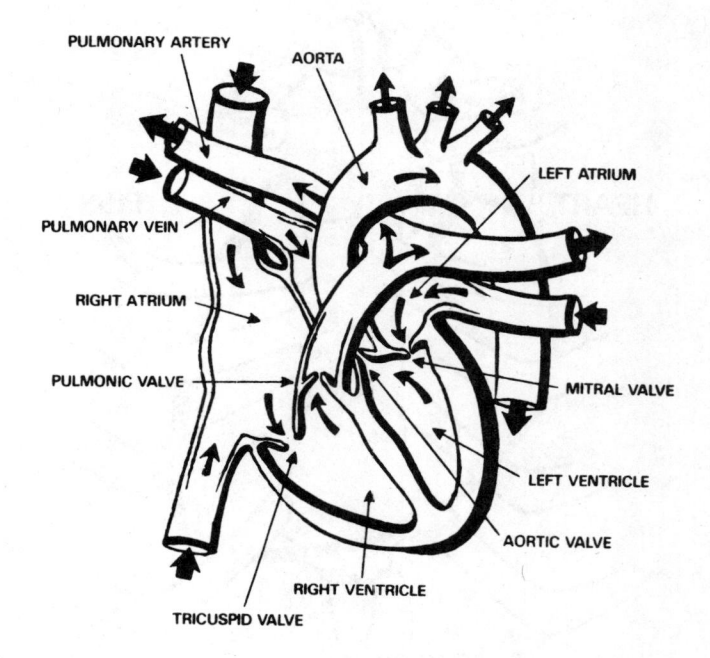

Figure 3

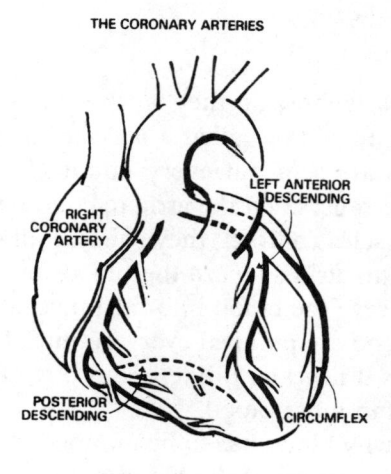

Figure 4

blood. The heart truly is a marvelous machine, but like other machines it needs preventive maintenance.

SUPPLY AND DEMAND—THE STORY OF A HEART ATTACK

John lay on his back staring at the cardiac monitor above his bed. Each time that his heart beat, a wave was traced on the screen. There were wires taped onto his chest, and an intravenous line was in his left hand.

How did it happen? Everything was going so well! He was only forty-five and about to become the youngest president in his corporation's history. What went wrong? He had never been sick a day in his life, and now he was in the hospital.

At least things weren't as bad as yesterday. Driving to work, he felt a terrible crushing pain in his chest and broke out in a sweat. At first he thought it was indigestion, but coffee and donuts had never done that before. Maybe it was the cigarettes. No matter what, it should settle down in a few minutes—but it didn't. At work things got worse, and he vomited. Maybe it was an ulcer? A call to his doctor only complicated matters. He was advised to call an ambulance and go to the hospital. If he hadn't felt so bad, it would have been embarrassing. After that, it was all a blur until today—shots, oxygen, blood tests, X rays, EKGs, something about a heart attack. I could have died! I'm too young. What happened? What's going to happen?

As a cardiologist, John's story is an all-too-frequent one to me. Let me share with you some of the things I tell people like John when they ask, "What happened?"

Hardening of the Arteries

Most Americans have heard of "hardening of the arteries." It is usually thought to be related to aging and found in old people. In truth, this problem can be found even in young people. It is this process that is responsible for heart attacks in most people. The medical term for hardening of the arteries is *atherosclerosis*. It is a degenerative process in the walls of blood vessels. Over a period of time there is a gradual buildup of material that causes narrowing of the inside of the blood vessel. Often this buildup is in one spot rather than uniformly throughout the blood vessel. The result is a local block or dam in the bloodstream. Now, only a limited amount of blood can get past the blockage. This also means that only a limited supply of oxygen can be delivered by the blood to the area beyond the block. Remember that oxygen in the blood is needed for muscles in the body to do their work. When significant blocks exist in a blood vessel, it is possible for the supply of oxygen to be inadequate for the demand (*see* figure 5).

HEART OXYGEN BALANCE

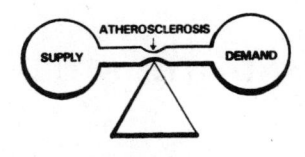

Figure 5

The heart is especially sensitive to these blocks. Because of all the work it is doing, the heart normally takes most of the oxygen out of the blood each time it passes through the coronary arteries. When more oxygen is needed for more work, the flow of blood must be increased. When atherosclerosis is present, the flow is restricted and the supply of oxygen may not be able to meet the demands. It is much like a farmer irrigating his crops. If the water valve is open, all of the plants get enough water. If the water valve is closed halfway, some of the plants will not get enough.

Atherosclerosis is a slowly occurring process over an extended period of time. It may begin early in our lives. When the blood vessels of young men killed accidentally or in wars have been examined, early changes have been noted. On that basis it would appear wise to begin to be concerned about hardening of the arteries even at a young age.

When examined under a microscope, the atherosclerotic lesion, or *plaque* as it is called, contains many elements. Fat, in the form of cholesterol, scar tissue, cellular debris, and calcium usually are present. The exact mechanism that causes this process is still not known, although there are many recognized factors that will speed up the process.

Atherosclerosis seems to involve certain blood vessels more than others. The vessels in the abdomen, legs, and heart are particularly involved. Although atherosclerosis may be developing for many years, it is not until the buildup reaches a significant level that problems may occur. It is generally believed that the buildup must narrow the blood-vessel diameter by 50 percent before there is trouble. When the narrowing reaches this degee, the blood vessel can be seen in cross section to be blocked by 75 percent (*see* figure 6).

In summary, atherosclerosis causes a dam in the river. This dam affects the supply of oxygen to the tissues downstream. If the supply of oxygen is inadequate to meet the demands, problems can occur.

What Happens During a Heart Attack

Imagine you are driving your car and you suddenly run out of gas. The engine would sputter to a stop. There is a similar situation during a heart attack, but fortunately the heart usually does not stop working. Although

CROSS SECTION

ORIGINAL SIZE OF BLOOD VESSEL

SIZE OF BLOOD VESSEL WITH BLOCK

ATHEROSCLEROSIS

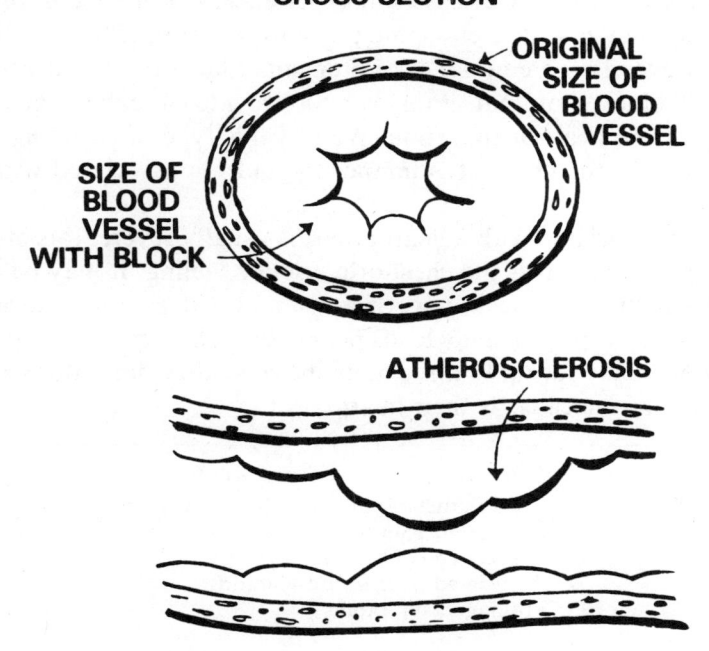

Figure 6

at least one and sometimes all three of the coronary arteries may have significant blocks, it is normally just one blood vessel that causes the problem. This vessel becomes totally blocked off, and no blood can get past the blocked area. The part of the heart supplied by the blood vessel suddenly has no oxygen. Without oxygen the heart cells cannot function and they die. It is the death of part of the heart muscle that causes all the problems of a heart attack.

The reason that the blood vessel suddenly blocks off seems to be related to the blood-clotting system. Pictures made of coronary arteries soon after a heart attack show that most of the victims have a blood clot at the location of the narrowed coronary artery. In fact, recent research has been directed at dissolving this clot and restoring blood flow. Some of the early results have been very exciting. The terms doctors use when a heart attack occurs usually are *coronary thrombosis* or *myocardial infarction*.

Symptoms of a Heart Attack

Whenever we injure a part of our body, we usually stimulate a painful response; the heart is no exception. There is a spectrum of pain that people with coronary-artery disease can experience. On one hand, the heart temporarily may not have enough oxygen for its work. This usually happens with exercise or emotional excitement. The coronary artery is not completely blocked off, but simply cannot provide enough oxygen for the demands of the heart at that time. We call this type of pain *angina pectoris,* or pain in the chest. It is temporary and not associated with heart damage.

The pain associated with a heart attack is usually severe. It is often like a crushing weight across the chest or a viselike feeling. It may be accompanied by pain in the neck, jaw, or arms, and it does not go away. The persistence of the pain usually leads people to their doctor or hospital, yet most people delay for up to three hours because they don't think or want to believe that the cause is their heart.

COMMON SYMPTOMS OF HEART ATTACK
1. Severe crushing or squeezing chest pain
2. Associated pain in neck, jaw, or arms
3. Associated cold sweats
4. Associated nausea and vomiting
5. Prolonged symptoms

Other symptoms sometimes accompanying a heart attack are shortness of breath, cold sweats, nausea, and vomiting. We all are different and have different responses to pain. Some people do not feel pain as much as they feel a fullness in the chest or a tightness. Others simply have discomfort but cannot characterize it any more than that.

Effects of a Heart Attack

Knowing what happens during a heart attack and also knowing something about the heart's function help us to understand the consequences of a heart attack. As you might expect, when part of the heart muscle is destroyed, the muscle is not as strong. The weakness of the heart muscle can lead to poor function of the pumping mechanism, resulting in a problem called *heart failure.* Congestion in the lungs can develop, causing shortness of breath. The blood pressure also may be affected and shock can occur. Fortunately, we have enough heart reserve so that many people recover from a heart attack and lead normal lives. The dead area of heart muscle becomes a scar, and the overall heart function remains close to normal.

Another serious problem, especially during the early hours of a heart attack, is a change in heart rhythm. The delicate electrical system of the heart becomes disturbed, and extra beats begin to appear. There may be a

Common Medical Problems

dangerous change in rhythm called *ventricular fibrillation*. This problem can be fatal and is usually the cause of sudden death. Even this can be treated, however, with cardiopulmonary resuscitation (CPR) and the use of electrical cardioversion by a trained person. Ventricular fibrillation is most likely to occur during the early hours of a heart attack. It is for this reason that it is important to seek medical help quickly if there are symptoms of a heart attack.

Other problems that might follow a heart attack include alteration in the function of a heart valve, especially the mitral valve. The valve may become leaky and thus produce heart failure. The sac around the heart can become inflamed and cause chest pain as well.

COMPLICATIONS OF HEART ATTACK
1. Heart failure
2. Shock
3. Heart rhythm irregularities
4. Inflamed pericardial sac
5. Abnormal valve function
6. Death

Each of us has known someone who died of a heart attack. Death usually occurs because of an abnormality of the heart rhythm, but severe problems with the pump function, and even rupture of the heart muscle, are other possible causes. Since the majority of deaths occur outside the hospital, emphasis has been placed on earlier recognition of the symptoms of heart attack, in order to get people to go to the hospital sooner. Heart-rhythm problems can be treated very successfully by life-support units. Most cities, and even smaller communities, now have personnel trained in advanced cardiac life support who can go out from the hospital to bring heart-attack victims back to the hospital. Additionally, large numbers of people are receiving training in cardiopulmonary resuscitation (CPR). Finally, many hospitals now have developed specialized areas for early cardiac care. These specialized units can significantly reduce the number of deaths occurring after a heart-attack victim makes it to the hospital. All of these modalities should help decrease the number of deaths caused by heart attack.

RISK FACTORS—THE WARNING SIGNALS

Mary was anxious as I entered her room. She was lying in bed with a bandage over her right groin. During the heart catheterization that morning she had been mildly sedated, but the medication had worn off and the stress was evident. She was fifty, a two-pack-per-day smoker, and thirty pounds overweight. Because of stress in her marriage, she had been smoking more heavily in the past year. She had been having pains in her chest for six months, but no definite cause was found even after several diagnostic tests. Mary had just undergone *coronary angiography* to find out if the symptoms were from heart trouble. Fortunately, everything was normal. But what should she do to be sure that she did not develop heart disease in the future?

We have examined the causes and results of a heart attack. What is more important is how to prevent the problem in the first place. Over the years, public-health investigators have been concerned about what might cause heart attacks. To get this information, entire communities have been studied over many years. What has emerged from these studies are certain factors that seem to predispose a person to a greater risk of heart attack. These factors cannot predict exactly which persons will have a heart attack; they simply predict the chances that a problem will occur. Some are considered major and others minor. Some can be changed, while others cannot.

Unchangeable Risk Factors

The risk factors over which we have no control are age, sex, race, and heredity. Hardening of the arteries takes time to develop. It is no surprise then that the older we get, the more likely we will have a problem with blood-vessel narrowing. It should be remembered, though, that one in four heart-attack deaths occurs before the age of sixty-five.

Blacks have a 50 percent greater chance of having high blood pressure than whites. High blood pressure, we will learn shortly, is a major risk factor for heart disease. Males have a higher incidence of heart attack than females. After menopause, women begin to have more problems with heart disease, but men continue to be the leaders. The reason for this lesser risk in women has not been explained.

Family history is also important. Some families seem to have premature hardening of the arteries. This does not mean, however, that a heart attack can be predicted in the children of a person who has had a heart attack. Our genes may simply influence other risk factors, many of which, fortunately, can be changed.

Changeable Risk Factors

The changeable risk factors can be grouped into major and minor ones. The major factors are high blood pressure, smoking, elevated blood fats (especially cholesterol), and diabetes. The minor factors are obesity, stress, personality, and life-style.

High blood pressure, or hypertension, usually causes very few symptoms by itself. It can be detected by measurement using a cuff around the arm and a stethoscope. In the United States, over 35 million people are estimated to have this problem. Statistics clearly demonstrate an unfavorable relationship between untreated elevation of blood pressure and the possibility of a heart attack. It is thought that elevation of the blood pressure may lead to injury of the blood-vessel wall, which then leads to hardening of the arteries. Since high blood pressure is so silent, it is important to have a periodic blood-pressure check to detect the problem early. There are many medications that can effectively lower the blood pressure and thereby decrease the risk.

Smoking is another major risk factor. It alone can increase the risk of a heart attack three to five times. The more cigarettes you smoke, the greater is your risk. Smoking begins early in our society and is a habit that is difficult to break. Many people are aware that smoking is bad for their lungs, but they often are unaware of its association with heart disease. It is cigarette smoking that carries the major risk. Cigar and pipe smoking do not carry as high a danger. The good news about smoking is that things get better if you stop. Over time the risk decreases to close to the level of nonsmokers.

We are what we eat! The diet of many Americans contains too many calories with too much saturated fat, cholesterol, refined sugar, and salt. This type of eating can lead to acceleration of hardening of the arteries. It has been determined that the measurement of total blood-cholesterol values can determine the risk for heart attack. **Elevated cholesterol** values can increase the risk at least four times that of a normal person. The general principle is the lower the better. Even persons with high-normal values should work on getting their cholesterol levels down. Part of the blood-cholesterol level is related to our diet, so it is important to be careful of what we eat. Changing our diet can definitely decrease blood-cholesterol levels. Reducing the intake of calories, cholesterol in foods, and saturated fats can help us significantly.

I should point out that recently some researchers have found a "good" cholesterol in the blood. This cholesterol is related to what is called *high density lipoprotein* or HDL. When levels of this cholesterol are high, the risk of a heart attack is decreased.

Diabetes also seems to be associated with hardening of the arteries. This abnormality is related to an intolerance in our ability to handle sugar normally. Being overweight may aggravate this situation. The problem usually is detected by blood and urine tests, since the blood sugar becomes elevated and ultimately spills into the urine.

The risk of having a heart attack is not simply the sum of the risk factors. Two or more present in the same person makes the risk many times greater. It becomes important then to detect all of the risk factors in each person in order to minimize the overall risk.

Less-serious risk factors are those of obesity, stress, personality, and life-style. We live in a country blessed with abundance. We eat constantly and our bodies show it. Most Americans are overweight and overfat. We reside in a high-technology society geared to time and productivity. We work hard and play hard. The clock often rules our lives. From early childhood our days are scheduled, and we seem to have constant deadlines. We learn to be efficient, but we often are not at peace. In fact, many times we don't know what to do with ourselves when we stop running. Each person responds differently to stress, but the fact remains that long-term stress may produce physical illness. We will say more about this later.

Certain personality types also seem to be more likely to have a heart attack. The personality known as Type *A* is an example. This person lives a twenty-five-hour day. He cannot rest and is driven. He is responsible, works hard, and accomplishes much. In our society he often is the type of person whom we consider successful—until he has his heart attack.

Risk factors that cannot be changed
- Age
- Sex
- Race
- Heredity

Risk factors that can be changed
Major
- High blood pressure
- Smoking
- Elevated blood cholesterol
- Diabetes

Minor
- Obesity
- Stress
- Personality type
- Sedentary life-style

Life-style also may have some role in heart disease. After high school it is downhill for most Americans as far as exercising is concerned. Being sedentary may have an unfavorable effect on our circulation. Its effect on other risk factors such as blood pressure and obesity makes it at least a contributing factor.

In summary, many things may predispose us to have a heart attack. Some are more significant than others. It is important for us to learn about these things that increase our risks since many of them can be changed through diet, exercise, and medication. When these steps are taken, our risk for a heart attack is minimized.

PREVENTIVE MAINTENANCE—DECREASING THE RISK
Medical Evaluation

Information about what causes heart attacks is clearly beneficial, but how do we put it to use? For many people, particularly those with many risk factors or suspected heart disease, a medical evaluation is necessary. Some of the risk factors can be detected only by blood tests and a physical examination. If you have never seen a doctor or see one infrequently, it would be wise to check with him about screening you for problems that could lead to heart disease. On the basis of your medical history and examination, prudent recommendations can be made. The earlier problems are detected, the better the chances of minimizing your risks.

The taking of a medical history usually reviews those symptoms known to be produced by hardening of the arteries. It also includes a record of known risk factors and family history of heart disease. A dietary history or exercise history might also be necessary, as well as a rundown of stress at work or home.

The examination could be quite revealing, even in a person with no symptoms. A simple blood-pressure and pulse reading will provide an idea of your resting cardiovascular status. Height and weight can be determined and compared with ideal body weight. An eye examination will help to define blood vessel changes, possibly related to high blood pressure or diabetes. The eye exam is the only way that the blood vessels in the body can normally be directly visualized. A heart and lung examination will detect underlying abnormalities and provide information necessary for recommendations on exercise. Skin deposits sometimes suggest underlying blood-fat abnormalities. The musculoskeletal examination helps with recommendations about the specific type of exercise that should be performed.

After the history and physical examination, certain blood studies would be needed. As we already mentioned, blood sugar and cholesterol are important. Other fats, such as triglycerides and high-density-lipoprotein (HDL) cholesterol, provide useful information. Some physicians measure low-density-lipoprotein (LDL) cholesterol since elevation of this type of cholesterol is unfavorable. Because these blood studies are often influenced by dietary intake, it is usually best to obtain them after a twelve- to fourteen-hour fast in a stable metabolic state. You should not be in the middle of a crash diet or having your blood test the morning after a gourmet anniversary meal.

An additional procedure that often is suggested during a screening examination for heart disease is an exercise test. For persons over the age of thirty-five, it probably is prudent to undergo one of these tests if an exercise program is planned. The test may be used to look for the presence of significant coronary narrowing in persons without symptoms, but it is less reliable in this circumstance. It is most reliable for use with those people who have suspected heart disease.

An exercise, or stress, test is usually performed on a treadmill or bicycle. A person walks, runs, or rides these devices at specific levels of effort for specific time periods. The electrocardiogram (EKG) is monitored continuously during and after exercise to detect changes in heart rhythm or wave form. The EKG also provides a means to measure the heart rate throughout the exercise and into the recovery. Blood-pressure recordings are also taken at intervals. The test provides information about the current fitness level of the individual, as well as screening for possible coronary-artery disease or heart-rhythm problems. If it is performed to maximum effort, the individual maximal heart rate can be obtained. This heart rate becomes important in individual exercise prescription. The results of these tests can be used for comparative studies to document improvement in fitness as well as heart-rate and blood-pressure responses after entering an exercise program.

Once a medical evaluation is complete, you are on your own. All of the information about your heart will be of little value unless it is put into action. It is the time for self-discipline and the development of good habits. Nothing is more difficult than changing habits, especially those of eating and exercise. The results take time to be seen, and perseverance is required.

Diet

Our bodies are like machines. We take in food as fuel and burn it up. If we take in more fuel than we burn up, we will store the excess as fat. We measure the energy we burn in terms of calories. For most of us a diet will require a reduction in the calories we eat. The benefit ultimately will be a reduction in blood-fat levels and achievement of ideal body weight and body fat for our size. If we exercise regularly in addition to dieting, we will facilitate this process since we will burn even more calories.

A healthful diet does not simply mean fewer calories. The specific types of foods that we eat must also be modified. Since high salt intake seems to be connected in some way to high blood pressure, it may be prudent to decrease the total amount of salt that we eat. The diet normally eaten in the United States contains significant amounts of salt. We also will need to reduce the amount of fats (particularly saturated) as well as cholesterol in our diet. Dairy products should be scrutinized: It may be necessary to switch from whole to low-fat milk and to switch from butter to polyunsaturated margarine. Total egg and ice cream consumption may need to be reduced. Cooking oils and shortenings used for baking and frying should be reviewed to determine whether or not they are the preferred polyunsaturated products. Most companies now list on the face of their product packages the type and amount of fat content to help in the selection of proper foods. Since animal fat in meats is also a problem, it generally is wise to eat smaller portions of meat, with fat trimmed, leaner meat, and more veal, fish, and poultry.

All of the effort involved seems to be worth it since altering the diet has definitely been proved to lower the blood-fat level. In animals, lowering of blood fats has also been associated with an improvement in the blood-vessel blocks. It is hoped that this result will also occur in man. Since the atherosclerotic process seems to start early and progress over the years, the sooner we start the better. Changing the diets of children has even been suggested by some specialists.

Exercise

Regular exercise is the other habit we need to develop. We will discuss this further in the next section of this book, but a few comments can be made here. It has not been absolutely proved, but there is strong suggestive evidence that regular exercise is beneficial in decreasing our risk for heart disease. Exercise certainly has a favorable effect on some of the risk factors: Blood fats decrease, and even a tendency to lower blood pressure has been noted. More calories are burned, so there is less chance of obesity.

With exercise the heart and lungs become more efficient in their function. The heart muscle in a sense is strengthened. It pumps more blood per beat and gets the job done with less heartbeats per minute. The heart simply doesn't have to work as hard. Some marathon runners are so efficient that their pulse is only forty beats per minute, which is half the normal number. Most people who exercise regularly develop a sense of well-being. They feel good and feel healthy. Their bodies become finely tuned, rather than running on half their cylinders. Some persons become even more fit than when they were much younger.

Any good exercise program will include warm-up and cool-down calisthenics. These help to keep the body limber and prevent injuries. They also help to warm up the heart for hard work. Remember to do them!

A few final tips. Wear proper clothing. It should be loose fitting and allow body ventilation. Good shoes are a must, especially if you become a jogger. Avoid exercising in extremes of temperature and after heavy meals. Don't overdo! Go slowly and add variety to your exercise to keep it interesting. If you don't have the motivation, or have constant interruptions in your exercise schedule, consider an organized exercise program in your community, which will force you to fit it into your schedule. Don't compromise.

Remember that you have a responsibility to yourself and your family to take good care of your body.

Heart Attacks
Section II. Developing a Personal Heart Strategy

Larry Losoncy, Ph.D.

In the first section you learned about the physiology of the heart—its structure and function—what happens when the heart and its complex parts do not perform properly. Dr. MacNeil discussed diverse preventive means to avoid having a heart attack in the first place. As he pointed out, once a heart attack has occurred, the damage is permanent.

In this second section, we will discuss in further detail what you can do to help yourself to prevent heart disease. Some of this advice involves various types of physical exercise, but just as important is your mental/spiritual health. You will learn what causes stress and about the terrible effect it has on your body, especially your heart. You have within yourself the capabilities of conquering this number-one killer disease—if you will but use them.

I have watched my father in his advancing age learn about his heart and how to take care of it; he has shown me that a heart attack can be a blessed warning. I mean to stay healthy so as not ever to have heart disease or a heart attack. But only God knows how we will die; even the healthiest persons must age and die physically. What we do in the meantime is to live in healthy ways and hope for fullness of years, not try to achieve an impossible fountain of youth.

You need not agree with all that follows in this section. While much of it consists of practical wisdom gained from the experience of others, much of it also reflects my own attitudes and beliefs. What is important is that you think about *your* attitudes and beliefs and that you develop a strategy that works for you to stay healthy and "be of good heart."

EXERCISE, EXERCISE, EXERCISE

The heart's friend is exercise. Our bodies are made to work. The less physical work we do, the more exercise we need to make up the difference. When nearly everyone worked in the farm fields or at some other kind of physical labor, the idea of exercising didn't seem logical. Who needed exercise after splitting wood all day? Why exercise after roofing a house?

As a young man I often accompanied my grandfather through his day of work on his farm. I would begin helping with the animals in the morning, carrying water and food, taking the cows to pasture, and fetching the eggs. Then there might be vegetable gardens to hoe, apples or corn to pick; sometimes there would be field corn to shell in the hand-driven shelling machine. There were always things to be hauled, errands to be run, animals to be tended.

I learned that even on a relatively small farm, the work never ends. I would be exhausted long before the day ended and long, long before Grandfather got tired! Grandfather was well over seventy years of age! He never needed exercise, nor did his neighbors! But as our civilization has developed to the point where most of us work without exerting ourselves physically, we find exercise to be very logical indeed.

Our bodies are so made that physical exercise is *good* for them; lack of physical exertion is bad for our bodies. Exercise provides the needed physical exertion. We now know enough about exercise to distinguish four broad families of exercises. They are: calisthenics, isometrics, anaerobics, aerobics.

Calisthenics are the limbering up and toning kinds of exercises. They help the muscles stretch and they firm the body. These include such things as arm flaps, bending, stretching; they also include the warm-ups athletes do before competing, dancers do before performing, and so forth.

Isometrics are the exercises that pit muscles against muscles. An example of this kind of exercise is to stand in a door frame and push out against both sides with the arms. Push-ups are isometric; even to press one finger against another is to use muscle against muscle.

Anaerobics are those exercises which, in addition to exerting the body muscles, force the heart and lungs to extra effort, but not on a steady basis. These exercises are also referred to as the "stop and go" exercises. They include such things as racquetball, baseball, softball, trampolining, football, tennis if played leisurely, and gardening or mowing the lawn.

Aerobics are those exercises that push the heart and lungs to work harder in a continuous and steady manner for sustained periods of time (usually at least twenty-five minutes), thereby increasing oxygen use in the body. In this category are such things as brisk walking, jogging, swimming, and bicycling.

Effects of Exercise

What effects does exercise have on the human body, especially on the heart? In general, when done properly, exercise keeps the body trim and firm by strengthening muscles (keep in mind that the heart is a muscle); it increases the burning of calories. It produces feelings of relaxation.

Calisthenics, in particular, are designed to condition the body by strengthening the muscles. Stretching and contracting are the way muscles work and when muscles work, they grow strong. Calisthenics stretch the muscles by design; various kinds of calisthenics stretch muscles in various places of the body. This stretching strengthens or tones up the body tissue since it takes tough, tight muscles to hold up sagging body tissue.

Isometrics also strengthen muscles but in the opposite way from calisthenics. That is, isometrics press muscle against muscle, which strains the muscle, causing it to contract or cramp. Calisthenics stretch muscles, while isometrics contract muscles. Just as the stretching of muscles is followed by the contracting, so in isometrics the contracting of muscles is followed by their stretching or relaxing. Isometrics, because they put so much pressure on the muscles, build up muscle tissue much more than calisthenics. They harden the body, as wrestlers and boxers and weightlifters can confirm. On the other hand, isometrics hurt, leaving us with many more aches, whereas calisthenics generally leave us with pleasant feelings in the muscles.

Calisthenics and isometrics are the exercises most used for the prevention of sagging. Stomach muscles are especially likely to sag from years of overeating. Each time we eat or drink, the muscles of the stomach wall are stretched. The more food and liquid we take in at any given time, the longer these muscles stretch and the more difficult it becomes for them to return (contract) to their normal length. Eventually these muscles can become like rubber bands that have been stretched too often. They become weak and elongated, which allows the flesh to sag instead of being held up properly.

Calisthenics and isometrics are of some value to the heart in that they help counteract overweight and body sagging by strengthening the muscles, helping the body tone, and providing us with good, relaxed feelings in our muscles and also about our overall image.

One of the convenient things about calisthenics and isometrics is that they can be done almost everywhere and almost anytime. Even at a business meeting it is possible to push against the table with a hand or foot (isometric) without being noticed. During coffee break a little stretching would be acceptable; waistbends can be done anywhere except, of course, when the boss is watching!

Calisthenics and isometrics could generally be thought of as muscle exercises, whereas the other two kinds, anaerobics and aerobics, can be thought of as heart-lung-circulatory exercises. The heart, of course, is a muscle, too, and like all muscles the only way to strengthen it is to use it. However, stretching and pushing will not serve to use the heart. The only way to exercise the heart is to make it pump harder and faster.

Anaerobics, while causing the heart to beat harder and faster, do so only briefly, on a stop-and-go basis. To swing a bat and run down the first-base line will surely get the heart beating at near top speed, as the gasping base runner so well knows. But once at first base the runner stops, so that the exercise lasts only a few seconds. Leisurely tennis also tends to be start and stop. While muscles certainly receive great benefit from anaerobic exercise—just as in calisthenics and isometrics—it seems doubtful that anaerobics help the heart-lungs-circulation in any major way.

Aerobic Exercises: Heart Strengtheners

It is important to strengthen the heart because the stronger the heart, the more chance it has to rest. Aerobic exercises are the only known way for us to strengthen our hearts. Why is this? How is the heart strengthened?

Consider the fact that as a large muscle, all the heart ever does is beat, pumping blood through the body with each beat. While the muscle exercises shape up the body so that the heart's work is easier, heart exercises strengthen the heart so that doing its work will take fewer beats. If a heart takes eighty-five beats per minute to pump the blood, let's say, then a program of aerobic exercise that strengthens the heart by making it work harder and faster during the exercise time might make the heart strong enough to do its work in seventy-five beats per minute. Doing its work in fewer beats is the way the heart rests. The only way! And so a stronger heart means a more restful heart.

When I began jogging, I was convinced that it would be boring. Further, I doubted that any great benefits, other than perhaps a slight weight loss, would result. My resting heart rate was almost eighty-five beats per minute; I suffered from constant fatigue, needing more than eight hours of sleep each night and a nap most days. I was always out of energy.

Within two years, after jogging three times each week, my resting heart rate dropped to seventy beats per minute; I lost twenty-five pounds; I could get less than eight hours of sleep and still have plenty of energy all day long. I came to realize that a heart that can beat less but still do its work is a rested heart. My energy level continues to climb because *I* truly rest when my *heart* truly rests!

For the heart to do its work in 10 fewer beats per minute would mean 600 beats fewer per hour or about 14,400 fewer beats per twenty-four-hour day! That's a lot of rest!

The heart needs to work hardest when we exercise and easiest when we are completely at rest. That is why sleeping is so good for us: It rests the heart. At rest our blood circulates more slowly because the need to cleanse the blood and take in new oxygen from the lungs is diminished. So the heart has a cycle of work and rest built into each day: working hard during the working-waking hours and resting during the resting-sleeping hours. When a heart does not slow down very much during rest, it is a danger sign that the heart is weak, needing more beats to do its job even when there isn't very much work. A weak heart produces a weak heartbeat, much like any other pump. And so the strategy for resting the heart once again comes down to strengthening it, so that during the resting cycle it can truly rest. That's where aerobic exercise fits in.

Aerobic exercises push the heart to work harder for sustained periods of time. A sustained period of time would be for more than three or four minutes without stopping. The longer the heart is challenged by this type of exercise, the stronger it gets in rising to the challenge. For the heart to really benefit from aerobic exercise, no less than twenty-five minutes every two or three days is required. Probably, aerobic exercise lasting longer than an hour begins to be of doubtful value.

Aerobic exercises do more than merely strengthen the heart, although that is their greatest benefit. Because aerobics (running, intense walking, swimming, jogging) increase our use of oxygen, not only the heart but also the lungs get a good workout. Especially important is the fact that to breathe deeply and intensely for a long period of time results in more efficient lung function, with the ability to take in greater quantities of air. And so the second major benefit of aerobic exercise is better, healthier lungs.

The third effect of aerobics is that they strengthen the blood vessels. By exercising steadily and hard, the blood pressure is increased, the blood flows faster, and the blood vessels are challenged to expand and strengthen. In this respect, it is as though our circulatory system were like a garden hose lying in the warm sun not getting used. After days and days of this, the hose would become soft, limp, nearly useless. When water is run through the hose, especially at high pressure, the hose is no longer limp but resistant. So, too, with our circulatory system. Using it is good for it. Aerobics allows us to use it.

Aerobic exercises strengthen the heart, the lungs, and the circulatory system. They do so by forcing them to work harder, creating good side effects. The heart itself is able to beat less often, by being stronger, and thus to rest. The lungs become strong, making the work of the heart easier. The blood vessels open up and become stronger, more elastic, and distensible.

The fourth effect of aerobics is the strengthening of muscles, just as is the case in calisthenics, isometrics, and anaerobics.

Whoa!

Most people, when they begin to realize what a bargain aerobic exercises like jogging, walking, swimming, or dancing can be, begin to get excited. The first impulse *I* had about jogging was to run out on the track without warming up. Then I would zoom around, passing the experienced joggers like a new car speeding down the highway. How exhilarating! A new jogger already surpassing the pros! Of course, after a mile or so of such nonsense the new whiz suddenly felt like dying. And the pain afterward from all those abused muscles made me wonder where I hurt the most.

Fortunately, my friends loved me enough to slow me down and help me learn to run for the long haul. Now I run four miles in forty minutes without panting or straining or aching. As a forty-one-year-old I am jogging at a good pace. The tendency among forty-year-olds is to run for their life, often to the point of blisters, sore ankles, damaged knees, bruised bones; sometimes people risk dehydration, frostbite, or heat exhaustion by overdoing it. "Why not just a few more laps? Why not run a little harder? Why not go a little faster? Why not one more fast break?" These are the questions you should not be asking, questions that the new, excited convert to aerobics often does ask but answers the wrong way.

I used to try to run three miles in twenty minutes because that was all the time I would give myself. Eventually I realized that twenty minutes of aerobic exercise brings little benefit, since the heart and lungs need to work for sustained periods of time to get significantly strengthened—more like thirty to forty minutes or more. I also realized that I was running too fast, trying to get many miles clocked, and thereby neutralizing any benefits by the harm of straining and tearing. Now I give myself time to run properly—like the old-timers who jog year after year with satisfaction instead of frenzy.

At the beginning of summer many people find themselves swimming too long the first few times out, only to become sore, exhausted, discouraged, sunburned. Do not overdo it! Too much is even more dangerous than none at all. The secret to aerobics and to getting all its wonderful benefits is to do the exercises *regularly* and in *moderation*.

The heart needs to be challenged at a steady manageable pace. That means keeping the heart beating at a faster, stronger rate for at least twenty-five minutes. "Faster, stronger rate" *does not* mean racing the heart or pushing it to exhaustion. For most runners the steady pace means jog, walk, jog, walk. Gasping for breath is not a steady pace; pushing the blood pressure too high is not helpful, only dangerous. Exerting to the point of cramps (caused by lack of oxygen, usually) is no good. A *moderate,* steady pace: That's what it's all about!

How to Get Started?

Are you convinced that exercise of various kinds is good for your heart? Are you ready to start? Here are a few rules of thumb about getting started:

1. Start with calisthenics and isometrics, and start with *a small amount.* These exercises will help get your muscles working. Better to exercise moderately several times each day than for a long time once a day.

2. Choose anaerobic and aerobic exercises that seem most enjoyable and best suited to you. The more enjoyable they are, the easier it will be for you to do them regularly. If you like to swim, choose swimming. If you like tennis, choose tennis. If you like taking brisk walks or think you could get to like walking, try that. Start moderately and build up gradually. Never keep going until you are exhausted, overheated, out of breath, near fainting, or hurting all over.

3. Use a mixture of exercises. This keeps you from wearing out or straining one set of muscles. It also helps all of your body to develop.

4. Do not begin any program of exercise without consulting your physician if you have any medical condition, are over forty, have had heart trouble or high blood pressure in the past. Also, consult your physician if you begin to feel sick once you have begun a new program of exercise.

A Good Rule of Thumb

Nearly everyone who exercises agrees that it is never wise to push one's self to the limit. The most benefit from most exercises comes when we give it approximately 80 percent of our effort, and that much only after warming up, building up, being in shape. A runner-jogger, for example, will get all the benefits from running at 80 percent of the speed he or she is capable of running. More than that does no more good (it could do some damage); less than that does less good. Even golfers consider a good shot one that goes 80 percent of the distance they could hit the ball if they swung all out with a particular club. So the rule of thumb is 80 percent. Easy to remember, easy to do.

You may have noticed in this chapter that we have favored aerobic exercises over the other three families of exercises. This is because only aerobic exercises actually strengthen the heart, lungs, and circulatory systems.

I was suspicious of "propaganda" on the part of aerobics enthusiasts. Joggers and aerobic dancers, it seemed, were too gung ho about making converts, too rosy about the benefits. It may seem to you, the reader, that I am now guilty of the same thing in stressing the benefits of aerobics, especially since I didn't even recognize the word itself until a few years ago. If I seem to be pushing an ideology, please forgive me.

The other exercises, however, do have great benefits, as we mentioned, and should also be used. To do only aerobic exercises is not as good for the body as doing a variety or mixture of exercises.

It is important to remember, too, that aerobic exercise helps the lungs. When we remember that the heart must pump our blood through the lungs in order for us to get oxygen before the blood starts its journey through the body, we can realize that any difficulty in the lungs will put an extra load on the heart. So it is important, in any program of helping the heart, to help the lungs. Aerobics does this by getting the lungs to work harder and become healthier.

The final message of this chapter is: Happy exercising, happy breathing, and happy heartbeats!

STRESS—VERY NERVOUS PEOPLE

We are a relaxing people: picnics, weekends at the lake, parties, golf, getaways, beer blasts, pills, drugs, hobbies, television, saunas, just to name a few of the things on which we spend millions, perhaps billions, of dollars searching for relaxation. Stress produces the opposite of relaxation, and to be sure, too much stress can help bring on heart trouble. Stress contributes to all sorts of illnesses. Healthy strategies for avoiding heart trouble necessarily involve strategies for avoiding, minimizing, and coping with stress.

Stress, fundamentally, provokes total-survival reaction. Total, in that the reaction to stress is physical, mental, emotional, spiritual. When we are threatened, the instinct is to survive, usually by running. This means more adrenaline pumping through the body, more alertness in the eyes, quickened heartbeat and reflexes, higher blood pressure, tighter muscles in the abdomen, heightened mental activity, and various other forms of "red alert" or "battle stations" throughout our entire body.

Some of the stress-causing events and situations for most of us are:

>Moving
>Getting married
>Getting divorced
>Getting sick
>Being caught in a storm
>Losing a loved one in death
>Fighting with loved ones

Imagine that the human being is like a diving bell. The diving bell needs to be pressurized from within in order to withstand the pressures on the outside. For people, the pressures on the outside are stress. The pressurizing from the inside could be called anxiety, or stress reaction. Just as the diving bell needs more and more pressure on the inside to withstand increased pressure from the outside as the diving bell goes deeper so, too, we need a stronger and stronger stress reaction as the stress upon us becomes greater.

Some of the signals from our body which indicate that stress is increasing and becoming too severe are:

>Indigestion
>Loss of appetite
>Headaches
>Fatigue
>Exhaustion
>Insomnia
>High blood pressure
>Aches and pains in our muscles
>Nausea
>Heart spasms or flutters
>Sore neck, shoulders, back

Feelings that often accompany too much stress include:

>Helplessness
>Hopelessness
>Anger

Restlessness
Being keyed up
Feeling cooped up
Frustration
Boredom
Fright
Worry
Depression

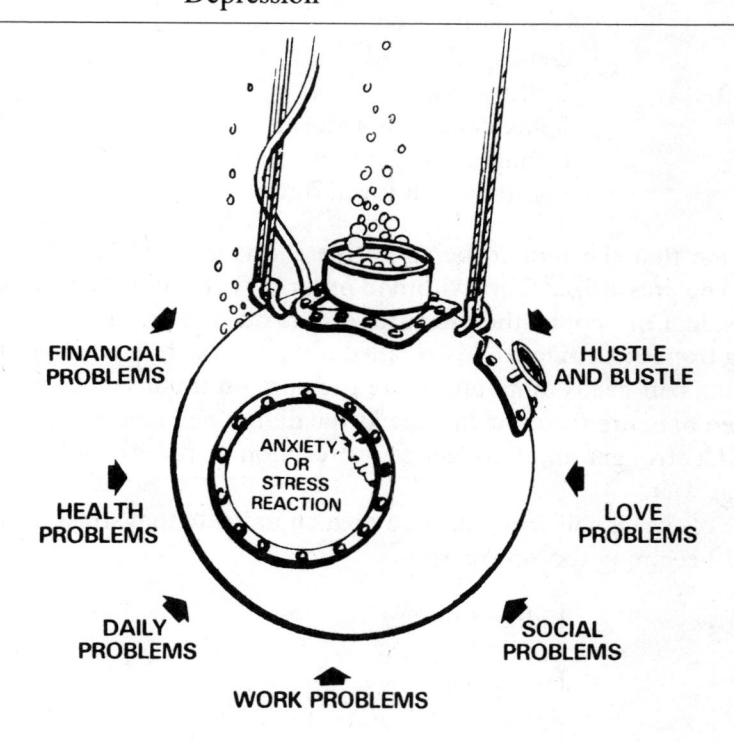

The human being reacts to stress from the outside with pressure on the inside known as anxiety, or stress reaction.

Little problems become big problems when we are under too much stress. Sometimes this is especially true of our relationships. Signs of stress that show up in relationships include:

Getting impatient with people
Interrupting what others are saying
Arguing and fighting
Feeling irritated by the requests of others
Resenting people who love us
Wanting to get away or go away from our family and friends

Common Medical Problems

Lashing out
Feeling the urge to attack

Does Stress Really Make People Sick? Can Stress Hurt My Heart?

Too much stress for too long a time produces the signs and feelings just described. Eventually, the damage gets worse and, yes, we *do* get sick because of too much stress and, yes, it can hurt our heart.

Stress is considered significant as at least a partial cause of many diseases and illnesses, including heart disease, cancer, colds, and ulcers. Too much stress contributes to these diseases indirectly because of the unhealthy things people under too much stress do, such as alcoholic drinking to excess, smoking, eating of unhealthy foods, overeating, losing sleep, stopping exercise, and not taking time off to relax.

Stress also contributes more directly to these diseases, many believe, because of the changes in body chemistry that stress reactions provoke. Foremost among these seems to be that of producing more adrenaline, which in turn causes changes in the body's immunity system.

Another effect of increased adrenaline output is stimulation of the heart, something quite necessary for survival in the face of danger. In the days when we needed to run fast at a moment's notice should a wild beast or hostile tribe appear, increased levels of adrenaline, which got the heart going quickly, were a blessing. Now, however, prolonged stress just gets the heart going and going, making rest for the heart next to impossible.

Stress comes from good events as well as tragic events, because even good events cause us to change how we live; even good events upset the routine, bring us reason to be frightened or sad. For example, getting married is a happy event, but it usually means leaving home (sad) and sharing life with a new person (frightening) forever (venture into the unknown). Weddings and the weeks leading up to them are very, very stressful.

As an organist and vocalist, I used to provide music for as many as one hundred weddings each year, sometimes three or even four on the same weekend. The stress that weddings put on the families of the bride and groom was obvious all too often. This stress seemed to spread, too, until sometimes the whole wedding appeared to crackle with static. I remember the photographer who became so stressed out that he literally pushed me aside in his desperation to get a good picture; he pushed me right off the organ bench and climbed up on the organ I was playing, and then stood on the organ! I thought he might break my fingers with his feet! He would never have done anything like that in his right mind, but as the stress rose, he was hardly aware of how obnoxious and ridiculous his behavior had become.

Getting promoted is another good example of a happy event that is stressful. A promotion is good news because it implies confidence in an employee by management. Promotions usually mean more pay and better working conditions—all good news. But promotions can be very stressful in that new skills and new demands are required in a new role. Old friends sometimes are lost, old forms of support are unavailable, and familiar routines often end. In addition, promotions often mean moving to a new town or state, setting off more stressful events, such as change in finances, change of work, taking a mortgage, change in residence, change in schools, and perhaps several others.

Warning Signs

Signs that we are not coping well with stress include anxiety, loss of interest in activities and friends, fears and worries about things we do not normally worry about, inability to concentrate, exaggeration of minor problems, indecisiveness, feelings of hopelessness and helplessness. Also, our sleep becomes disturbed with frequent dreams, nightmares, waking up, tossing and turning. There often are headaches, loss of appetite, aches and pains. Other physical signs of too much stress include redness in the face, nausea, and digestive problems. Some people get the urge to eat too fast or too much; others drink too heavily.

As a therapist one of my first clients was under great stress and seemed to show all the signs: uncontrolled drinking of alcohol, uncontrolled anger and shouting, uncontrolled fits of eating (to the point of gluttony), uncontrolled gambling, inability to sleep, and so forth. The most unnerving symptom of his stress, however, was that when he became angry at me in therapy, his face would turn bright red and then swell up and become deep purple!

Usually with too much stress we do poorly in our relations with other people: We become impatient, cut people off when they are talking, become easily irritated by others, feel the urge to get away and to be left alone, feel resentful. Often we lash out at others, yell at them, sometimes even feel the urge to attack them.

Coping With Stress

Coping with stress is not easy, but it is necessary. The only ways to reduce stress, of course, are to solve the problems or get away from them. This is not always possible, however, and so the question becomes one of

Common Medical Problems

> SUMMARY OF THE SIGNS OF STRESS
>
> *General:* anxiety, loss of interest in activities and friends, fears, inability to concentrate, exaggeration of minor problems, indecisiveness and feelings of hopelessness and helplessness. Disturbed sleep, headaches, loss of appetite, aches and pains.
>
> *Physical:* redness of face, digestive problems, urge to eat or drink too much too fast, restlessness, irritability, feelings of anger and depression, trouble sleeping, trouble relaxing.
>
> *In relationships:* impatience with people, cutting them off in the middle of what they are saying, irritation with requests of others, difficulty being with those you love, urge to get away from family, associates or friends; resentment; lashing out at others verbally or physically; urge to attack or actually attacking others.

how to cope in the meantime. Coping successfully with stress means nullifying the effects of stress. The basics in such a plan are:

    Proper diet
    Rest
    Sleep
    Exercise
    Venting

Proper diet means not only eating the proper fruits, vegetables, meats, and getting the proper vitamins, minerals, proteins, and carbohydrates, but also eating *regularly* at the same time each day and not drifting into the stuff-starve pattern of eating that is so common with stress. Stress tends to play havoc with the appetite, making us ravenous one minute but not hungry at all the next. It also tends to tempt us to skip meals, especially breakfast, because we are in a rush. Sometimes we eat on the run, which may mean junk food.

Rest is essential to reducing stress. It is essential for thriving as a human being. It is certainly essential to a healthy heart. Rest includes sleep, but we need to rest at other times each day—not only when we sleep. A proper plan of rest includes a little period of rest morning, afternoon, and early evening, even if that means only a few minutes to put down our head, lie on the couch, close our eyes, enjoy a little coffee, read the paper.

Sleep needs to be of good quality. Restless, worried, fitful sleeping is probably more tiring than helpful. So, if you are having trouble sleeping, we recommend that you sleep for shorter periods of time. Eight hours of sleep may seem impossible to a very stressed person. But four two-hour periods of sleep may look a lot more attractive.

We recommend using an alarm clock to wake yourself up *before* you think your stress will wake you up, which puts *you* back in command. Get up and enjoy a little reading, worrying, perhaps a walk or shower, and then go back to bed for another period of enjoyable sleep.

Venting is another part of coping with stress. Venting means feeling what you feel, worrying about what worries you, expressing your feelings, raging, screaming, "letting it out." For some, this means talking, for others walking or pacing, for some it means thinking with a wrinkled brow, chewing fingernails, wringing the hands.

I have always found prayer to be a good way of venting because not only do I speak about my worries and problems to God, but I begin to realize that He is in a position to either do something about what I cannot control or to sustain me in the midst of what I fear.

The heart benefits from our coping successfully with the stress that might otherwise damage it. But notice: The very things that help us cope with stress also build up the heart! Proper diet, rest, sleep, and exercise make for a strong, thriving heart!

It must also be pointed out here that if the steps described in this chapter are not helpful almost immediately, it would be wise to seek professional help. Your physician will need to check for physical problems and possible organic causes of your symptoms. Sometimes medication will be indicated to help with sleep, digestion, or calmness, or to lower high blood pressure. In every case of severe anxiety, a physician should be consulted immediately, especially if there is nausea, vomiting, bleeding, or pain.

Sometimes a professional psychotherapist should be considered, too. This person is trained to get at the deeper emotional problems underlying stress, as well as to help with proper relaxation techniques and a better understanding of relationships, conflicts, and anxiety. The often-quoted rule of health certainly applies here: An ounce of prevention is worth a pound of cure.

The best way to deal with the bad effects of too much stress is not to be under too much stress in the first place. This comes from a well-ordered, purposeful life, the topic of our final section. A "good heart" physically speaking comes about most often when we have a good heart spiritually speaking. Of the two, we believe a good heart spiritually is what matters most, since even the healthiest person cannot escape death and must deal with the ultimate meaning of life and the ultimate destiny of the human spirit.

When the Lord says, "Be of good heart," what does He mean? We believe that being of good heart means more than having a sound ticker. But we also believe that often enough when we have our lives "together" in the deeper sense it is possible to live within reasonable limits of stress and to be healthy.

THAT SPECIAL DIMENSION—BEING OF GOOD HEART

The ultimate in relaxation is peace, inner peace. Perhaps more than any other single quality, our world lacks inner peace in the turbulent eighties. The turmoil and armed conflicts that cover the globe today reflect turmoil and conflict within the hearts of people—a loss of purpose and meaning that affects even children.

What Is Life For?

A healthy perspective sees the purpose of life to be the building up of people. Sometimes this building-up process means supporting others in their growth. This is what parents and teachers do. Sometimes it means loving others when they fail, forgiving them when they injure us, affirming them when they do something perfectly rotten. This is called *reconciliation* and is what all of us are called to do.

Sometimes the building up of people as the true purpose of life means a commitment to the healing of others. While physicians, psychologists, clergymen, nurses, psychiatrists, and psychotherapists do this professionally, we all do it in one way or another when we enter into the sickness and suffering of people.

Service to others is another way of building up people. We are here to love one another. Love, to use a biblical example, means "washing feet." It translates into action—tangible deeds. The building-up process always includes and results in the development of *self*. We are intended to grow and develop and to help one another as we do so.

Persons: The Highest Value

Persons are of the highest value, as opposed to money, power, fame, achievements, possessions, and "things." If people tend to have their heart where they have their treasure, then perhaps today that would mean I will be thinking about what I *own*. If I have a cabin as a retirement home, that is what I will be thinking about and planning for. If I own a hotel in New York or a bank in the business district, that is what I will think about, work at, worry over, organize my time and energy around. A healthy attitude, however, should include the concept that the good of other persons—the growth of self *and* others—most merit the spending of our time and energy. This is so because as persons we are of greatest value.

If we love one another, we are able to care not only about other persons but to forgive them and reconcile with them when things go sour.

Reconciliation

The call to reconciliation is a special form of healing of the human spirit, for it declares we are not rotten even when we do some terrible act—but lovable!

Reconciliation to another's good graces says I am worth loving at a time when even I don't think so. It says *you* are worth loving when you think you are not. This insistence upon reconciling through forgiveness is the source of peace—inner peace—for such a step assures us of our goodness and lovableness in the eyes of our fellow humans and it pleases our Father in heaven. The commitment to love, care about, and have harmony with other persons—all other people, regardless of who or what they are or have—furnishes hope for the future and peace for the present.

Overcoming the Guilt Trip

When my clients discover they are suffering from tremendous guilt, especially from such actions as abortion and adultery, then the remedy ultimately involves looking ahead and recommitting to love specific persons in their lives. Guilt keeps us shackled to the past. Without a future there is no reason to hope, to live, to love—no way out of our guiltiness.

When a person is filled up with love, there is a meaning and purpose to life. Hope springs forth. Growth as a person begins. We get filled up with what is good and purposeful to such a point that there is no room left for hate, despair, or bitterness. A way of life emerges, characterized by service to others, fellowship, and community. This health of the body is not the final concern. Good health of the human spirit and good human relationships are the deeper and more lasting results. The whole person is the concern.

How Does One Get Started?

Good, wholesome living is not merely a self-help program or a positive-thinking approach. It is a *response,* a *celebration* of the life and love given us—a logical consequence of initiatives bestowed on us.

If you believe in prayer, your first response may be to pray. It is a conversation, sometimes in external form, such as when we pray together with others. Sometimes we pray—or meditate—in the inner stillness of our mind.

Sense of Self and Self-Worth

The loving of others in effective, meaningful ways is so paradoxical! To serve others is to get off our own self-centeredness and to get our attention directed toward others. The paradox is that every time we do so, there follows a deeper, truer sense of *self!* This sense of self includes both a sense of our limits and a feeling of our own worth, as well as a sense of our purpose in life.

The hurry-up person who is dying of tension and overwork will learn, if he really thinks about it, what work is too much—he'll find that a sense of peace, purpose, perspective always emerges when one devotes some private time to studying his own feelings and emotions.

A sense of self also emerges if one accepts his own strengths and weaknesses in order to plan more realistically and be comfortable with limits. This sense of limits is called *mortality*. Yes I have—we all have—limits. I have only so much strength and so many skills. I can do only so many things in a day. Worst of all, I will grow old and die someday. My life is limited. I am mortal. Better this way than not at all! Have you ever considered not existing—never having been in body or spirit?

Consideration of that option (never having been) reveals that limits are not so devastating. And, as Churchill reportedly said about growing old, "It's not so bad when one considers the alternative!"

It is important that we begin to develop a sense of our own worth. Feeling worthwhile is not always easy. Living up to our valuation is not so easy, either. Most of us live beneath our own evaluation. That's why we do the very things that bring on heart trouble, such as overeating, underexercising, eating and drinking unhealthy or damaging substances, putting ourselves into stressful situations for no good reason, and generally refusing to take care of our bodies.

So, spend some part of each day alone—meditating. Be sure to "collect" yourself before you begin, laying aside for a few minutes other worries and considerations, or else presenting the problems to God as to a counselor.

Try to arrange this quiet time at the same hour each morning and evening, until it becomes a habit. Many people meditate while they walk or jog; some even express their thoughts out loud on the trail!

Paradoxically enough, as we spend this quiet time with ourselves, as we calm down about illness and death, we heal better. We live not only better, but longer, for we live with *all* of life.

How do we obtain that special dimension: being of "good heart"? For me that special dimension is a personal God. It is up to you, reader, to find that special dimension yourself.

May you live your life to the fullest and learn to be happy in the meaning of your life.

10
Pain

David P. Armentrout, Ph.D.

Pain is something we have all experienced. It comes in various forms, sometimes sharp and swift, sometimes throbbing and long. We don't usually think about it much—that is until we experience it. Even then the attention we give it is brief and limited. We squeeze the finger that we smashed with the hammer, take the aspirin for our headache, and in the case of more severe injury, limit our activity and take our medication until the healing is complete and the pain is gone. The problem is, the relief doesn't always come.

Brent had worked hard for what he had. As president of his own company he was respected; moreover, he enjoyed his work. The headaches were small nuisances at first, and the stronger medication seemed to help—at least for a while. That was more than three years ago. The pain had continued, he was unable to concentrate, and finally resigned his position. Now most of his time is spent at home. He likes to stay in his room with the lights off. The pills and the shots don't seem to touch the problem; he has become a prisoner of his pain.

Kathy couldn't really say when it started, it just seemed to have crept up on her. She was married and had had her first baby before she noticed an occasional stiffness in her knees. By the arrival of her second child the periods of pain were more frequent, she found herself dropping things, and at times she would find herself emptied of energy. At those times all she wanted to do was collapse into a huddle on the floor and cry. Years after the diagnosis of arthritis had been made, her struggle continued.

Pain can arise out of almost any physical problem. Bones may be slightly deformed at birth and press on nerves, causing pain. Injuries may heal leaving scar tissue that does the same thing. Even surgery to relieve chronic pain has the potential of continuing or even adding to the problem as the nerve pathways seek to reestablish themselves and as additional scar tissue is formed. In addition to these potential producers of chronic pain are such diseases as arthritis, which bring with them continuing damage to the body—and pain. It is easy to see that chronic pain can involve almost any area of the body from the top of the head to the bottom of the feet. It is little wonder then that chronic pain is a major health problem.

No matter what its original source, the pain can grow and grow until it is a major problem in itself, at times eclipsing the tissue damage that gave it birth. When this happens, and pain holds you in its ugly grasp, it can begin to squeeze the life out of you, leaving little more than a shell of existence. You can go on to experience a range of emotions (anger, frustration, fear, depression) that further rob your life. And if that weren't enough, these same emotions can turn and actually increase the pain.

In the past ten years there has been a renewed awareness in the scientific and medical worlds to this reality of chronic pain. Prior to this change, the very way pain was viewed and understood had the potential of adding to the problem. Let me explain.

If you had been hurt in biblical times, the understanding of the tissue damage or injury may have been limited, but the nature of the problem with pain may have been better understood. Over half of the Hebrew words for pain found in the Old Testament come from the root word *chûwl,* meaning to "twist and twirl, to writhe in pain or fear," especially in childbirth. Some of the words are translated simply as a "throe," which Webster defines as a "desperate or agonizing struggle." If you were suffering with chronic pain in those times, it would have been understood that your pain was the total of the state of your mind, spirit, and body. The emotions that you experienced were not merely a response to pain or preparation for it; they were an integral component of your pain, woven inseparably through it.

If you had the misfortune to wait to have your pain until the Scientific Revolution was well underway, however, your experience would be somewhat different. Knowledge of the anatomy and physiology of the body had mushroomed. Because of this your injury would probably receive better treatment, but not your chronic pain. As the nerve pathways for transmitting pain signals to the brain began to be understood, pain was separated from the emotional and spiritual state. This separation grew to the point that pain was viewed, and therefore treated, as coming from *either* a physical *or* an emotional source. If your tissue damage fell within the realm of the identifiable and understood, and if the level of pain you experienced matched what was expected for that particular type of injury, your pain would be seen and treated as "real." If you should have the misfortune of having pain that came from a less easily diagnosed source or, if you appeared angry and depressed and the pain exceeded the expected level, your pain would be viewed as being of the "less than real" kind and would be treated as being emotional.

This separation of mind, body, and spirit in relation to pain continued down into the middle of the present century. The effects of this point of view dramatically influence the way pain is treated.

There is much that we can learn about our pain, its management, and control. As we explore these facts and methods, it is important to keep in mind that such exploration is meant to supplement expert medical care. While the medical care you receive may be able to alleviate much or even all of the disease or body damage responsible for your problem with pain, there are other factors that have an effect on the pain you experience. We will continue our exploration of pain together with an examination of the emotions of pain.

THE EMOTIONS OF PAIN

Anyone who has lived with pain knows that you can never say that pain is pain is pain. It is like a river: at times running and racing, smashing through rapids; sometimes deep, wide, and frightening; or, dwindling to an almost imperceptible trickle. Among the most important factors in the changing faces of pain are the emotions of pain. The pain and the emotion that you experience are not separate things.

Scientists have finally come full circle and now recognize what the Bible has shown us, and what anyone who knows pain could easily tell us. Emotion is intimately related to pain. We respond with emotion to the presence of pain, to its impact—and finally it turns and becomes a part of the pain itself.

Billie had gone to bed that night feeling good. It had been a full day and she was glad to be able finally to collapse into sleep. When she awoke it was back. It had been awhile since she had felt the burning in her joints, but without question it was there again. As she dragged herself out of bed, her stiff body complained and the pain continued to grow through the day. At first she tried to push it from her mind. She had things to do and places to go and she wasn't about to let this get in her way; but she couldn't get the thoughts out of her mind.

It was different this time, it was in both knees instead of one. "Is it getting worse? Will I become helpless and crippled? How long can I continue to care for my children the way I want? Will my husband turn away from me? Will I become deformed and ugly?" On and on the questions raced through her mind as fear of the dreaded pain and what it meant continued to fill more of her life. The morning stretched into days.

As the pain continued, another emotion joined the constant state of tension and anxiety—anger. Small things piled up, it took so much more energy just to accomplish the routine tasks of living. Frustrated with herself, her lost abilities, her lack of energy, her pain grew as the level of tension and pressure grew within her.

These are the emotions of the acute stages of pain, the flare-ups. Often beginning with denial, this period typically involves anxiety, tension, anger, and fear. The pain problem is increased in several ways by these emotions. First, it requires us to cope with one more thing. The anger and fear become problems that have to be taken care of in addition to the pain itself. Second, our bodies respond to the presence of these emotions with an increased level of muscle tension. This increase in muscle tension can produce additional pressure to already damaged and painful areas. Tension on inflamed joints or around damaged vertebrae can easily cause additional pain. Finally, the muscles can become chronically tightened or contracted and produce spasms that are in themselves painful.

Thus we can see that these emotions can contribute directly to the pain with which we struggle. The relationship between anxiety and pain goes even further, in that the level of anxiety also acts like an amplifier for pain. The more anxiety and fear we have, the more pain we are likely to experience. This happens because the brain interprets the signals coming from the area of damage together with the emotional signals as pain. This affects the amount of pain perceived in our brain.

A single ray of light danced on the bed covers in the darkened room. The drapes remained tightly pulled, barely letting the errant ray get by. She resented its intrusion. Barbara wasn't asleep; in fact, she seldom felt as though she really truly slept. She never felt good, and it had been years since she was able to move about the way she would like. It seemed that her body just refused to cooperate. Ever since she had injured her back, the pain had prevented her from getting out much, and the few friends she had left, she seldom saw. Pain had blurred her empty days and nights into what seemed an endless stream of suffering.

Depression and withdrawal are not at all uncommon to the pain that accompanies any serious injury. Walk down the hallways of any hospital and you will see it happening all around you. In fact, scientists say that this is part of the final phase of pain. Quiet inactivity and withdrawal from a wide range of accustomed activity is an optimal strategy for promoting the cure and recovery of damaged tissue. When all goes well through this phase, a patient finds himself gaining in strength emotionally and spiritually as well as physically. Adjustments that need to be made are accomplished during this period, and at its end life resumes with full, even if altered, involvement. For many, however, some level of tissue damage remains, or if the damage is produced by a disease, it may reoccur, leaving them with the continuing presence of damage and pain. As the pain continues, depression is likely to grow.

We saw how Barbara had continuing pain after a back injury, and how her life continued to be a shadow of what it had once been. She had reached a point of depression and emptiness in which the dancing of sunlight was resented as an intruder. Her pain had become intimately linked with depression and isolation. As more and more meaningful areas of her life were surrendered, the more her depression increased. The more frustrated and dissatisfied with her life she became, the more her depression grew. The more spiritually and emotionally empty she became, the more intense Barbara's depression became. Her depression had begun in grief over lost abilities and was continually fostered and aggravated by pain and even her exhaustion. More than once she had to struggle deep within herself to keep from "accidentally" taking too many of the pills on which she relied for some relief from pain.

If anxiety and fear are like a pressure cooker for problems of pain, depression is an echo chamber. The signal of pain booms through one's emptiness.

In the battle of pain, our emotions often become the ally of the enemy. They must be brought back into proper perspective if we are to win the fight, but this is not always easy to do. Our pain and its allies, as we shall see, place us in prisons as strong as any made of steel.

THE PRISONS OF PAIN

The grasp of pain is far-reaching and tight. Its influence and ability to exert control over us is nothing short of amazing. Without realizing it we become locked in the prison of pain.

The Prison of Loss

Chronic pain is frequently accompanied by a variety of losses. There can be any degree of physical loss ranging from the loss of use of a knee to the loss of control over the movement of the entire body through paralysis. In other chronic-pain situations there may not be a total loss of function, rather there is a decrease in mobility. Walking, writing, lifting, bending, and other movements become painful and difficult. No matter which one or which combination of losses you have, a change in life-style is forced upon you.

Our physical functioning is a vital part of our self-concept, so when a portion of our physical being is impaired, we not only have to change our style of living, but the way we view ourselves has to be adjusted. Some of the losses may involve our sense of femininity or masculinity and carry a still greater impact. Surrender to these losses, discouragement, depression, and pain come quickly and quietly. It can happen without your ever realizing that it has taken place, leaving you captive to your losses.

The Prison of Learning

We do much of what we do out of habit, or in other words because of what we have learned. This brings a sense of order to our lives and in most cases serves us well, but not with problems of chronic pain.

Anxiety and fear are powerful forces in the process of learning. When fear and pain are involved in an activity, we will do almost anything to avoid it. You may have known someone who just about falls apart if it starts to rain when they are driving. Having had a bad accident in which they were injured may have been the original source of the problem, but now the slightest reminder of the event is all that's needed to make their body tighten with fear and emotional arousal.

Pain from an activity can severely restrict your willingness to attempt it again. Even if there were to be a change, or a change would become possible, the pattern of avoiding the activity would prevent you from discovering it. In effect the patterns of reduced activity lock you in; you become a prisoner of what you have learned.

The inactivity itself is likely to multiply and add to your problem with pain as well. The less you do, the more strength and capacity you begin to lose. Your muscles begin to lose tone, and you find yourself able to do less and less. Even small amounts of exertion begin to cause pain, and your activity is therefore restricted further. The key to increased freedom, when pain has locked you into inactivity for a long time, is slowly and systematically working until you reach the level of limitation imposed by tissue damage. We will discuss this in more detail later.

The Prison of Love

Chronic pain and limitations in abilities force changes in the way you view yourself. Sadly, one of the common things that happens is the loss of areas of involvement that were important, without their being replaced. The vacuum that is left does get filled. As time passes activities related to your problem of pain fill more and more of your life. The doctors you see, the latest treatments available, the pattern of pain you are experiencing, the medications you take and their side effects, hospitalizations, and so forth, take up more and more of your self-definition. As before, you share with others the content you have available from your areas of involvement. Only now what you have to share is much more limited, and is of less interest to others.

These changes can have a traumatic effect on a relationship in which the commitment to each other and love and care have grown weak. The loss of additional mutuality may be enough to finally kill a marriage; yet, this is not what typically happens. More often, a new set of complementary involvement develops. The bond of love and commitment continues as strong as ever, but the areas of sharing become more limited and the level of dissatisfaction within both partners increases. The ways you express love, the things you talk about, the ways you learn to feel good about yourself, all begin to revolve around this new state of life involvement—pain and its associates.

The patterns that are formed tend to keep you as you are. Bringing about change on your own would be something like trying to nominate a Democrat at a Republican convention. If your spouse has learned to show his love for you by asking how you are feeling, by getting your medicines for you, and so forth, his behaviors will tend to keep you focused on and shackled to your pain. The changes that you wish to make must be mutually undertaken; otherwise the patterns of expression, attitude, and expectation are likely to sabotage the best of your efforts. The relationships that develop in the presence of chronic pain actually come to make improvement more difficult, locking a person into a prison of love.

We have come to know the enemy well. Armed with a knowledge of your pain, what affects it and the prisons it can bind you in, we are ready to engage in battle, to win in our struggle with pain.

GETTING A COACH

One of the problems I have found among people who are fighting a battle with chronic pain is that they are fighting alone. Some have seen a long string of different physicians in their attempts to end their pain once and for all. On the average they have consulted from six to seven different types of specialists, to say nothing of the number of visits they made to each doctor. Needless to say, hundreds of hours have been spent along with thousands of dollars. In their desperate search for an answer, they would visit a doctor, try out his recommendation, and if it didn't work, they would try another doctor, or rely completely on their own ideas of what constituted good treatment. With chronic pain, however, depending on themselves seldom produced the desired result, and at times worsened their suffering.

I was listening to the news as I drove home from work a short time ago, when I heard a discussion of why one of the top female tennis players had changed coaches. The reporter went on to say that since the change, the tennis player had vastly improved her game. It struck me as somewhat funny that one of the best tennis players in the world would need to have a coach. Surely she knew as much about the game as he did. She knew, however, that her knowledge of the game was not enough to stay on top. She needed someone who could watch her closely, who could help her identify where the problems were, and guide her in making the necessary changes.

If you have suffered from pain for several months to a year, you may well need a medical "coach," a physician who can consistently work with you, coordinate the involvement of other specialists, and attend to all the complexities of chronic pain.

Having a physician to coach and guide you through your problem of pain can help you in many ways:

—He can help you relieve many unwarranted fears and worries.
—He can help you to avoid harming yourself through self-treatment.
—He can help you evaluate "miracle cures."
—He can help you understand and face the realities of your pain.
—He can help to identify activities that would be harmful and guide you toward increasing your level of physical capacity.
—He can search for and identify pathology that can be corrected on a continuing basis.
—He can assist you with medication to relieve your pain, while closely watching you to insure that you don't get into additional problems with it.
—He can help you identify emotional components of pain, and help you to get assistance in dealing with them if needed.
—He is in a position to coordinate the work of other specialists whom you may need to see about your pain.

A physician may not have all of the answers or be able to remove all of your pain, but you need to find a competent professional who can not only diagnose and treat you, but who can also guide you through the entire course of your problem. Facing a chronic problem of pain without this kind of help is like engaging in battle without armor or weapons.

Don't be afraid to ask around and check out references. Not every physician can or should command your trust and respect. Your task then is to find a doctor who has the temperament and skill to work with you toward winning with pain.

REBUILDING BODIES

Why is it that athletes seem to recover from painful injuries so much faster than you and I? The answer is probably obvious to us all. They have spent many long hours training and fine tuning their bodies to run smoothly and precisely. When there is an accident or illness, their bodies already are at peak health and strength, and they are prepared to bounce back. Even if we are not athletes, when we keep ourselves healthy, our muscles in good tone, and when we have developed good levels of stamina, we have a greater capacity to withstand injury and illness. On the other hand, the more we allow our bodies to fall into disuse, the more we deteriorate and the more we can expect difficulty when we are injured.

Chronic problems of pain not only tend to restrict activity, but also narrow your focus, causing you to lose sight of what is happening in the rest of your body. Think back over any long bouts of flu or other illness you may have had. Can you remember what it was like when you finally were able to get out of bed again? Can you remember how weak you felt, how much strength you had lost, how your once-strong muscles protested when you forced them to walk up even a single flight of stairs?

With chronic pain, we have already noted that there is a strong tendency toward inactivity and withdrawal. The impact on your unused muscles can be dramatic. People with only a slight amount of damage, propelled into increasing inactivity by their pain, find it difficult to walk. The pain of unused muscles blends indistinguishably into the pain that originally produced the withdrawal. A cycle of growing incapacity sets in, and an increase in the level of pain and discomfort comes after less and less exertion. Even the worst of problems, however, have some promise of improvement.

An individually tailored exercise program can do much to increase the level of function in the area of injury and serve to strengthen the body overall. A careful measurement should be made of the degree to which an exercise can be done without causing tiredness or an increase in pain. Then an estimate of the desired level to be attained for each exercise should be made and a program laid out of gradually increasing levels during a certain time period.

You may want to consult with a physical therapist, exercise specialist, or utilize your own knowledge. Check with your physician about the body areas you are working on as well as the specific exercises. Let him help you determine what your limits realistically are and what level you should work toward. Remember, your goal is not to return to the way you functioned at eighteen; it is the progressive restoration of stamina and strength to your weary and weakened muscles.

Chronic pain builds a stronger and stronger prison as time passes, increasing the limitations already imposed by your injury or disease, but remember, the imprisoning grip of pain *can* be broken.

RELAXATION AND REST

Relaxing is one of those things you assume you can do perfectly well because it seems like such a common, everyday matter—and to some degree you are probably right. You'd be just as correct saying that you had full control over your muscles; but compare the control you have with that of even a mediocre gymnast. I have marveled at the precision of gymnasts as they slowly and smoothly suspend their body from a pair of rings with their arms outstretched, perfectly still.

Hours of practice went into the development of that kind of control. It takes practice as well to truly be aware of the tension in your muscles and then to relax them. But why is this level of control even worth talking about? For most of us there has never been any particular reason to focus on the level of tension in our muscles. We think that we relax because we recline or go to sleep. The few times we do take notice are when our body shouts an alarm through a headache or aching neck or sore back. It is only when the tension has reached a high level and been maintained for a prolonged period of time, long enough and intense enough to produce pain, that we pay attention to the level of tension that is present in our muscles. Relaxation skills are important for everyone, but especially for those struggling with chronic pain.

First, relaxation skills can provide you with a tool for coping with the intense pain typical of flare-ups. The effectiveness of this method is best seen in the pain of childbirth. Pain can completely take over, consuming the woman, making the labor and delivery process an excruciating ordeal. When a woman has been trained in relaxation skills, she exerts a great deal of control during the period of increasing pain, minimizing the difficulties experienced by the unprepared mother. This type of preparation for childbirth so improves the course of labor and delivery that it is almost standardly recommended. There is less pain experienced, the delivery goes smoother, less medication is required, and even recovery can be hastened.

A second reason for working at acquiring the skill of muscle relaxation is that it counteracts chronically tight muscles, taking the pressure off sensitive joints and body areas. In breaking the cycle of tension/pain, the level of pain overall can be reduced and kept under better control.

Finally, the utilization and practice of relaxation skills is an effective method of bringing fear and anxiety under control.

In addition to relaxation skills there is another related area that needs attention. The demands placed upon your body by injury, disease, and/or pain will often increase your physical need for rest. Rather than to keep going, you need to learn to listen to the genuine needs of your body and provide for additional rest. Pushing yourself beyond your limits will only spell additional problems for you, and very likely will add increased pain to your already heavy burden.

In accommodating rest into your schedule, there is at least one precaution that should be followed. You should keep your rest periods relatively brief and as few as your body will permit. The reason for this is that you need to protect your body's natural waking/sleeping cycle. Very long naps may make it difficult to fall asleep later at your normal bedtime. Disruption of your sleep cycle with accompanying tiredness can easily make your pain problem worse.

The combination of highly developed relaxation skills and sufficient rest can be a powerful ally in your battle against pain. With them you increase the amount of energy available to you and limit the input of chronic muscular contraction. Control of these factors is essential if you are to win with your pain.

THE POWER OF CONSISTENCY

One of the major problems faced by people with chronic pain is overcoming inconsistency in the level of their day-to-day activities. When I was in college I was able to stay up most of the night studying for exams and then "crash" for several days of rest. My body bounced from one extreme to another. I would go from a great deal of physical exertion to almost none with only a relatively small price to pay. Today my body and mind simply couldn't take it. If someone were to tell me to run five miles or they would kill me, I probably could do it. Afterwards, however, I would either feel as if they had or wish that they would. My body has not been prepared for that level of exertion; I simply do not have the strength and resilience required.

There appears to be a cycle in chronic-pain problems of periods of inactivity followed by overexertion. After being "tied down" or "cooped up" for some length of time, boredom and frustration set in. We reach a point where we feel that we can't tolerate such a style of life any more and we determine to live a "normal" life at any cost—and the cost is often much higher than anticipated. Spurred on by frustration, we push ourselves far beyond the capacity of our body, resulting in a period of increased pain and inactivity.

You have already seen that through a slow, gradually increasing program of exercise, the resilience of your body and tolerance for activity can be increased. The same principles apply to the amount of activity you undertake in any given day.

Once again, before you attempt to increase anything, you must have a good idea of what your present level of activity is. The simplest way to do this is to keep an accurate record of how much time you spend each day sitting, standing and reclining.

Once you set a goal for increasing activity, you should move slowly and systematically toward it, increasing or decreasing the particular type of activity in small steps. If you move through the change too quickly or if the goal you set is unrealistic, your body will tell you through increased pain and/or tiredness. The message it gives you, however, will not be catastrophic since you have moved in small steps. Your physician can help you to set realistic goals and even guide you in the size of steps you should take. Talk to him about what you are doing, taking with you the record of your actual activity for him to evaluate. When he sees how you are working to maximize your capacity, and have objective observations to work with, he will not only be pleasantly surprised, but he will also be better able to guide you in your endeavor.

MEDICATION—HELP AND HINDRANCE

Throughout our lives we have been trained to treat pain chemically. If our head hurts we take aspirin. If our stomach hurts we take an antacid. The dentist injects chemicals into our gums so that drilling our teeth doesn't hurt. There are few who advise giving up all of these "helps." In fact, there is a host of chemical compounds that can be given to relieve the variety of acute pains we experience. At the most severe end of the scale, the pain problems associated with a terminal disease or injury, mixtures of the most powerful pain relievers known are likely to be given. In such cases there is no concern about two major medication problems: habituation (the body's adaptation to the presence of the chemical, causing it to lose its effectiveness); and addiction (the development of a state where the body requires the chemical, either physically of psychologically, to function). The medicines that help us with acute problems of pain have the potential of turning into our enemies when we have a problem with pain that endures over months and years. Let's take a look at how this happens.

If you have ever smoked or known someone who has, you are familiar with an excellent example of how habituation and addiction develop. The child who sneaks out behind the garage to try his first cigarette is in for an unpleasant surprise. Contrary to what his "cool" peers or the enticing commercials say, his body responds violently. The offending smoke hurts his eyes and causes them to water, the taste is foul, and as his lungs scream for air, he finds himself coughing uncontrollably. His face feels hot and flushed and he becomes dizzy. He may become queasy and nauseated. After years of smoking, however, he can deeply inhale the smoke into his lungs and hold it without the smallest protest from his body. He can breathe the stuff through his nose as if it were pure oxygen. His body has become accustomed to the presence of the chemicals and has learned to ignore them (habituation). Should he try to stop smoking or even go a short period without, he finds that his body and emotions start complaining as loudly as they did when he first started. He has developed a physical and emotional need for the cigarettes (addiction).

When you have taken pain medication, or mood-changing medicine like Valium, for an extended period of time, the same kind of thing can happen. Medicines that were once effective at minimal dosages, must now be taken more frequently and in larger amounts to get the same effect (habituation). Life may seem to fall apart or the pain feel intolerable when you go even short periods of time without your medication (addiction). But for those with chronic pain, the long-term use of some medications can have additional, unwanted impact. Some of the medications, like Valium, not only have addicting potential, but they can also have the side-effect of depression, and we have already seen that depression itself *adds* to your pain. High dosage levels of some medications add further to your difficulty by reducing both mental and physical capacity. Most of the problems arise out of the long term use of narcotic and synthetic narcotic pain relievers and drugs taken to reduce anxiety.

The majority of hospital pain units systematically attempt to reduce the patient's dependence on pain medication, getting them as close to drug free as is feasible. The obvious exceptions to this are the drugs taken to treat other disease processes, for example insulin for diabetes. Those with long-term problems of pain are often surprised at how much better they feel after their systems have been cleansed of the offending chemcials.

Not all people can be removed from their medications, however, and at times new ones will be needed. One in this latter category is medicine that helps with depression. Such medicine has been shown to be of help in many chronic pain problems, although it is still not fully known whether relief is due to the effect on depression, pain, or both.

If you have been on medication for relief of pain for any length of time, it would be wise to carefully assess yourself. Has the amount of medication you take increased? How well do you get along when you don't take the medication? Have those who are closest to you noticed any changes in your mood or personality? As you consider these indicators you also might want to talk the situation over with someone close to you for verification of your conclusions.

Should you suspect any difficulty at all, do not try to correct the matter on your own. Withdrawal from some medications requires the supervision of a physician. This is another of the areas you will need to work on with your medical coach. Your physician/coach can help you escape the prison of habituation and addiction. He can help you find the level where the benefits from the medicine are maximal and the dosage is minimal. For many, complete or nearly complete freedom from medication is possible.

GIVING UP THE GOOD BAD

Change is a funny thing. One of the characteristics of it is that after you have gone so far, the things that pushed you to change lose their power, while another set of things pulls you back toward where you started. Tiring of the problems in my work I once decided to change jobs. I felt good about the decision and began making plans for the change. The closer I got to making the change, the larger the problems of the new situation looked. At the same time I began to remember more and more the good things about the job I was in. The dissatisfactions that had been pushing me to change had weakened and the positives of the old job had taken over and started to pull me back.

We could conceivably be pulled back and forth indefinitely. The closer to the dissatisfactions we get, the more they push us to something new. The further from them we get, the more the positives of the old try to pull us back, making us little more than a frustrated yo-yo. When I considered the job change and decided to stay with my job, I weakened the pull of what I thought were the negatives. Sometimes people with chronic pain must consider the positives that can quietly, but ever so powerfully, pull them back into their old pattern.

This may come as somewhat of a shock to your thinking, because with problems of pain, you are not likely to have spent a great deal of time thinking about the positives that a pain problem has for you. Believe it or not there are some.

One group of patients I worked with struggled with this for a while with interesting results. The first reaction was one of outright denial and rejection of the idea that there could be anything good at all from having a pain problem. In fact one or two got downright mad at me. But a twinkle came in the eyes of one of them when he shared "Well, it might not do anything for you, but it helps get me out of going over to my in-laws every week." At that they all laughed and began to realize that pain had come to serve some purpose in their lives as well.

Through our pain problem we may get preferential treatment from family and friends. People trying to do things for us, give us attention that we might not have otherwise gotten and so on. Pain can be a convenient way of getting out of something you don't want to do. No matter who you are and how distasteful your problem may be, there are bound to be some "good bad" things involved in your problem. This is not to say you are tricky or deceitful. All it means is that in your life situation, your pain has had effects other than those you are used to thinking about. If you are to win your battle with pain it is important to look at your life and see what form these "good bad" things have taken. Identify them and then go on to other areas of life where pain is not involved. This will take away the power the "good bad" exerts in holding you locked in a prison of pain.

REBUILDING LIVES

The more your pain forces you to withdraw and become isolated, the less involved you become with sources of reward, satisfaction, challenge, and stimulation; you become barricaded from the source of many of life's joys and satisfactions.

Does pain have to be a barrier to meaningful, purposeful living? Does it have to empty the joys and satisfactions out of your life? Not at all. There have been many who have gone ahead and blazed the path for you. Many of them have found themselves in a position where they were excellent candidates for pain captivity, yet they not only managed to escape, but also forged out new lives that touched many others.

One young man was sent by his country to fight in Vietnam. A strong, muscular, athletic young man when he left, he returned minus both legs and one arm. He had every right to sink into absolute despair and stop living—his country would take care of his needs. But Max Cleland fought back and he fought for as much function and mobility as he could get. Physical therapy was more than a treatment for him; it became a way of life. He had earned the right to be taken care of by the Veteran's Administration. Instead, he continued to rebuild his life and was appointed by President Jimmy Carter to head the agency.

There are countless numbers of people in pain who have not settled for a mere shell of existence. Some are so successful that those around them are not even aware of the battle that is being waged and won. One of the great masters of painting is believed to have done his exquisite work in spite of deforming arthritis in his hands. One of his paintings was a self-portrait and in the beautiful detail of the masterpiece, you can clearly see the gnarled and painful joints of advanced arthritis.

We could continue a litany of the great and near great whose lives have contributed to the lives of those around them and generations to come, but this is not where we need to focus. All around us there are literally thousands waging the same battle as you, and winning. Some have been able to continue at old activities and work by making adjustments, while others have had to totally change the content of their lives to accommodate the realities of their situation. All continue to wage their winning fight with pain.

It is important to face head-on the question of what you are to do with your life. Not everyone is able to return to income-producing work, although many will be able to do this quite well. For some it will mean entering meaningful, purposeful retirement.

We are living in an era when change is almost routinely faced. Your neighbor may have to go back to school because the plant where he worked for fifteen years has become automated and his skills are no longer wanted. In fact, we are being told by journalists, economists, and many others that we are entering an age in which retraining will be a continuing and expected part of our lives. We already see this in many fields. Medicine changes so fast that physicians are required to take a specified number of courses each year to be able to continue their practice. Those who work in any of the new "high tech" fields have constant learning and retraining built into their lives, because the technology continues to go through explosive change.

For you there may even be a hidden blessing to your pain problem. Many chronic pain sufferers qualify for governmental assistance. Certain agencies can offer help in adapting your home to your physical needs, provide assistance in retraining or returning to school, or many other special services. Help is also available from local human service agencies and from foundations. Don't let simple lack of information keep you from available help. Here again, you can turn to your coach and ally, your physician. If he does not know what is available, he will be able to refer you to a social worker who can guide you through the confusing maze of agencies and organizations. He can also help by providing you with the documentation you may need. Don't allow yourself to fall into a trap that will make your battle harder—being too proud to utilize the resources that are available.

A life that is filled with nothing more than your pain, your losses, and emptiness cannot sustain you. The Bible tells us that people perish without a vision. The purpose and vision that you formerly held for your life may no longer be realistically available to you. If so, you will need to let go of it. Until you do, it can be like a giant weight, keeping you from moving ahead toward a new vision of life.

Here are a few steps that you can take to begin the rebuilding of your life.

Evaluate. Take a good look at yourself. What are your skills, abilities, and talents? Are there things that you did years ago, but have forgotten about? In making this evaluation, don't rely on yourself alone; depression can at times rob you of true objectivity and cause you not to see all that is there. Ask your husband or wife what they think your abilities are. You might even want to let a vocational rehabilitation specialist help you in evaluating yourself.

Dream. When we reach adulthood, many of us limit our growth because we put dreaming away as "kid stuff." In fact many of our dreams and desires grow out of natural abilities and talents that God gave us. You may have lost touch with them if you have not continued to let yourself dream.

Plan. Once you have some idea of your abilities and have cultivated your desires into a dream, you will need to start making concrete plans: "What does it take to get where I want to go? What resources will I need to make it? Who else will need to be involved if I am to make my dream a reality?"

Divide and Conquer. It is not unusual for a dream to seem unreachable because it is too far off or too big. When the Russians launched their Sputnik satellite, the United States committed itself to a very large dream; they purposed to place a man on the moon. In hindsight, that may not seem that big a dream, but consider that at the time the best that the United States was able to do with the largest of its rockets was to place a fifty-pound device into space. That's a long way from the tons of payload that would be needed to put a man on the moon. We all know that the dream came true. It was accomplished by dividing the dream and plans into small steps. These were then tackled one by one, and each solution moved them a small step closer to the dream. The same applies to you. Your dream may seem just as far away as landing someone on the moon, but you can divide your dream into small solvable pieces, which one by one will get you where you want to go.

Rebuilding your life is one of the strongest steps you can take toward winning with pain. In the face of your pain you can have emptiness, which will add to the suffering you carry, or you can have meaning and purpose. Hurt and exist—hurt and live; the choice is yours.

THE POWER OF WORDS

"Think you can, think you can't, either way, you're right." These words attributed to Henry Ford couldn't be more true. The power of the words we speak, to others or deep within where only we can hear, is tremendous.

Psychologists have shown consistently that the expectations which you develop shape the course of a large portion of your life. In fact, the self-talk that fills our heads is thought by some to be a major contributor to depression. The power of our words, spoken and unspoken, is a major force in all of our lives. If it is important in shaping what the average person does, it is even more so for anyone with a major burden to overcome, like chronic pain.

Long before modern man began to understand these principles, the Bible made it clear that the words that come out of our mouths are a powerful influence. We read that the tongue has the same kind of power over us that the rudder has over a ship in setting the direction it goes (James 3: 4). The Bible does not limit this influence to setting direction; it goes as far as to say that we have the power of life and death in our tongue, depending on how we choose to exercise it (Proverbs 18: 21).

Any way you look at it, the truth is the same, your words, both spoken and unspoken, can drastically affect your ability to be successful in your battle with pain. Self-talk not only can hold you back, it can actually increase your suffering.

One of the most common objections raised to the prospect of changing our internal conversations is the belief that the things we say are "true" and "realistic" and that to say otherwise would be dishonest with ourselves. In actuality, the constant stream of discouragement, disbelief, and disparagement limits your vision so that probems are *all* that you see. It may be true that there are limitations and obstacles, but the whole realm of new purpose and solutions is obscured by such a negative stream of verbiage. Changing your self-talk is not denying reality, but expanding the way that you are willing to look at it.

Our self-talk is an automatic part of our life. You don't sit down in the morning and plan out what you are going to say to yourself that day. It is a learned pattern that comes through your mind so readily that you most often would not even know that it was there. Because it is such a strong pattern, you may wish to get help from a therapist who has a knowledge of the principles of learning. There are, however, several things that you can do to help yourself.

1. *Listen to yourself.* The first step is to begin to pay attention to the kinds of thoughts that run through your mind during the day. What

Common Medical Problems

effect do they have on you? Do they make your life easier or harder?

2. *Keep count.* After you have gotten used to listening in on this internal conversation, begin keeping a record of the number of self-defeating, deprecating, or doubt-filled statements you make to yourself each day. You can do this by keeping a diary on note cards or simply by using an inexpensive counter, like those used by shoppers. Counting will make you more sharply aware of each time you begin to use destructive self-talk, and this awareness prepares you for the next steps.

3. *Don't hold on.* During the course of any given day a great number of thoughts will flash into your mind. Some you dismiss because they are silly, objectionable, or otherwise unwanted. Others you consider for a short time, such as which dress you want to wear, while still others you hold on to, bringing them up over and over again, such as deciding whether or not to sell your house and move to a new one. Once you have become aware of your destructive self-talk, you will need to dislodge it from your mind each time you become aware that it is there. At first this will be a little difficult, but it will budge if you keep after it. As soon as it returns, and you can be sure that it will, push it out again. Continue doing this and gradually you will notice that the thought leaves much more easily and quickly.

4. *Substitute.* Now that the old thoughts are on the way out, you will need to replace them. Actively build into your mind words and ideas that build you up. Instead of, "There's no use," fill your mind with, "It may be hard right now, but I'm going to make it." The Bible has some solid advice in this area as well when it advises you: "Whatsoever things are true, whatsoever things are honest, whatsoever things are just, whatsoever things are pure, whatsoever things are lovely, whatsoever things are of good report; if there be any virtue, and if there be any praise, think on these things" (Philippians 4:8 KJV). Remember, the power of your own words can make or break you, and you have a say in which it will be.

5. *Be patient.* Old habits don't just lie down and die, they fight for life; so be patient with yourself, knowing that by persisting with your efforts at building a new pattern, you will succeed.

Putting your own word power behind you gives you one more solid ally and removes one more obstacle in your fight to win with your pain.

REBUILDING RELATIONSHIPS

Pain is so much more than flesh and bone. We have discussed already the fact that pain is also an emotional experience—that pain can be multiplied and extended by our own emotional feelings, and that it can turn around and produce emotional responses within us. The tentacles of pain also reach out and can alter our most important relationships. The impact of a chronic pain problem can be seen between husbands and wives, brothers and sisters, parents and children.

In your struggle with pain, you will find that the battle is much easier to wage from the support of a solid relationship. If pain has caused difficulty in an important relationship—and it very well may—you have only your own strength to sustain you. But by rebuilding and renewing your marriage, for example, you mutliply your ability to wage war on pain.

Stop and reflect on ways in which living with pain has affected you and your loved ones. In working on this problem it is important to establish or keep up good communication, and you may need to consider professional counseling to get you started. The most powerful changes come through working, talking, and communicating with your loved ones in order to build the kind of life you desire.

BUILDING A TEAM

We have explored together the nature of pain, the way it can become a life problem, and have outlined some of the specific steps we can take to win in the battle against it. But each of us faces unique problems with pain. For some, there is a new life ahead just with the implementation of one or two of the suggestions that have been covered; for others, the problem is too overwhelming, too deeply entrenched, too consuming to win on our own.

Any way that you look at it, pain is a team problem. The size of the team will be up to you, but to win, you will need someone on your side. The first two members of your team are your spouse and your physician. As you proceed with the evaluation of your problem and begin to work on making changes, you can choose whether or not to add additional people. We have seen that the contribution of a psychologist can be of value and you may wish to have the help of a social worker in locating available resources.

One of the resources that is available in a number of locations across the country is the pain unit. These are multidisciplinary treatment programs designed to evaluate and treat pain in its chronic, complex form.

The advantage of such a treatment program is the number of treatment resources that are combined in one single setting. The treatment is usually condensed into two to six weeks, and there is both psychological and medical inputs. In such a program you are evaluated, a program of increasing activity and exercise can be designed, you can receive individual and family instruction, and there is a professional staff available to help you with planning and to assist you in locating the resources of other agencies.

The pain unit also offers an array of treatments that are not available in all communities. These include such procedures as nerve blocks (the injection of substances into nerve pathways to block the transmission of pain signals to the brain), transcutaneous stimulation (an electrical device that bombards the skin in carefully selected areas with mild electrical signals which can alter the perception of pain signals), and a variety of physical therapies. Some centers are equipped to offer acupuncture, hypnosis, vocational evaluation and counseling, and therapeutic swimming facilities.

Pain units are not for everyone or for all problems of chronic pain though. There are many individuals who can make significant changes in their problem without having to utilize such a vast number of resources. If the team you work with is in your home community, they will be able to continue to follow your progress over a long period of time, whereas distant pain units are not as accessible. Also, the expenses involved in treatment at pain units are higher.

If you are able to restructure your activity and life with the assistance of a small treatment team, so much the better. For those of you who cannot do this, pain units offer a good alternative. They might just offer the kind of environment you need to win your individual battle with pain. If so, the investment is worth it.

SOMETHING MORE

Where do you reach when you're at the end of your rope? What do you draw on when you know for certain that everything within you is already spent? These are questions faced by many of you who have had pain as part of your life for a long time. The answer has a lot to do with how well you are able to mobilize yourself and other resources toward the goals we have been discussing.

In working with chronic pain we have come to realize that there is another dimension to the problem—a spiritual dimension. This is affirmed by such noted experts as Dr. C. Norman Shealy, a pioneer in the treatment of chronic pain. He attests to the importance of spiritual factors in winning the war with pain, even though his treatment center bears no particular religious affiliation. I have found this to be true in my own efforts to help people in their struggle with pain. In fact, it's hard for me to write about pain and talk about some of the things that you can do to help yourself, without discussing the real source of change that I have seen in myself and my patients: the power made available to us by God through His Son, Jesus Christ.

There are many facets of your relationship with God that come into play, but in a limited discussion like this I can only mention a few. First, God can intervene directly in your life in the form of emotional and physical healing. At times, depressions are lifted, fears dissolved, and marriages are reborn. Second, He has provided guidelines for growth and release from the prisons we find ourselves entangled in, including pain. Scripture tells us about the power of our words, how they carry in them the power of life and death for our own lives as well as others. We are told that we are incapable of bringing our tongues under the kind of control that is needed by ourselves. We need Him (*see* James 3:8). His Word also reminds us that we are created for purposeful, meaningful lives, but points out that He is the one who has laid the path out in front of us (*see* Ephesians 2:10). Without an understanding, a vision, of where we are headed, we begin to lose hope, to shrivel emotionally and spiritually, and in many senses we die.

God also has made it clear that we are not islands unto ourselves, we are not self-sufficient. He created us with varying gifts and talents, which we are to use fully. He created us to utilize all of our strengths, but not alone. There is an emptiness within each of us that can only be filled by a relationship with Him through His only Son. That's the way he made us—creations who thrive on fellowship with their Creator.

Our interdependence goes even further. We need to draw strength from God Himself, and also from those human beings He has placed closest to us. We draw from them, and in return we pick them up when they fall and they draw from us.

There's another important aspect of our relationship with Jesus that is relevant to problems with pain. In such a relationship, pain and suffering can be turned so that it serves us instead of destroying us. It can deepen us, make us stronger in our minds and spirits. It can sensitize us to the priorities of living.

For those of you who do not know Jesus personally, the way is simple and the invitation always remains open. All that is required is that you recognize your inadequacy and sin and ask Jesus to come into your life, to be your burden bearer, your guide and source.

Problems of pain require a team, and the most powerful results can be expected when Jesus Christ, the Son of the living God, is the head and Lord of your team.

> ..."But God is faithful [to His Word and to His compassionate nature], and He [can be trusted] not to let you be tempted *and* tried

and assayed beyond your ability *and* strength of resistance *and* power to endure, but with temptation He will [always] also provide the way out—the means of escape to a landing place—that you may be capable *and* strong *and* powerful patiently to bear up under it.

1 Corinthians 10:13 AMPLIFIED

11
Headaches
Joan Miller, Ph.D.

DISCOVERING THE MESSAGE AND CAUSES OF YOUR HEADACHE

More than 40 million Americans suffer enough from chronic headaches to discuss them with their physicians. Up to 90 percent of the adult population has experienced at least one headache. Headaches affect not only the sufferer, but also those who live and work with the one in pain. Most headaches can be prevented, or at least reduced in intensity, by the techniques which will be discussed here.

Headaches are symptoms. Like a fever, they are part of your body's feedback system, alerting you to a problem. Ignoring the headache's message or covering it over with pain-relieving medication is like capping a bad tooth. Such a coping style may work temporarily, but the headache will return to remind you that the problem has not been solved. And if you persist long enough in ignoring the message, your body may have to get your attention with an ulcer, dermatitis, heart problem, or another stress-related disease.

Be grateful to your body for giving you a headache! The headache, your friend, points out the need to make a change, so that your body can stay healthy and function effectively. It is up to you to discover the causes of the headache and to design a program for freeing yourself of headaches.

Headache History. To begin your road to recovery, you will need to collect information about your headaches in order to discover contributing factors. You may have different types of headaches with a variety of triggering mechanisms. The "Headache Survey," located in the back of

Common Medical Problems

this section, pages 295–299, will assist you in the search for clues to the development of your headaches. You may want to answer the queries right now. It is not aimed at helping you get a headache, so don't fret over your answers!

As you read on, the significance of your answers to the survey will become evident. After altering your patterns of thinking and behaving, you will notice that some of your answers will change.

What are the causes of your headache? Headaches result from pressure, inflammation, or damage to cells near the pain receptors in the head. The nerve endings can become irritated from tense muscles, swelling of blood vessels, or inflammation of tissue linings.

It is important to recognize and alleviate as many of the contributing sources as possible. Often the same headache may have more than one cause. The following are the most common causes of headaches.

1. **Inherited predisposition.** "Headaches run in my family; I'm stuck with them." You may have inherited a tendency toward getting headaches. In attempting to cope with stress and problems, you may develop a headache while other people develop gastrointestinal difficulties, hives, allergies, or heart problems.

2. **Family influences.** If headaches run in your family, you probably also learned to model your coping pattern after your family members and, therefore, may develop similar ailments. Thus the source of your headaches may be more of a *learned* habit pattern rather than an inherited predisposition.

3. **Tension.** When you find yourself in a stressful situation, you normally experience tension in your system. After your muscles are tight for a while, they get strained and tired. Eventually the tension may affect the blood flow to the brain, and you will then develop a headache.

4. **Food.** A significant number of people develop headaches when they fail to eat properly, or when they eat certain foods which may be toxic to their particular systems. Headaches can also occur during withdrawal from caffeine. A headache, therefore, might be signaling you to balance your nutritional intake.

5. **Environmental factors.** Headaches can come as a reaction to cold drafts, intense heat, high altitudes, high humidity, change in air pressure, pollen, chemicals, and/or pesticides. Formaldehyde is one such environmental influence which causes headaches in some people. This is found in particle board, plywood, and insulation. Mobile homes are particularly prone to high formaldehyde levels.

6. **Physiological causes.** These include a high fever, vision problems, teeth or bite problems, hormonal imbalance (during pregnancy or pre-

menstruation period, or from birth-control pills), sinus or allergy reactions, a disease or infection, or a concussion. Less frequently, but yet possible, you can develop a headache as a symptom of a cerebral hemorrhage, meningitis, or a brain tumor.

7. **Weekend headaches.** This headache, occurring on Saturday or Sunday, may have several causes. You may have had too much pressure from work on Friday. You may oversleep and skip breakfast, thus causing a headache which comes from a decrease in the glucose level of your blood. If this is the case, eating a minimal amount of food at the normal breakfast time should relieve the headache. Other weekend conditions include: the increase of family conflicts; smoking more or drinking more coffee; overexcitement or boredom; and insufficient sleep.

TYPES OF HEADACHES

Most headaches can be categorized in one of several distinct patterns. These include: (1) *tension headaches;* (2) *dilation headaches* (migraine, cluster, hypertensive, fever, hunger, hangover, and toxic poisoning); and (3) *traction* or *inflammatory headaches* (infection or diseases of the eye, ear, nose, throat, sinus, teeth, or jaw; and mass lesions as in tumors and cerebral hemorrhage). It is very possible to have a combination of two types of headaches simultaneously or sequentially.

1. **Tension Headaches.** The most common headache (about 90 percent) is the tension or muscle-contraction headache. Three times as many women get tension headaches as do men. Forty percent of tension-headache sufferers have a family history of headaches.

In tension headaches, the muscles of the head, neck, and scalp tighten, and the blood vessels constrict, causing pain. The headache is the brain's way of saying, "Relax! Give the muscles a rest, and let the blood flow normally."

Tension headaches can occur on both sides of the head, in the forehead, at the back of the head, or in the jaw area. The head usually feels as though you have a band around it, which is being tightened. The head can also feel as if there is a pressure within which might cause an explosion. Tension headaches do not usually throb; they will more likely ache, and there may be tenderness of the scalp and neck. There may be a burning or tingling sensation. Nausea, although not usually common, can occur, especially if the pain becomes severe. A tension headache usually lasts a few hours, but it can last longer.

Tension headaches can develop in anticipation of an unpleasant occurrence, during an emotional upset or conflict, after a stressful or fatiguing event, or from poor posture. Worrying about getting a headache can even cause a headache. Other specific influences include squinting in bright light, holding a telephone with your shoulder, typing or sewing for too long, wrinkling your forehead while worrying, and wearing high heels.

The emotions generally associated with tension headaches include worry, anxiety, fear, pent-up anger, and/or depression. Sometimes the headache provides a useful excuse to avoid a task or to get help. Experiencing tension headaches can often lead to insomnia, tiredness, irritability, and eating disorders.

Almost all tension headaches can be alleviated and/or prevented by following the exercises outlined in this book, including relaxation, pressure-point massage, and changing your thinking processes. In addition, taking a leisurely hot bath often helps relieve a tension headache. Although medication is rarely necessary, circumstances might warrant an occasional aspirin. Additionally, counseling may be appropriate to learn skills of conflict resolution, stress management, and other coping skills and goal setting.

2. **Dilation Headaches.** In these headaches, the blood vessels swell (dilate), inflame, and exert pressure on the nerves around them, causing pain. Headaches of this type include *migraine, cluster, hypertensive, fever, hunger, hangover,* and *toxic poisoning*. With dilation headaches, the brain is saying, "Make changes so that the blood vessels can return to their normal size."

Symptoms of Migraine Headaches. The pain often localizes on one side of the head. The temple area is usually tender. Migraine sufferers experience intense throbbing and constant pain, and the neck may become stiff and achy. The pain is generally so severe that the sufferer cannot carry on normal activities. The migraine is sometimes accompanied by nausea or vomiting and a loss in appetite. Bending over makes a migraine worse. The headache may last a few hours, although it often lasts a full day or longer. When the attack is over, the victim will feel exhausted for hours or days.

Occurrence of Migraines. The migraine occurs most often after a stressful situation, such as following a vacation, or on the morning after a trauma of the day before. It can wake the person up in the middle of the night. Migraines can, however, also occur during the stress itself.

A migraine can be triggered by something as simple as rays of sunlight, physical exercise, sitting in a stuffy or smoky room, or watching television in a dark room. It can also come after eating certain foods, such as milk products, chocolate, wheat, nuts, citrus fruits, spicy food, pork, or alcohol (*see* complete list on page 289). Migraines can also be brought on by going without eating for an extended period, as is true when one oversleeps or fasts. They can also be triggered by withdrawing from caffeine. Weather changes or high altitudes can cause a migraine in some persons.

Effect of Drugs and Chemicals. Drugs which can stimulate a migraine include reserpine, nitroglycerin, estrogen, and too much ergotamine. Even car exhaust and certain odors can trigger an attack. Migraine headaches can occur from changes in hormonal levels, such as during ovulation, menstruation, pregnancy, and menopause, or as a side effect of birth-control pills. Ironically, some women who usually get migraines become free of them during pregnancy.

It is estimated that about 70 percent of migraine sufferers have a family history of such pain, indicating the possibility of a hereditary predisposition and/or an environmental influence. As children, most migraine sufferers experienced headaches, nausea, and/or car sickness.

Personality Traits of the Migraine Sufferer. Traits associated with migraines include being meticulous, compulsive, and perfectionistic. Migraine sufferers often are ambitious, hardworking, and conscientious; they become overly concerned with setting and meeting goals. They are usually highly energetic and often very intelligent. Delays and failures trouble them deeply. They are usually demanding of themselves and others, eager to please, and sensitive to criticism. Not all migraine sufferers have these personality traits, nor do all individuals with these traits have migraines. In some cases, these personality traits can be abandoned fairly easily by acknowledging their counterproductiveness. In other cases, it might be necessary to enlist the help of a therapist, because the personality traits and habit patterns may be very deeply ingrained and attached to issues of self-acceptance.

Types of Migraines. There are two kinds of migraines: the *common* and the *classic*. The common migraine accounts for about 80 percent of all migraines and affects men and women equally. More women are affected by the classic migraine, and its symptoms are usually on one side of the head (while the common migraine can be on both sides). Unlike the common migraine, the frequency of classical migraines diminishes as a person gets older since, with aging, there is a general loss of elasticity of artery walls.

If you are a common-migraine sufferer, your warning phase, if any, will be a generalized vague, uneasy, or irritable feeling.

If you are a classic-migraine sufferer, you will have a warning of from ten to thirty minutes, during which time the blood vessels constrict. The preheadache symptoms usually occur on the opposite side of the head from where the throbbing will occur later. You may see streaks of light, zigzagging lines, blotches of darkness, blurring, or other visual distortions. Your speech may become slurred and/or indistinct. Numbness or

Common Medical Problems

tingling may occur in your hands and feet. You might experience nausea or tremors and will probably feel weak, tired, confused, restless, and irritable. It is best to lie down and relax in a dark room as soon as possible when the warning comes.

The dilation and inflammation phase is similar for both the classic and the common migraine. The blood vessels in your head become larger, the tissues around the blood vessels become inflamed and chemical irritants collect. The headache throbs with increasing severity. You feel tense, short-tempered, and confused. Your voice becomes low, perhaps even inaudible. You may accumulate fluid in your ankles and face. You may experience heavy perspiration, increased urination, constipation, and/or diarrhea. Sounds and bright light become especially irritating. During this phase, it is best to cool your forehead and warm your hands and feet to help reverse the dilation of the arteries in your head. Since the pain seems unbearable during this phase, medication may be necessary.

Later—sometimes after a full day—a dull, steady headache replaces the intense pain. During this time, you may suffer from a stiff neck, tenderness, exhaustion, and tension.

Cluster Headaches. Another dilation headache, with pain as unbearable as the migraine, is the cluster headache. Ninety percent of cluster headaches occur in men, and these men usually range in age from twenty to forty.

The excruciating pain of a cluster headache occurs behind one cheek and eye and stretches to the back of the head and neck. Sometimes it pierces the other side of the head. If you suffer from a cluster headache, you may experience tearing, heavy perspiration, or nasal congestion. The headache usually throbs and aches, and it reaches its intensity very quickly. The pain often feels like a knife stabbing in your head.

Cluster headaches can occur in the middle of the night every night during the period of the attacks. The headaches can occur several times in a single day, or daily over a period of time up to two months. They then disappear for months or even years. The headaches often occur in the spring and/or fall. Usually a cluster headache lasts between ten minutes and four hours. Occasionally the headache can last continuously for a long period of time. Alcohol, nicotine, histamines, or nitroglycerin often trigger these headaches.

The cluster-headache sufferer may share the personality traits which are often true of migraine sufferers. Vigorous exercise, such as running, swimming, tennis, or lifting weights, can reduce these headaches.

Hypertensive Headaches. Another dilation headache is the hypertensive headache, caused by elevated blood pressure. This headache normally starts in the morning and diminishes on its own during the day. It produces blurred vision, drowsiness, and even confusion. When the blood pressure goes down, the headache decreases.

Miscellaneous Dilation Headaches. Other dilation headaches include those resulting from fever, hunger, environmental conditions, strenuous sexual activity, a head injury, exhaustive exercise, overconsumption of alcohol, and poisons, such as carbon monoxide. Although the causes of these headaches are different, the response of the blood vessels is similar to that for migraine and cluster headaches. The intensity, however, of these miscellaneous headaches is usually less.

3. **Traction and Inflammatory Headaches.** These headaches are stimulated by organic diseases or infections, such as meningitis, strokes, phlebitis, arthritis, or neuralgia. Other headaches may be associated with inflammation in specific areas, such as eyes, ears, nose, throat, sinus, teeth, or jaws. Although rare, headaches can also occur within the brain itself, such as from mass lesions, including tumors and cerebral hemorrhages. In these cases, specific medical treatment should be sought for the underlying disease or infection.

Sinus Headaches. An example of an inflammation headache is the sinus headache, which results from increased pressure, caused by inflammation of the mucous membranes in the sinus cavities. A stuffy nose and sometimes a fever may accompany the pain. If the pain is in the forehead area, it is worse in the morning; if it is in the cheek area, it usually gets worse in the afternoon and diminishes at night. Sinus pain is usually dull and aching. It often occurs more in cold weather, after drinking alcohol, during the menstrual cycle, during sexual excitement, or as a result of an allergy attack or a cold. The pain becomes worse when bending over, coughing, sneezing, or lifting a heavy object. Nausea or vomiting are seldom present. Many people label tension or dilation headaches as sinus headaches, and therefore treat them incorrectly.

Allergy Headaches. Very similar to sinus headaches are allergy headaches, caused by reaction to such environmental conditions as pollen and molds. Nasal congestion and watery eyes usually accompany an allergy headache.

Eyestrain Headaches. Another traction headache can occur from eyestrain and is therefore located behind the eyes. It may come after prolonged reading, reading at an improper distance, watching television in a dark room, or reading in poor light. If these headaches persist after altering the conditions, then your eyes need to be examined.

Jaw-related Headaches. A final traction headache may be associated with the jaw or temporomandibular joint. Pain resulting from this problem usually occurs in front of or behind the ears. Your temple area may also be tender, and you experience pain when you chew. You may experience a clicking sound when you open your jaw. This ache can result from clenching or grinding your teeth, or having a poor bite because of teeth or bone structure. If these aches persist, consult an orthodontist, who can often make an adjustment (which is sometimes as simple as grinding or capping).

Remember that your headache may come from several sources and may appear only under overlapping conditions, such as stress, nutritional imbalance, infection, and exhaustion. It is, therefore, important to become aware of all the potential causes for your headaches, and try to correct as many as possible.

MEDICAL OR PSYCHOLOGICAL CONSULTATION

After you have been examined by your doctor, and been reassured that there is nothing seriously wrong, practicing the exercises in this section of the book will bring significant relief.

Generally, dilation, traction, and inflammation headaches require medical advice. Specifically, *seek medical advice if:*

- Your headaches persist and become chronic, or get worse.
- The headaches come on suddenly and severely, especially if associated with a stiff neck.
- You experience a "different" kind of headache from what you have had before.
- You experience extreme vomiting.
- Your vision suddenly dims, or you notice a distinct deterioration of your sight.
- You have a fever.
- You feel mentally confused, lose your memory, or can't concentrate.
- You have a seizure or a convulsion.
- Extreme sleepiness or insomnia accompanies the headache.
- You repeatedly awaken in the middle of the night, or wake up early with a headache.
- You have morning headaches, which disappear on their own within an hour.
- You have difficulty with your speech or have a hearing loss.
- You experience numbness, clumsiness, and/or weakness in your arms or legs.
- Your throbbing headaches get worse as you get older.
- Your headache comes on by coughing, sneezing, or straining.

Possible Tests and Treatment. Your physician can determine any physiological or metabolic problem. In addition to a neurologic examination, diagnostic tests can include: an X ray, electroencephalogram, blood tests, CAT scan, and a spinal tap. Your physician can prescribe drugs, if appropriate, suggest physical therapy, or perform trigger-point injections. In more rare situations (as for a tumor), your doctor may find it necessary to suggest radiation therapy or perform surgery.

Possible Medication. Drugs which your physician may recommend include preventative as well as pain-reducing medication. These drugs fall in many categories. An analgesic medication is pain relieving and can be as simple as aspirin or as powerful as codeine. Tranquilizers calm you down while antidepressants help relieve your depression. Vasoconstrictor drugs (like ergotamine and caffeine derivatives) cause swollen blood vessels to return to normal, while anti-inflammatory medication suppresses inflammation. Antihypertensive medication counteracts high blood pressure; antihistamine drugs block the effects of histamines, which can cause headache-associated symptoms; decongestant drugs cause swollen membranes to shrink; and anticonvulsants are used to minimize convulsions. These three medications also have a sedative effect. Additionally, hormones may be prescribed when appropriate. In all cases, your physician will need feedback from you regarding the medication's effectiveness and/or side effects. Finding the correct medication for you may require several medication changes.

Need Other Advice? In addition to medical attention, you should *seek psychological advice if:*

- Your headaches are integrally tied with stressful situations that you have not been able to resolve.
- You are unable to relieve yourself of anger and/or intense resentment.
- You become aware that your headaches serve a secondary gain (that is, you get them when you want to get out of doing something or to get someone's sympathy).
- You feel your headaches are long-standing reactions to authority, or to fearful or unpleasant situations.

Your therapist can help determine your underlying emotional issues and help guide you in resolving them. You may also be taught biofeedback, which can assist you in learning to alter various bodily functions, including muscle tension and blood flow.

If you have been unable to locate in your area a physician or therapist who specializes in headache reduction, get in contact with The National Migraine Foundation at 5252 N. Western Ave., Chicago, Illinois 60625.

Headache Log. Keep a record of the occurrence of your headaches.

You thus can begin to isolate patterns that lead to your headaches. When the headaches occur, you can then make the appropriate changes to rid yourself of the pain. You may, for example, experience headaches after eating certain foods. You can then alter your diet and note whether there is a reduction of the incidence of headaches.

Note the date and time the headaches occur and their intensity. Write down the circumstances during which the pain occurs, and what you have eaten or not eaten before it began. List any drugs you took and/or time spent in relaxation, and the results of your actions.

As you fill out the log, your awareness of your own bodily responses will increase. You will also notice your progress as the result of the various exercises. Share the information from your "Headache Log" and the "Headache Survey" with your doctor.

Remember, you are the most important person in determining the precipitating nonmedical causes. You also become the expert in reducing your pain because it is your own experience.

The following pages outline suggestions and exercises to practice on your road to freedom from head pain. After following these suggestions, your headaches should diminish. If you then experience a headache, you know it is indicating a new area to investigate and resolve. As you continue to take charge when headaches threaten, you will find a more energized and enjoyable life!

TRANSFORMING YOUR LIFE

Your life is made up of a series of events, including the headaches you experience. By altering some of your perceptions, attitudes, and responses, you can reduce your headaches.

For instance, how much wasted time has been spent worrying, and thus causing needless headaches? You can reduce worrying by attending to the constructive activities of planning and being genuinely concerned about a situation. When you can't do anything about something, you can focus your mind elsewhere, and trust yourself to handle the situation if it does happen.

Boredom headaches can be relieved by creating more enthusiasm and optimism in your life. You can believe in yourself, tap your own wisdom, and maximize your hidden potential. People who think they can, *can!* As you move out of your comfort zones, you will feel more of your own natural power. However, as you take risks and stretch your wings, be sure to be realistic about your limits:

> Blessed are they who bite off more than they can chew.
> Even more blessed are they who know when to spit it out.

Many headaches occur when we feel stuck and unable to solve a problem. You can become flexible, unique, and creative in your problem resolution. Don't hold on to ineffective habits of behavior, styles of communication, and patterns of thinking. Be willing to consider alternatives if the solution isn't working.

Some headaches come when we take ourselves or the world too seriously. So, don't forget to laugh! Laughter is therapeutic in releasing tension as well as creating a fresh view.

Headaches can be created when we feel lonely. Therefore, get and give enough emotional hugs. Whereas it used to be said that three hugs a day were essential for mental health, by now (due to inflation), it takes fifteen hugs a day to remain sane! Hugs can be physical or verbal as in: "Thank you"; "It's nice to be with you"; "I like you"; "I feel happy when we're together." People who make positive physical contact with other people tend to have lower blood pressure and less tension and thus, by implication, fewer headaches.

CALMING DOWN

In calming yourself down and creating more happiness, it is important to realize you don't have the power to change anyone else. You can influence people to change, but *you* can't do the changing for them. *The only person you can change is yourself.*

When undesirable events happen, you can change your perceptions and attitudes to prevent yourself from getting overly upset and developing a headache. As you practice setting more realistic goals and making fewer demands, you can experience your own power to transform your life!

LETTING GO OF A HEADACHE

Trephination used to be performed on people who complained of chronic headaches. The procedure included drilling a hole in the person's head to release the evil spirit, which was supposedly causing the headache. The procedure was viewed as successful because the person didn't report any more headaches!

Most people view a headache as an enemy to attack, ignore, or squelch, but you now know that your headache serves as part of a feedback system. Therefore, fighting or suppressing it will, at best, bring only temporary relief and, at worst, lead to more physical ailments. We will next look at alternative actions that will produce more permanent relief.

This first exercise is especially effective for reducing tension headaches

Common Medical Problems

CHART 1
THE DEVELOPMENT AND CONSEQUENCES OF EMOTIONS

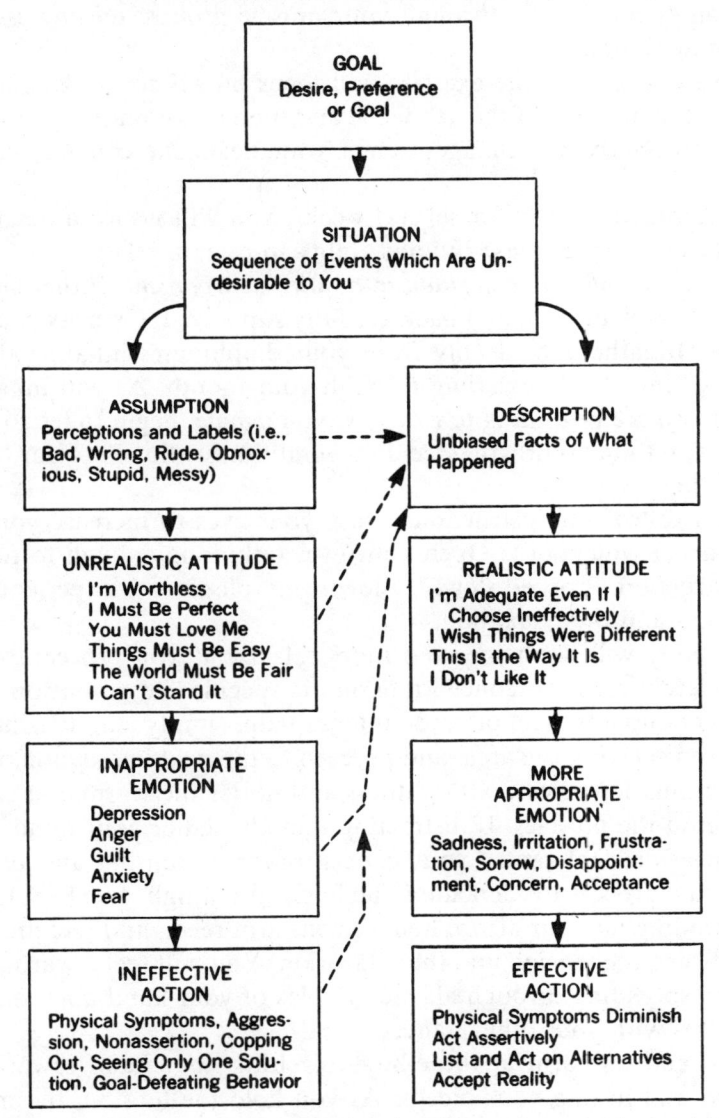

```
┌─────────────────────┐
│        GOAL         │
│ Desire, Preference  │
│      or Goal        │
└──────────┬──────────┘
           │
┌──────────▼──────────┐
│     SITUATION       │
│ Sequence of Events  │
│ Which Are Un-       │
│ desirable to You    │
└──┬───────────────┬──┘
   │               │
┌──▼───────────┐ ┌─▼──────────────┐
│  ASSUMPTION  │ │  DESCRIPTION   │
│ Perceptions  │ │ Unbiased Facts │
│ and Labels   │ │ of What        │
│ (i.e., Bad,  │ │ Happened       │
│ Wrong, Rude, │ │                │
│ Obnoxious,   │ │                │
│ Stupid,      │ │                │
│ Messy)       │ │                │
└──────┬───────┘ └────────┬───────┘
       │                  │
┌──────▼────────────┐ ┌───▼────────────────┐
│ UNREALISTIC       │ │ REALISTIC ATTITUDE │
│ ATTITUDE          │ │ I'm Adequate Even  │
│ I'm Worthless     │ │ If I Choose        │
│ I Must Be Perfect │ │ Ineffectively      │
│ You Must Love Me  │ │ I Wish Things      │
│ Things Must Be    │ │ Were Different     │
│ Easy              │ │ This Is the Way    │
│ The World Must    │ │ It Is              │
│ Be Fair           │ │ I Don't Like It    │
│ I Can't Stand It  │ │                    │
└──────┬────────────┘ └───────┬────────────┘
       │                      │
┌──────▼────────┐ ┌───────────▼────────┐
│ INAPPROPRIATE │ │ MORE APPROPRIATE   │
│ EMOTION       │ │ EMOTION            │
│ Depression    │ │ Sadness, Irrita-   │
│ Anger         │ │ tion, Frustration, │
│ Guilt         │ │ Sorrow, Disappoint-│
│ Anxiety       │ │ ment, Concern,     │
│ Fear          │ │ Acceptance         │
└──────┬────────┘ └───────────┬────────┘
       │                      │
┌──────▼────────────┐ ┌───────▼──────────────┐
│ INEFFECTIVE       │ │ EFFECTIVE ACTION     │
│ ACTION            │ │ Physical Symptoms    │
│ Physical Symptoms,│ │ Diminish             │
│ Aggression, Non-  │ │ Act Assertively      │
│ assertion, Copping│ │ List and Act on      │
│ Out, Seeing Only  │ │ Alternatives         │
│ One Solution,     │ │ Accept Reality       │
│ Goal-Defeating    │ │                      │
│ Behavior          │ │                      │
└───────────────────┘ └──────────────────────┘
```

or the tension component of dilation, inflammation, and traction headaches. By experiencing it, you will gain more insight into your headaches, which will facilitate designing your program of relief.

Relaxation is important for feeling healthy, for reducing tension and pain and/or for promoting healing. Since a portion of any pain results from tension, relaxation is usually able to assist in reducing headaches, as well as to prevent future head pain.

The first part of the exercise makes it easy for you to learn how to relax. The procedure, which was first developed by Edmund Jacobson, M.D., leads you systematically through your muscle groups, tensing and then relaxing the muscles.

The second part of the exercise will focus on acknowledging and listening to the message of the headache and then to committing yourself to making any necessary changes. Then your headache can stop nagging you.

As you practice daily for several weeks, you will notice a decrease in headaches and an increase in your ability to remain relaxed.

Get into a comfortable position in a quiet environment. Either sit or lie down, so that your neck and back are fully supported. Uncross your arms and legs. Breathe very deeply from your diaphragm, inhaling through your nose and slowly exhaling through your mouth. As you inhale, tell yourself you are beginning to relax. As you exhale, begin to let go of any tension. Continue to breathe deeply several times, allowing your body to relax more.

As you follow the instructions, close your eyes to increase your concentration on your body. Open your eyes only long enough to read the next instruction. Proceed slowly, allowing ample time to experience both the tension and the relaxation.

Your body will get heavy and more relaxed as you proceed. As you tense different muscles, concentrate on the specific site of tension. If you begin to cramp a muscle or cause intense pain, simply stop tensing, concentrate on relaxing the area, and proceed to the next instruction. As you relax the muscles, release all tightness and notice the warm and calming sensation in the muscles. If distracting thoughts enter your mind, gently set them aside, and return your concentration to tensing and relaxing.

Begin the process by clenching one hand into a tight fist. Feel the tension spreading up your arm. Then let your arm relax, and feel the difference between the tension and the relaxation. You will feel a warm, tingly sensation spreading through all the muscles of your hand and your arm. Repeat this with your other hand.

Next, bend one arm at the elbow, reaching your hand toward your shoulder, and flexing your biceps. As you hold the tension, the muscles will pull on the entire top of the upper arm. When you relax, the calming sensation will flow down your arm. Take a deep breath. Repeat the tension and relaxation with your other arm.

Moving to your shoulder area, shrug your shoulders toward your ears. Lift them as high as you can and hold them tightly. Feel the pull of the large muscles across the shoulders. Then drop your shoulders and allow them to relax as much as they can. Then bring your shoulders forward, as

Common Medical Problems 283

if you're going to touch them together. Hold the tension. Relax and let the tension drain from the tight muscles in your shoulders. Then take a deep breath, and as you exhale, let pleasant relaxation stream through your body.

Moving to your face area, wrinkle your forehead by raising your eyebrows and tensing your forehead. Then relax. Pull your brow together by frowning. Then relax. Squint your eyes tightly and wrinkle up your nose. Then relax that area. Open your mouth wide and tense your mouth muscles. Then close your mouth and relax. Tense your jaw muscles by clenching your teeth together tightly. Then let your jaws go completely slack. Push the tip of your tongue strongly against the roof of your mouth, so that you can feel tightness in the throat muscles. As you drop your tongue and relax, you will notice your head and body becoming limp, calm, and more relaxed. Breathe deeply.

Next, push your head back as far as it will go, and concentrate on the tight muscles in the back of your head and neck. Then release the pressure. Bend your head forward, until your chin touches your chest, feeling the tightness in the back of your neck. Relax, as you return your head to a comfortable position. Turn your head to the right. After feeling the strain that that produces, release the tension and relax. Repeat that stretch to the left.

Concentrate on the chest area by taking a deep breath and holding it. Then exhale through your mouth. Notice the pleasurable relief throughout your whole chest. Breathe normally. Next, push your shoulder blades together tightly and arch your back. Then release and allow tension to drain away. Tighten up your abdominal muscles as if someone were going to hit you there. Then relax and focus on the surge of relief.

Notice that your hands and arms are limp. Your shoulders are resting naturally. Your face muscles are relaxed and wonderfully calm. Your breathing is easy and rhythmical. Your torso is heavy and pleasantly relaxed.

Now tighten the buttocks muscles. Then relax. Tense the upper thighs of both legs by pushing your knees down. Then relax. Focus on your calf by pointing your toes away from your head. Then relax. Next, point your toes toward your head. Then let your muscles in your whole legs go limp. Finally, curl your toes downward and arch your feet upward, as you feel the pressure under each arch. Then relax the muscles in your feet.

Now concentrate on your headache. Close your eyes after each instruction to increase your awareness. Look at your headache with the observer part of your brain. Where is it located? What is its shape? Is it round or square or like a blob? Is it flat or thick? Is it like a band, a tube, or a steel bar? Consider the intensity of your headache. Rate it on a scale from a zero for no headache to ten for excruciating pain. What color do you perceive your headache to be right now? Notice how heavy or light it is. What texture does its surface seem to have? Is it smooth, soft, rough, or prickly? Does it make any sound? Is there a thumping, a throbbing, a moaning, or screaming? Observe the temperature. Is it hot or cold?

Remember your headache is your friend. It tells you that something is not right in your body. What information or advice does your headache have for you? Listen to its message, continuing to breathe deeply but gently. What advice does your headache have for you? Perhaps it is saying, "Worry less"; or, "Take things less seriously"; or, "Relax more"; or, "Be kinder to yourself"; or, "Get more sleep"; or, "Eat better"; or, "Exercise more"; or, "Get a medical checkup."

Assure your headache that you will follow the advice that it has for you. Tell it that you'll take better care of yourself. Promise your headache that you will make any necessary alterations to improve your life. The headache then won't have to nag you anymore.

Thank your headache for letting you know that changes are necessary. Give your headache a hug!

Now, *observe your headache again.* Where is it right now? What shape and color is it? From zero to ten, how intense is it? How heavy or light is it? What's its texture? What temperature is it? What sound does it produce? Does it have any more messages for you? Take another deep breath, allowing more tension to leave and more relaxation and confidence to fill your body. Notice how much easier you breathe.

By now, you should notice that the headache has altered. It probably has become smaller. It should be less intense and cooler. It may be paler in color and lighter in weight. Does it look like a cloud or perhaps a little dot?

As the headache reduces, you feel more in control and clearer about what you need to do. You are grateful for having such a clear feedback system. Acknowledge again the advice that the headache has for you, recommit yourself to modifying your life. Take another deep breath and feel the calm, relaxed sensation. You are happy and confident that you are in charge of your life.

Remain in a relaxed position as long as you wish. When you want to return to your daily routine, gently breathe deeply again and visualize the oxygen awakening your cells. Take at least a minute to become aware of your surroundings. Your mind will be alert, and yet your body will remain relaxed. Consciously maintain this relaxed state, and continue breathing deeply. As you resume your activities, your mind will be clear and refreshed.

CARING FOR YOUR BODY

The best way to relieve a headache is not to get one in the first place! This requires staying calm by keeping your attitudes realistic; keeping your muscles flexible through exercise and relaxation; getting plenty of sleep; and being careful what you eat.

How you take care of your body determines how you feel. If you fail to treat your body well, it may respond to such abuse by developing headaches. While some people overeat, others do not eat enough, or they stuff themselves with junk food, and *then* get headaches.

If the following nutritional information is insufficient to aid in your achieving a proper nutritional balance, see a nutrition-oriented physician or a nutritionist.

Eat foods which are enjoyable as well as nutritious. All individuals need basic nutrients. These include: (1) proteins, (2) carbohydrates, (3) fats, (4) liquids, and (5) vitamins and minerals. Let's look briefly at each of these.

1. **Protein.** We find protein in meat, fish, poultry, milk, cheese, eggs, nuts, beans, peas, and greens. Protein builds, repairs, and protects the cells throughout the whole body, including the cells of muscles, blood, skin, hair, nails, organs, and brain. It also aids in making hormones, which control a variety of bodily functions (such as growth, sexual activity, and metabolism). Protein helps provide energy and heat.

Protein deficiency can cause low blood pressure, anemia, depression, and/or a lack of antibodies to fight off diseases and infection. When people are under physical or mental stress, they may require more protein than usual.

2. **Carbohydrates.** Foods such as bread, fruits, and vegetables contain carbohydrates. They provide the chief source of energy for all bodily functions, making carbohydrates necessary for digestion and assimilation of other foods.

Complex carbohydrates occur in unprocessed fruits, vegetables, and grains, while refined carbohydrates occur in white flour, sugar, and polished rice. Complex carbohydrates are superior to refined carbohydrates because they metabolize better and contain many of the nutrients which are lost in the refining process.

Sugar overuse. A particularly common carbohydrate abuse is the overuse of refined sugar products. Everyone is aware of the high amount of sugar in cake, cookies, and candy. Fewer people know that a twelve-ounce soda contains the equivalent of over eight teaspoons of sugar!

Sugar not only adds pounds (which, of course, causes the problems associated with overweight), but it also is hard to metabolize and causes a drain of vitamins, especially B vitamins. It is common when you feel sluggish to desire sugar. If you eat something sweet, it causes adrenaline to be released, which gives you a quick burst of energy; but after an hour or so, you have a downward crashing feeling. You feel low again, take more sugar, and the cycle continues.

Processed foods often contain hidden refined sugar in the forms of glucose, sucrose, maltose, fructose, or dextrose as found in baby food, cereals, salad dressing, ketchup, sauces, canned fruits, vegetables, soups, and even liquid medications. While many people can eat sugar in moderate amounts, it's preferable to eat sugar from natural sources, such as in fruit, rather than in its refined state.

Many individuals who go on a diet to lose weight experience a headache. The headache develops from a drop in the blood-sugar level, a lack of nutrition, the withdrawal from a particular food, or a deficiency of a specific vitamin or mineral. It is important therefore, to avoid a so-called crash diet and to review your diet with a nutrition-oriented physician.

Hypoglycemia. Some people get headaches from an allergy to sugar. Others develop hypoglycemia, another cause of headaches. Hypoglycemia (or low blood sugar) is a condition which is the opposite of diabetes. Insulin is normally secreted to prevent too much sugar from remaining in the blood. In hypoglycemia, the pancreas secretes too much insulin, which lowers the blood sugar to a subnormal level. Starchy and sweet diets cause the pancreas to work erratically and to secrete too much insulin. In addition, if a hypoglycemic is under stress, his/her adrenal gland doesn't send the message to the pancreas to turn off the insulin. Hypoglycemics also overproduce insulin after smoking or drinking caffeine or alcohol. They should not eat refined carbohydrates to increase the blood sugar. Fruit juices are also generally considered a poor choice because they provide a rush of sugar and should therefore be diluted if they are drunk. In more severe cases, even fresh fruit may be difficult for the system to process.

In addition to headaches, common symptoms of hypoglycemia include dizziness (especially before eating or when rising or bending), fatigue, lack of concentration, shakiness when hungry, anxiety attacks, loss of memory, menstrual problems, impotency, craving for sweets, and depression. Hypoglycemics need to eat six small meals a day which are high in protein. Additionally, they need to eat moderate amounts of nonfruity, complex carbohydrates as well as moderate amounts of fat. They may also need to restrict potatoes, corn, white rice, peas, and lima beans. If the symptoms persist, a hypoglycemic should seek advice from a nutrition-oriented physician or a nutritionist.

Salt Overuse. In addition to too much sugar, many people oversalt their food. The sodium buildup can trigger a migraine, which usually occurs six to twelve hours later.

3. **Fats.** We need a few teaspoons of fat each day, an essential for normal nerve and brain tissue and hormone development. Fats aid in the digestive process and keep our bodies warm. They help process some of the vitamins and, combined with carbohydrates, provide fuel for the body.

You can find fat in animal products, such as butter, eggs, bacon, cheese, and in vegetable oil made from corn, soybean, or safflower. Hydrogenated fats, such as are found in margarine and shortening, have been processed by extracting the water to make the fat more solid and to prevent rancidity. In the hydrogenation process, the vegetable oil, which originally was polyunsaturated, now becomes saturated and is therefore much more difficult to digest and is limited in its ability to help the system process other nutrients. It is thus less desirable than natural nonhydrogenated fats.

Avoid rancid fats, which can induce serious vitamin deficiencies. Fat becomes rancid when not stored properly under refrigeration. Such fats are found in bacon drippings, prepackaged pie-crust mixes, prepopped popcorn, or opened potato chips, and nuts.

A cousin of fat, *cholesterol,* is found in such animal foods as butter, cream, and egg yolks. Cholesterol is a normal component of most body tissues and is essential to forming hormones. Sources of natural cholesterol contain their own emulsifier to help the cholesterol break down in the blood. An unusual buildup of cholesterol usually occurs from eating processed foods or having metabolic disturbances created by excessive sugars and starches.

4. **Liquids.** Two-thirds of the body's weight is made up of water. Liquids, therefore, are essential in nearly every metabolic process, including digestion, circulation, absorption, and excretion. Liquids also help maintain a normal body temperature.

We lose approximately three quarts of liquid each day through urination and perspiration, depending upon our activity level and environmental conditions. We could lose as little as one quart a day with sedentary activity on a cold day, or as much as ten quarts a day in the desert. Many people become dehydrated when they don't replenish lost liquid.

We obtain our fluids in liquids and foods containing juices. It's better to eat these foods whole, rather than in juices, because the processing often destroys nutritional benefits.

We need at least a quart of liquid a day. Milk, fruit juices, and pure water are superior to processed drinks. Drink most of your liquids between meals, otherwise too much liquid can dilute enzymes and acids used in digestion.

Caffeine. Drinking caffeine creates problems for the body. Caffeine, a strong stimulant, constricts blood vessels and causes adrenaline release. This leads to increased alertness, sometimes making us feel edgy. It also speeds up metabolism and leads to the depletion of valuable nutrients (especially the B vitamins). As people become more stimulated, they are also more easily irritated and frustrated. This increased tension often leads to a headache. Caffeine also interferes with sleep, which results in exhaustion and stress. This can increase headaches. Other symptoms of "caffeinism" include depression, rapid or skipped heartbeats, diarrhea, stomach pains, heartburn, light-headedness, and frequent urination.

A throbbing headache can occur as a withdrawal symptom when the body is deprived of caffeine for a day. Other possible withdrawal symptoms (which can last up to two weeks) include drowsiness, lethargy, poor concentration, depression, runny nose, and nausea.

The headache sufferer should slowly eliminate caffeinated drinks, including coffee, tea, chocolate, and cola drinks. Substitute decaffeinated coffee, herbal teas, juices, and water. Some pain-reducing medicines contain caffeine and should be avoided by chronic headache sufferers. These include Anacin, Cope, Excedrin, Vanquish, Cafergot, and Fiorinal. Other medication containing caffeine should be avoided, as in certain stimulants, weight-control aids, cold or allergy drugs, and menstrual aids. When you no longer drink caffeine, you will discover your own natural energy and calmness.

5. **Vitamins and Minerals.** The final essential nutrients are vitamins and minerals. A full supply of vitamins and minerals are necessary for the health of all the tissues, cells, organs, and body systems. In order for the cells to reproduce normally, each vitamin has a specific function.

Vitamins A, D, and E are *fat-soluble,* while vitamins B and C are *water-soluble.* If the body gets too much of water-soluble vitamins, it simply disposes of them through the elimination system. However, if you take too many fat-soluble vitamins, they are stored up in your body and may cause a toxic reaction. Water-soluble vitamins can be taken in smaller doses, several times a day, to maintain a proper level of healthy functioning.

Headache sufferers often lack vitamin B, which is depleted under stressful situations. You will feel edgy without vitamin B. Therefore you might supplement your diet with the B vitamins and notice if you feel calmer.

Vitamins do their job only with the help of minerals. Unlike most vitamins, which can be manufactured in the body, minerals must be obtained from what we eat or drink.

It is better to meet your nutritional needs by eating fresh fruits and vegetables, eggs, poultry, and meat, rather than from dietary supplements. This may be difficult, depending on your time schedule, food availability, cooking skills, and interests. Rather than be deficient, however, supplement your diet with vitamins and minerals.

Improper growing, shipping, cooking, and canning can destroy nutrients. Preferably buy fresh, organically grown food to assure the presence of vitamins and minerals and the absence of toxins from the pesticides.

Suggestions for Food Preparation and Choice. Thoroughly wash (but don't soak) fresh produce. If the food must be cooked, cook it quickly to keep from destroying nutritional value. This can be done with waterless cooking, steaming, or stir frying.

Eat fresh (rather than canned) food, because the canning process destroys many nutrients and adds preservatives, which may have a toxic effect on your body and may cause headaches. Frozen foods usually retain more nutrients than canned. Avoid junk foods, including potato chips, candy, sugared drinks, and most breakfast cereals. Eat snacks (including dried fruits and unsalted nuts) which have been prepared without harmful chemicals.

It is usually better to eat several small meals daily rather than one large meal. Eat slowly and enjoy your food. Hurried eating can cause poor digestion and can trigger tension which may lead to a headache.

Food Allergies. As mentioned before, some individuals, allergic to certain foods, develop migraine headaches. Foods which are especially potent for triggering a migraine include: milk and milk products, including ripened cheese, yogurt, sour cream, and ice cream; chocolate; excessive caffeine; nuts and peanut butter; citrus fruits (including tomatoes); avocados; bananas; canned figs; wheat, as in fresh breads, coffee cakes and doughnuts; pods of broad beans (lima, navy, and pea pods); onions; spicy foods like pizza and foods with monosodium glutamate; brown vinegar; fermented, pickled, or marinated foods; processed meats (ham, bacon, hot dogs, luncheon meats, and sausage); chicken livers; pork; herring; and alcoholic beverages.

What Causes Your Headache? To determine which foods cause your headaches, first, simplify your diet by cutting out most of the foods on the allergy list. Then, one at a time, add them to your diet and observe your reaction. Particularly notice whether the food which causes a headache is fresh or processed. By regulating your diet, you may find eventually that a decreasing number of foods will cause an allergic reaction. Consult an allergist if you suspect a food allergy which you have been unsuccessful in regulating.

In conclusion, you are the person who ultimately benefits from being healthy. It is not your doctor's responsibility to keep you healthy. As you become more aware of the correlation between what you eat and how you feel, you will not only become healthier, but your headaches will also diminish.

STRETCHING EXERCISES

You can often prevent a headache by not becoming tense or by releasing tension as it builds. As you practice the following stretching exercises, you will notice your body becoming more loose and flexible.

When you do the stretches, concentrate on releasing tension. Turn off your racing mind and refuse to focus on distracting thoughts. Move slowly and smoothly into the stretches. Enjoy the refreshing easy movement of your body. Breathe deeply from the abdomen. Send oxygen into the muscle that you are stretching.

Sit in an upright chair with your back supported and straight. Take a deep breath. Slowly release it. Turn your head slowly to the right. Then turn it to the left. Experience the stretch as you move. Drop your chin toward your chest. Tilt your head backward, and then sideways toward each shoulder without raising your shoulder. Roll your head slowly twice to the right, and then twice to the left. Take a deep breath.

Push your forehead backward with the palm of your hand as you resist by pushing your head forward with your neck muscles. Pull your head forward with your hands behind your head, as you push your head backward. As your right hand pushes on the right side of your head, tilt and push your head to the right. Repeat on the left side. Then relax and breathe deeply.

Holding your head level, roll your eyes toward the ceiling, then look down toward the floor, then look as far as you can to the right, and then to the left. Rotate your eyes in a full circle counterclockwise. Then roll them clockwise, stretching the muscles. Gently let your eyelids fall shut. Take a deep breath and experience the pleasant sense of relaxation.

Shrug your shoulders by bringing them up toward your ears and tensing the muscles. Then let the shoulders drop. Place your hands on the back of your neck, so that your elbows are facing away from your shoulders. Expand your chest by stretching your elbows backward, as if you could touch them behind your back. Place your hands on the opposite shoulders, crossing your elbows as if hugging yourself. Feel the strong pull in your shoulder blades.

Next, roll your shoulders by moving your shoulders up to your ears, rolling them back, pushing them down, rolling them forward, and then letting them return to normal. Repeat that roll again, only in reverse, by moving first to the front, then down, back, up, and then to their normal resting place. Let go of the tension and take a deep breath. Move your neck and head around and stretch in any direction you wish. Notice how your head can move more easily. Take another deep breath.

Raise your arms and bend them at the elbows, bringing the fingertips together in front of your chest. Push your arms out with a strong thrust and stretch. Repeat this ten times. Let your arms fall loosely beside you and feel the tension go out of the shoulders, as you breathe deeply.

Extend your arms overhead. Grasp your right hand with your left and slowly bend to the left, using your left arm to gently pull the right arm over your head. Then repeat, bending and stretching to the right.

Clasp your hands behind your head and slowly pull your head and neck down, so that your chin touches your chest. Further the stretch by bending forward at the waist. Return your head to normal and breathe deeply.

Straighten your legs out in front of you. Slowly rotate your feet from your ankle five times in one direction and then five times in the opposite direction.

To stretch your back and waist further, stand up and unlock your knees, so that they are slightly bent. Bend at the hip and reach slowly toward the floor, stretching the back and leg muscles. Do not overextend yourself. Return slowly to standing position and raise your arms overhead and reach toward the ceiling. Stretch alternately with one arm and then the other, as if reaching for the ceiling. Return your hands to your side. Then interlock your fingers behind your back. Slowly bend forward with your head moving toward your knees and your arms raising behind you toward the ceiling. Return to normal standing and breathe deeply.

Finally, lie down and breathe slowly. Allow your whole body to relax for as long as you would like before returning to your daily routine with renewed energy. Notice the refreshed and invigorated feeling your body experiences, as the muscles have let go of their tension.

Regular Exercise. In addition to stretching, it is important to keep yourself healthy by exercising regularly. It is best to choose a type of exercise that you can enjoy doing, whether it be swimming, calisthenics, jogging, yoga, playing racquetball, or tennis, or merely walking. *It is generally recommended to exercise at least fifteen minutes four times per week to a point which increases your heart rate to about 70 percent of its maximum output.* (A simple formula for figuring your individual exercise heart rate is to subtract your age from 220 and take 70 percent of that figure.) Your particular physical condition might preclude vigorous exercise, and thus, if in doubt, your program *should be cleared by your physician.* Remember: exercise is an excellent investment in preventing headaches.

RELAXATION, WISDOM, AND CONFIDENCE

The following exercise will further increase your ability to relax. Find a comfortable position in which your back and neck are fully supported. Uncross your arms and legs and breathe deeply from your diaphragm, allowing your body to relax. As you inhale through your nose and exhale through your mouth, say silently, *Calm and tranquil.* Notice the pleasant sensation as you allow tension to flow out of your body.

Mentally survey your body for any tension. When you find a tight muscle, relax it, allowing the tension to drain away. Envision each part of the body as you release any tension.

Focus on your scalp and forehead; your eyes and nose; your cheeks, tongue, mouth, and jaws; your neck and shoulders; and your chest. Visualize the tension gliding down your arms to the tips of your fingers, and then slowly dropping away from your body. Concentrate on relaxing your upper back; your lower back; your stomach and abdomen; and your thighs, calves and ankles; and your feet and toes.

Turn off all tension as you become pleasantly calm, loose, and limp. Continue to breathe deeply. Fill your body with refreshing air, allowing the oxygen to calm the whole body. Exhale the carbon dioxide completely.

Allow your relaxation to deepen as your entire body is releasing its tension. First, think about your hands. Mentally see them relaxed and free of tension. Silently say to yourself, *My hands are feeling warm.*

Imagine your arms as you say, *My arms feel heavy.* Next think, *My feet are pleasantly warm, and my legs feel wonderfully heavy.*

Concentrate on your breathing: *My breathing is slow and even.* As you envision your body, say silently, *My heart is beating slowly and regularly.*

My forehead feels cool. My mind is calm and tranquil, as my body relaxes.

Notice your mind has become quiet; your anxieties have vanished. You have a pleasant sense of well-being. Say to yourself, *I feel quiet and peaceful.*

Think of the tranquility of your total mind and body and say, *I can sense my own calm feelings.* This calmness, like a weightless blanket, spreads slowly over your body, beginning at your head and moving downward to your toes.

In your imagination, go to a pleasant place. It may be to the ocean, an open field, the top of a mountain, or a forest area. View yourself there enjoying the fresh air and sunshine. You are at peace and have no worries. The sun and gentle breezes caress your body. Inhale the smell of your pleasant surroundings. In your mind observe the vivid colors in the scenery. Hear the pleasant sounds.

Take a minute to contemplate any problem you might be experiencing. Listen to the wise part of you, as you formulate a solution to your problem.

Think to yourself, *I'm grateful to God for creating me to be just as I am. I can maximize my potential best only when I am healthy.*

Probe deeply into your thoughts: *What would I like to do in my life? What would make my life more meaningful? How can I make life more interesting and fun?*

Pause and breathe deeply. Recognize a sense of true confidence in yourself. You like being you. You have no self-doubts. You remember the kind of things others have said to you. Smile and allow the love and support of others to help you feel affirmed.

As you breathe deeply again, ask yourself, *What would I like to focus my attention on and accomplish?* Observe the clear assurance that you can attain whatever you set as a goal. You feel capable.

Notice your energy and power. Visualize yourself making decisions more quickly. Experience the confidence you have in your own wisdom and power.

In your imagination, give yourself a hug. You are your own best friend. Out of your love for yourself can grow the ability to project your love to others. They do not have to return the love, and yet, if they do, you can accept their love because you are lovable. You feel a smile forming. Your world is friendly.

As you take another deep breath, your body feels as if it is overflowing with love, power, and confidence. You feel joyful and energetic. You are clear about what you want to do for yourself, as well as how to extend your love to others.

Remain in your relaxed position as long as you like. Then take a minute to become slowly aware of your surroundings. Return to your routine feeling relaxed, refreshed, and confident!

GOING TO SLEEP

Anxiety can prevent sleep, which leads to tension, which leads to headaches and more insomnia—a vicious cycle, indeed! The following is a description of a process to facilitate your going to sleep.

First, stretch your muscles by straightening your arms and legs as tightly as possible. Then let them drop and relax. Next roll on your side and bend your top leg, so its knee touches the bed and its foot rests on the knee of the bottom leg that is straight. Place your lower hand on the raised knee. Stretch the upper arm back over your head until it touches the bed. Twist and stretch, so that both shoulders touch the bed. Repeat on the other side.

Now get into a comfortable position for sleep. If you lie on your back, place a pillow under your knees. Be sure the pillow under your head keeps your neck straight with your back.

Breathe slowly and deeply. Close your eyes and imagine yourself setting the hands of a large clock to the time you want to wake up. Concentrate on that time. Say silently to yourself, *I will wake up comfortably rested at that time. I will be alert and eager to have a wonderful day.*

Then think, *I will soon be pleasantly asleep.* Take three slow, deep breaths. Think to yourself, *I am very calm and comfortable.*

Squint your eyes tightly, being aware of the tension. Then let the eyelids relax. Relax the rest of your face completely. Notice any feeling of drowsiness.

Keeping your head straight, turn your eyes to the right and hold that position, feeling the tension. Let the eyes return to normal and feel the relaxation from the muscles letting go. Repeat this process to the left, to the top of your head, and then to your feet. Notice your whole head becoming heavier.

Say to yourself, *I'm getting very sleepy.* Breathing slowly and deeply, repeat silently several times, *Calm and sleepy. Calm and sleepy.* Your body is pleasantly relaxed. You are drowsy. You want to go to sleep. Your body is feeling very limp.

In your imagination, allow both of your feet to become very heavy, as you sense tension draining away. Let your calves become heavy. Then your knees. Then your thighs. Notice how heavy both legs are.

Relax your hips and let them become heavy. Then your abdomen. Your back. Your stomach. Your chest. Breathe deeply, allowing yourself to become comfortable and tranquil.

Common Medical Problems 295

Visualize your upper arms becoming heavy. Then your elbows. Your lower arms. Your wrists. Your hands and fingers are growing heavy and limp.

Focus on the tension draining from your shoulders. Let your neck get heavy. Then let your jaw relax. Your cheeks. Your eyes. Your forehead. Your whole head is heavy, calm, and pleasantly drowsy.

Your worries disappear. Your eyelids are heavy. You can't stay awake any longer. You feel yourself drifting away.

You must lay this book down because even it feels heavy. You will then count very slowly backward from 100, saying each number: 100, *calm and relaxed:* 99, *calm and relaxed:* 98, *calm and relaxed.* . . .

EPILOGUE

If your doctor has reassured you after examination that there is nothing seriously wrong you now have information that can help you reduce the frequency and intensity of your headaches. To succeed, you will need to: *investigate causes; practice the relaxation and prevention exercises; alter your nutritional intake;* and *change your attitudes, thought processes, and habits.*

Remember: A headache is a friendly feedback message to alert you to take better care of your body and be kinder to yourself. Listen to its message and take the necessary steps to remedy the problem. You are ultimately in charge of your recovery from headaches. You are the one who has the most to gain from freeing yourself of headaches.

As you become healthier, you will discover how energetic you can feel—and how exciting your life will become.

HEADACHE SURVEY

1. How many headaches do you usually have per week?
    a) 1 or less
    b) 2 or 3
    c) 4 or 5
    d) Daily
    e) Headaches constantly
2. About how many headaches have you had during the last six months?
    a) 2 to 5
    b) 6 to 10
    c) 11 to 20
    d) More than 20
    e) Headaches constantly

3. Your headaches last between:
   a) 0–4 hours
   b) 4–8 hours
   c) 8–12 hours
   d) 12–18 hours
   e) 18–24 hours
   f) More than 24 hours
4. The intensity of your headache is usually:
   a) Barely noticeable
   b) Mild and weak
   c) Moderate and uncomfortable
   d) Severe and distressing
   e) Excruciating and intolerable
5. Your headache is usually located in the:
   a) Forehead region
   b) Left temple region
   c) Right temple region
   d) Base of the skull
   e) Back of the neck
   f) Whole facial area
   g) Other
6. The location of your headache pain is essentially the same from one headache to the next.
   a) True
   b) False
7. Your headaches often seem to be related to (mark as many as are relevant):
   a) Emotional factors
   b) Fatigue
   c) Stressful situations
   d) Changes in the weather
   e) Lighting
   f) Food or drink
   g) Lack of food
   h) Menstruation
   i) Chemicals
   j) Drugs
   k) Other
8. How does your headache affect your daily routine and life?
   a) No interference
   b) Some interference
   c) Great interference

Common Medical Problems

    d) Confinement to bed
    e) Need for immediate medical attention
9. The pain usually comes on:
    a) Abruptly
    b) Gradually
10. Mark the characteristic(s) which describe your headache pain:
    a) Over the entire head or face
    b) Throbbing
    c) Deep, steady ache
    d) Mainly on one side
    e) Tight band around head
    f) Stabbing
    g) Other
11. If the headaches are different, how do they differ?
    a) Kind of pain (such as stabbing vs. throbbing)
    b) Location of the pain
    c) Intensity of pain
    d) Other
12. On a scale from 0 to 10, if 0 represents no pain and 10 represents the most pain you could possibly stand, how would you rate:
    a) Your worst headaches? 0 1 2 3 4 5 6 7 8 9 10
    b) Your usual headaches? 0 1 2 3 4 5 6 7 8 9 10
13. At what age did you first experience headache problems?
    a) 1–6
    b) 7–12
    c) 13–18
    d) 19–25
    e) After 26
14. If you have been to a physician, the diagnosis was:
    a) Tension headache
    b) Migraine headache
    c) Sinus headache
    d) Eye-strain headache
    e) Other
15. Check all of the following medications which you typically take for relief or prevention of your headache:
    a) Fiorinal
    b) Cafergot (ergotamine tartrate)
    c) Sansert (methylsergide maleate)
    d) Inderal
    e) Aspirin

f) Antihistamines
g) Other
16. Can you tell that you are going to have a headache prior to the onset of pain?
   a) Always
   b) Usually
   c) Sometimes
   d) Infrequently
   e) Never
17. Which of the following family members have headaches?
   a) Parent (one or both)
   b) Brother or sister
   c) Grandparent
   d) Uncle or aunt
   e) Children
   f) Other
18. As a child did you often experience headaches, nausea and/or carsickness?
   a) Often
   b) Sometimes
   c) Never
19. Which, if any, of the following foods seem to contribute to your headache?
   a) Spicy food
   b) Chocolate
   c) Milk products and/or eggs
   d) Eggs
   e) Alcoholic beverages
   f) Other
20. Are you presently taking extra estrogen as in birth control pills or menopausal medication?
   a) Yes
   b) No

For each of the items below, indicate how often the symptoms are associated with your headache by marking the appropriate letter:
   a) Always
   b) Usually
   c) Sometimes
   d) Infrequently
   e) Never

Common Medical Problems

21. _____ Buzzing, ringing, or roaring in your ears
22. _____ Heightened sensitivity to odors
23. _____ Pressure from within the head
24. _____ Nausea, vomiting, and/or inability to eat
25. _____ Sensation of wearing tight cap or a tight band
26. _____ Sensitivity to light
27. _____ Scalp tenderness
28. _____ Tearing of eyes
29. _____ Nasal congestion or drip
30. _____ Tightness in the back of the neck
31. _____ Heightened sensitivity to sound
32. _____ Loss or blurring of vision
33. _____ Double images, or strange visual patterns

References

Headache Reduction

Brainard, John B. *Control of Migraine.* New York: W. W. Norton, & Co., Inc., 1977.
Diamond, Seymour, and Jose Medina. *Headaches.* Summit, N.J.: CIBA, 1981 (booklet).
Faelten, Sharon. *No More Headaches.* Emmaus, Pa.: Rodale Press, Inc., 1982.
Hills, John R. *What You Can Do About Headaches.* Wellesley, Mass: Tufts-New England Medical Center, 1978 (booklet).
Kurland, Howard. *Quick Headache Relief Without Drugs.* New York: William Morrow and Co., Inc., 1977.
Lance, James W. *Headache: Understanding, Alleviation.* New York: Charles Scribner's Sons, 1975.
Prudden, Bonnie. *Pain Erasure: The Bonnie Prudden Way.* New York: M. Evans & Co., Inc., 1980.
Saper, Joel, and Kenneth Magee. *Freedom From Headaches.* New York: Fireside (Simon & Schuster, Inc.), 1981.
Speer, Frederic. *Migraine.* Chicago: Nelson-Hall, Inc., 1977.
Turin, Alan C. *No More Headaches!* Boston, Mass: Houghton Mifflin Co., 1981.

HEADACHE LOG

DATE	TIME BEGAN	HEADACHE INTENSITY*	HEADACHE LOCATION	HEADACHE TYPE**	PHYSICAL/ EMOTIONAL STATE***	PRIOR FOOD INTAKE	MEDI- CATION	MINUTES RELAXED	TIME OF RELIEF	INTENSITY OF RELIEF*

*INTENSITY OF HEADACHE AND RELIEF

Numerical	Intensity	Reaction
10	Extreme; excruciating; intolerable	Incapacitating; agonizing; unbearable
7-9	Severe; distressing; annoying	Concentration difficulties; miserable
4-6	Moderate; uncomfortable	Distracting but tolerable
1-3	Mild; just noticeable; weak	Bearable
0	No headache	Relieved

**HEADACHE TYPE Select: Tension, Migraine, Sinus, Hunger, Hangover, Eyestrain, Cluster, Fever, Premenstrual, Weekend, and/or Other

***PHYSICAL/EMOTIONAL STATE Select: Menstruation, Physical Exertion, Weather Change, Overslept, Insomnia, and/or Other Anger, Tension, Guilt, Depression, Fear, and/or Other

Part IV

Common Emotional Experiences

We all experience grief in our lives at times of loss or bereavement. The authors very helpfully present the fact that grief needs to be worked through thoroughly in the weeks and months following the death of a loved one, or loss of any other highly prized factor in one's life. Completed mourning is a necessary prerequisite to future happy living.

Uncompleted grief can lead to postponed reactive depression—where the next chapters take up the issues. Neurotic and endogenous (chemical) depression are also described, and their distinguishing features and causes are well-summarized. Many recommendations for the treatment and prevention of depression are given.

A shorter but almost parallel section on anxiety follows naturally. Types and causes of anxiety are summarized, and treatment and preventive measures are also described. This whole section should be read by anyone with loved ones suffering from grief, depression, or anxiety in order to be as supportive and encouraging as possible. The section ends with a brief summary of the main features of a nervous breakdown.

12
Grief

Burrell Dinkins, S.T.D., and Larry Losoncy, Ph.D.

INCOMPLETED GRIEF

> *For the moon never beams without bringing me dreams*
>   *Of the beautiful Annabel Lee;*
> *And the stars never rise but I see the bright eyes*
>   *Of the beautiful Annabel Lee....*

Annabel Lee is the beloved of the narrator in Edgar Allen Poe's famous poem of the same name. In it he tells of his love for a young woman—of her beauty, of how he dreams of her night after night. His precious, beautiful, loving bride is long since dead, however, having been stolen away from him by the chilling, killing, cruel wind of death, which came by stealth in the night when she was hardly more than a child.

What the poet has done is refuse to let his beloved be dead and gone. He tells us that still, to the day he writes, the moon never shines and the stars never come out but that he thinks of his Annabel lying cold in her sepulcher down by the sea. He expresses rage at the jealous angels who have stolen his only angel; and thus the tone of the poem is filled with his black, depressing grief. Most of all, he makes it clear that he will never let go of his love, even though she be dead. Since he refused to let her go he continues to grieve with the kind of grief that will never reach resolution, for he does not want it to be over. She is being held in limbo in his heart; she is gone from him but not all the way gone. She is dead, but not totally departed. She lives on in his heart and dreams, and he still loves her.

The poem is a good example of what ungrieved and incomplete grief embodies: depression, anger, brooding, reliving and rehashing, blaming, and even denial that the loved one is dead and gone.

Kay met her fiancé during orientation week in their freshman year of college. Both were popular and talented students. They were engaged at Christmas of their sophomore year. Everyone predicted success and happiness for this beautiful couple. Then disaster struck on an icy mountain road where he was killed in an automobile accident. Kay's family, friends, and classmates surrounded her with affection and concern. She had little time to think about what her loss meant to her emotionally. Along with her deepening depression she made excuses to stay away from friends. She was asked to go out on dates. She accepted some of the invitations to have something to do, but she was unable to have a good time. She usually refused to go out with the same person more than once. Her relationships became tentative. She went through the motions of studying and managed with her innate intellectual ability and previous work to get by in school. Basically, she had lost interest in living.

After a lecture on death and dying, Kay asked for an appointment with her professor. She wanted to talk with him about some of the symptoms of the "walking dead" he had described in class. She identifed herself as a person who had not realized the full impact of the death of her fiancé. Kay asked to talk more with her professor about her depression. She was beginning to identify some of the symptoms of emotional problems she had been reading about in a counseling book. Her major concern was her lack of responsiveness to men. When she described the events surrounding the loss of her fiancé, the professor asked her to describe her marital status (single, engaged, married, divorced, or widowed). She responded that she was technically single, but she felt widowed.

It soon became evident to her that she had developed a bond of commitment to her fiancé that was not broken by his death and burial. She related the history of the relationship and the tragic death. She was able to weep openly and begin the process of releasing her fiancé to his final resting place. The professor suggested that she not only continue the grieving process but that she also release herself from the promise to marry her fiancé. Her counselor also suggested that she make one last visit with the family at his grave to say good-bye to all the potential in-laws. Kay required no intensive therapy. She needed permission to grieve and some specific steps to take in letting go of her loved one. A few weeks later Kay dropped by the professor's office to tell him that she felt much better. Through the experience of painful grieving, she was released to enjoy dating.

The shadow of unresolved grief follows us always unless we have the courage to face the shadow and come to terms with it. As Freud said,

"The shadow of the deceased falls upon the ego of the living." If we refuse to face the shadow of the deceased loved one, something in us dies along with the loved one. Most often it is the capacity to deeply love another person. Grief is like a purging agent to clean out the powerful influence of the personality of the deceased.

Mike was a minister who served on the staff of a large metropolitan church. One of his responsibilities was visiting the sick in the hospitals. In a peer-reflection group he reported that a young man close to his age was hospitalized with terminal cancer. He found the visits extremely difficult and usually had to leave before completing what he would normally hope to achieve during a visit with a dying patient. He could not understand his emotional reactions to this patient. When asked by his peers, "Did you have a close friend during your adolescent years?" he replied that his father was a minister and the family frequently moved. This kept him from developing many close friendships, although during his high school years they did stay in one place. He then told the group about Jim and their close friendship. His expression was animated as he talked about the escapades of two buddies. Suddenly he stopped talking and became very quiet and looked sad. Someone asked, "What happened to him?" He responded, "He was killed in Vietnam and I do not want to talk about him anymore."

The subject shifted to what happened to Mike after graduation from high school. He reported that he was drafted along with other young men his age. He was sent to Germany after basic training, but most of his friends were sent to Vietnam. He was asked, "How did you learn about Jim's death?" He resisted answering but was encouraged to share what he could with the group. He related that he continued writing to his friend after arriving in Germany, but soon the letters were being returned to him by the military postal system. He thought his friend had been transferred out of his unit. One day as he was packing to go on maneuvers, a letter arrived from his mother with all the news from home. One of the sentences read, "By the way, did you hear that Jim was killed in a helicopter crash in Vietnam?" When asked about his reactions, he reported that there was no time to react because he had to leave on maneuvers with the other troops. He tried to put it out of his mind and had made himself not think or talk about Jim since then.

The group leader folded a piece of paper like a letter and handed it to Mike. He was asked to open it and read the same sentence he read ten years earlier when he first got the news about the death of his friend. Mike tried to please the person who handed him the paper by going through the actions, but kept his feelings to himself. Suddenly he became aware of the loss of a loved person whose death had not been grieved. It was as fresh as the day the loss was first experienced. First he showed shock and disbelief, then he burst into loud body-wrenching sobs which lasted for twenty to thirty minutes.

When Mike could talk again, he began to tell about his loneliness as a boy and how much having a friend in high school had meant to him. He went in and out of his sobbing as he talked. The group sat with him as he grieved. It was past time for the meeting to end so the leader suggested that they have a memorial service for Jim at the grave site. The following Sunday Mike's pastor friends gathered with him in a pouring rain to hold the service.

Mike's appearance was that of a person whose close friend had died only three days previously. The days and weeks that followed were depressing to him. He felt weak from drained emotions caused by intense grief. Through the support of his wife and his peers he began to rebuild his life—without his friend Jim, but with the capacity to feel close to other people. He reported to the group that his anxiety in visiting the young man who was dying from cancer had disappeared. He now looked forward to the visits as he walked through the "valley of the shadow of death" with the patient.

These two cases illustrate a widespread and badly misunderstood approach that many of us take toward the loss of a loved one, especially loss through death: We try not to grieve. Or, perhaps we allow ourselves to grieve for a few hours, a few days, or a few weeks. But, since life must go on, we go on with life before we have completed our grieving.

Grief may be imaged as a wound. When we love another person, we gradually invest more and more of ourselves in them. Should our loved one die, it is as though part of us—the part which we have invested in the loved one—is torn away. The result is not only the loss of the loved one but a large gaping hole in ourselves. The pain that we feel from this is what makes up grief: feelings of anger, sadness, guilt, fear, rage, denial, loneliness, depression. The wound is "bleeding."

Mike suffered such a loss; so did Kay. Since they had not healed from their wound, they continued to suffer from their grief wounds on the inside. Their grief was incomplete; they were unhealed.

In the Gospels Jesus says a very strange thing: "Blessed are they who mourn, for they shall be comforted!" Strange indeed, until we realize that the word "comfort" is an English translation of the Latin words *cum forte*. The loose translation of these two words would be "with strength." But *fortis* in Latin is a specific word, referring to that special kind of courage or strength that makes a good soldier good. Strength in this sense would be great courage, or "toughness." This kind of strong person does not easily frighten and would never be frightened again at the thought of battle, because he or she had already experienced hand-to-hand combat and lived to tell the tale. *Comfort* would then translate more accurately as "extreme bravery and strength," like that of the seasoned soldier. The sense of "Blessed are they who mourn, for they shall be comforted" would be that those who mourn can be happy knowing that in grieving their loss they have become even stronger and braver than before. It is in this sense that we approach the work of grieving. Not to resolve or complete our grief is to be permanently wounded, whereas to heal from our grief is to become stronger than ever. Mourning is a form of healing, a process unto life.

The poet who loved Annabel Lee did not know or did not choose the process of healing through deep grief. He tells us between the lines that he would rather live dead, clutching his Annabel Lee than let go of her and live alone and whole. His grief enveloped him like a perpetual thick fog, killing him from the inside.

THE ROLE OF VOWS IN LOVE AND GRIEF

Love and oaths of loyalty go hand in hand as lovers exchange their words of affection and determination to let no one come between them. "I love you and I always will," or "There will never be anyone I love as much as I love you," or "I swear there will never be anyone to take your place," or "I promise to be true to you forever," are statements frequently heard. These innocent and sincere words of commitment spoken between two sweethearts or friends help cement the bonds of a relationship. They may be the prelude to more formal declarations of loyalty such as wedding vows, when a couple promises love and fidelity to each other.

Vows and oaths reach deep into our being. They are intended to be fulfilled at all costs. They often continue in force long after the relationship has terminated. We may push the vows from conscious remembrance, but they keep coming back to influence future commitments of a similar nature.

Mary was in her fifth year of marriage and seeking counsel about her inability to feel close to her husband. She was asked to reflect upon her previous relationships with men. She started with her first engagement, but was asked to go even further back. She reported several casual dating relationships, then she spoke with great feeling about her boyfriend in the senior year of high school. She had gone to an out-of-town college to please her parents, and fifteen months after she left home, the boyfriend decided not to wait for her until she finished college. When asked what kind of promises they had made to each other, she stated clearly that she promised her boyfriend and herself that she would not let another boy get close to her. The counselor suggested that she had kept her word, even with her husband.

Mary was yet another example of ungrieved grief, even though the loss of her loved one was not to death. The grief was reinforced by vows of commitment to the lost boyfriend. In her next counseling session her counselor helped her say good-bye to the old boyfriend and to grieve what should have been grieved when the breakup occurred. There is no way to count the many persons who still hold to their vows of loyalty. They often refuse to develop another loving relationship or they give themselves only partially to their mate. It is as if another partner lives, in ghost form, demanding loyalty. There is a form of bigamy taking place, in that a love relationship is going on with the real-life partner but also with the absent partner.

Even more serious than vows to love someone always are vows that come out of disappointment and loss. These are words spoken in anger, guilt, and depression. The anger comes at the time of the loss, through death, divorce, or being "dumped." The one who suffers the loss may seek protection from further hurt with a vow against further vulnerability, such as "I'll never love another person."

James was in his third marriage and still unhappy. He was asked to reflect back to when he started protecting himself from being hurt. He reported that when his first wife left him for another man he swore that another woman would not hurt him. The counselor asked him if he swore this to God. He smiled and said, "Yes, with expletives added!" The counselor suggested he ask God to release him from his vows.

The choice between hurting and not hurting is not ours to make in moments of significant loss. Rather, it is only within our choice as to how deeply the hurt will reach in order to heal the brokenness. The refusal to grieve deeply when loss occurs spreads out the grief over a longer time—perhaps to our death—and amounts to covering over the loss rather than accepting it. The grief gets buried, not completed.

Guilt over a loss often encapsulates the grief, thus keeping it from being completed.

Christy continued to cry two years after the death of her husband. She received plenty of sympathy. She was almost addicted to people taking care of her. Her husband's insurance was enough to give her excuses not to work. She became very angry at the counselor's suggestion that her life had improved since her husband's death. Then she poured out her story about how unhappy she had been in the marriage, often wishing something would happen to her husband! She didn't have the courage to divorce him. But when death brought the fulfillment of her wishes, she was trapped in her guilt. The best way to disguise her guilty feelings (even to herself) was to cry. She vowed not to be happy again.

Guilt is a normal reaction to the loss of a person with whom we were close. We begin searching for answers as to the cause of the death. Often the finger comes back home to ourselves, whether deservedly or not.

Sue made no progress whatsoever during her first six sessions in therapy. She was drinking heavily, in danger of rupturing her chronic ulcer, depressed, angry, generally falling apart. The counselor was certain that guilt about something was at the bottom of her troubles. He decided to start all over again with a case history, asking the same questions about her age, address, when she got married, how many children she had, and so forth. This time another child showed up! During her first session she had listed all her children, living and dead, but now she listed a new child. This child had died twenty years before of an illness that Sue obviously thought could have been cured if only she had taken the child to the doctor sooner. This was her favorite daughter, and yet she had never shed a tear, as if to cry would mean unlocking the floodgates or guiltgates. She refused in any way to allow her therapist to lead her into her feelings about this daughter or the loss of this daughter, and broke off her therapy. Some months later Sue was hospitalized for a bleeding, fatal ulcer.

This was a case of a person who quite literally believed that the pain of grief, especially the feelings of guilt and sadness, were too awesome to feel. For Sue, death was less to be dreaded in her own case than was grieving at a deep and complete level. As she told her therapist, "I'll die before I let you get me to scream, cry, rage, or let go of my dead daughter."

Vows, be they explicit promises or internal resolutions, be they spoken during the ecstasy of love or at the loss of someone we love, have a powerful and long-lasting effect upon the vow maker. They bind us spiritually to the person we love. They also become or can become a substitute reaction for grieving at the loss of the loved one.

Vows are an important part of our lives. We use them to reinforce our life commitments. They should be carefully spoken if we wish to avoid emotional damage that comes from loss and grief over losses.

We have special occasions such as weddings in which to make our vows, but we have no rituals or ceremonies for releasing ourselves from vows. The need for release from our vows is essential when the relationship has terminated. We cannot *fully* terminate the relationship as long as the vows are active.

There are some ways to find release from vows. A general guide for gaining freedom from old vows is to make a request for release from the one who was the object of the vow in the first place. If it was made to another person, that person is the one who can most likely give permission to discontinue the vow. If the vow was made to God, then God should be the one toward whom the request is addressed. If the vow was made to oneself, then permission must be granted from within. Open and direct communication with the person in question is the first choice.

When the situation does not allow one to communicate directly, symbolic communication can be almost as effective. Write in letter style the history of the vow, the changes that have taken place, and the requests for release from the vow. Make believe it was mailed, but as you systematically destroy the letter, turn loose the vows made to that person. We have found this method to be effective with grieving over the death of a sweetheart or spouse. It can also be used to help complete the cycle of the relationship with a living person who might cause embarrassment in their reaction to such a request.

Vows are intended to be kept at all costs, but sometimes the cost is much too high. At other times the cost is foolish because the reason for making the vow no longer exists or functions. All that remains is the stubborn determination to keep the vow or die in some way. At such a point the person must ask, "Is my life worth a vow?"

Grief is a wound that requires mourning in order to heal. One way that healing is prevented is to let vows made to the loved one (or vows made to oneself at a time of loss) cover, block out, or otherwise encapsulate the wound.

LIVING WITH THE DEAD

Not to grieve is to get stuck in ongoing or continuing denial, anger, bargaining, and depression. We have no choice about getting hurt through loss, for loss comes to all of us in life; we also have no choice about being caught up in grief. The choice we do have is whether to grieve completely so that healing will come and we will be comforted and made strong. Attempts to block, deny, hide, or ignore our grief results in perpetual hurt by the uncompleted grief.

Denial is one way in which we are tempted to avoid grieving; so too is clinging to the lost loved one through vows and promises, tying some aspect or dimension of our present life to the memory or loyalty of the lost one because we cannot be as close to any new person as we were to the lost loved one. In the case of Mike, denial had been so complete that even Mike was surprised to discover his grief! That, of course, is what denial achieves: a kind of protection from pain.

Unfortunately for us, however, the "protection" does not make grief go away. It only prolongs the hurt and makes the wound fester as we go on living with the dead. Sue, in the following case study, was *fully* aware she was living with the dead, unlike some of the people in our earlier examples who were surprised to discover they had not let go. Sue, in fact, fully intended to visit with her father frequently for the rest of her life.

Sue came to therapy very depressed, with no apparent reason. She had never seriously dated, although she was nearly thirty years old. She wanted to get married but simply could not find anyone she really liked enough to start a romantic relationship. She had never had a steady boyfriend or even a close girl friend. The only man she had ever really liked was her father. He was the only "true friend" she could ever remember.

The routine background questions had already established that Sue's father died while she was still in elementary school. The death of her father had been pushed far back in Sue's life. After three sessions, she could still not establish any direction in her therapy. She wanted to be in therapy but did not know why; she was depressed but could not find any cause. She was neither happy nor unhappy. She lacked a sense of direction in anything she attempted.

The therapist finally looked up at her and asked, "Who is it? Who are you meeting in your dreams?"

Sue was dumbfounded: "How did you know?"

"Never mind. Tell me who it is!"

"Daddy." Out came the tears.

As Sue continued in her therapy, there emerged a story that illustrates what it is to live with the dead. When Sue was a little girl she and her father were very close, good friends. One day when she came home from school she discovered that her father had been suddenly stricken during the day, rushed to the hospital, died, and was already being prepared for burial. She had last seen her father alive and happy that morning. The next time she was to see him, he was in his casket. She stayed at a distance, afraid to go near.

Her mother, naturally, was hysterical along with the other family members and relatives. No one paid much attention to little Sue. She was on her own, half-afraid that Daddy was not actually dead and would be buried alive, half-convinced that she should pretend he was still alive. That way it would be as if he weren't gone and she could still talk to him and be happy with him.

Sue's father was buried in a cemetery between their home and the school to which she walked each day. She made it a point to go by his above-ground crypt each day to and from school and "visit" with him, telling him about what was happening and asking him questions just as she always had. Before long she noticed that he would come and visit her in her dreams.

When Sue grew up and left home for college she gave up the visits to the cemetery, though not in her dreams. Her dreams, it turned out, always ended the same way. Daddy would hold her hand and tell her he wished to go away to stay where he belonged, and he promised he would be happy there. Sue would plead with him not to go until she was ready, and he would reluctantly agree.

Sue was very aware that she was "living with the dead," or, more accurately, keeping the dead living with her. She was not angry and morbid like the poet who wrote about Annabel Lee, for her love was simple like a child's, and she had plenty of other loving people in her life. But what she began to discover in therapy was that by hanging on to her father and avoiding the final pain of letting go, she was also keeping his shadow between her and any other man with whom she might become close to and love. Even in her dreams a kind of bargaining was going on as to how and when she would let go of him.

We have said that to love someone is to invest a part of ourselves in them. The very beginning of life is such an experience, in that each one of us begins as part of our mother and for several years after birth are emotionally merged with her. "Unmerging" is painful in the most fundamental sense, even though we must do so in order to be individuals. From that point on, we find it good to be alone and good also to be with those whom we love. When we actually "fall in love" we find it much better to be together in love than to be alone. Unmerging in the sense of loss becomes painful, even overwhelming. Some of the words we use for "unmerging" when in love reflect this pain: boyfriends and girl friends call it "breaking up," married people call it "splitting up." Lovers call it tragic . . . the end . . . bad news . . . curtains.

Loss is somewhat different according to who is lost and when they are lost. The infant who loses a parent loses a loved one, but not in the same way as a child, adolescent, or adult who loses a parent; the loss of a loved friend is somewhat different in childhood than in adolescence or adulthood; the loss of a fiancé is somewhat different from the loss of a spouse; the loss of a spouse at the beginning of marriage is somewhat different from loss later in marriage.

For example, the infant who loses a mother loses the center of life, because for the infant under two years of age, the mother is the emotional center of gravity, the very love and nurture essential to thrive.

Children who lose a parent struggle often with the special guilt of blaming themselves for the loss and for becoming close to a new parent figure. Adolescents grieve both the lost parent and the good years ahead that might have been had the parent lived. This, too, is the case when a fiancé is lost or a spouse is lost early in marriage. The griever experiences the loss of a person, the special relationship, and all the fantasized expectations of a new life with the loved one.

In some cases when the relationship was not going well at the time of the death or divorce, we have found the grievers to have more grief over the happiness they did not have, the "lost years" so to speak, than at the actual loss of the person. They grieve because they feel cheated.

As Elisabeth Kübler-Ross has discovered, grief involves denial and isolation, anger, bargaining, and depression. Guilt, sadness, and panic go with these strong emotions. So does a sense of relief that it is over or that we did not die. The first and natural instinct is to protect ourselves from the hurt, the full shock, the deep pain of loss. If the "protection" succeeds, instead of grieving through to completion and letting go of our loved one so that the hole in ourselves can heal, we cover up the wound, block the grief process, and hold on to the loved one in some way. The cases we have described so far all have one fact in common: The grievers managed not to let go, carrying their dead ones forward with them in life, whether consciously or unconsciously. They paid the fearful price; they were unable to heal. Like a person dying from an undiagnosed terminal illness, they too were slowly dying by refusing to let go of their dead. They were not blessed for they had not mourned and could not be comforted, made strong, be healed.

We will now turn our attention to the question how does one heal from grief. First, we will discuss how to seek healing from ungrieved or incompleted grief, and secondly how to grieve well at the time of loss.

LETTING HISTORY BE HISTORY

We believe grief to be a healthy, though painful, reaction to loss. It is the natural and useful means whereby we find release from the attachment to persons, places, or things that have been significant to us. It is the withdrawal of ourselves from an emotional investment that has either ceased to produce positive dividends for us, or has been taken away from us. The refusal to release ourselves from someone or something that has been taken from us blocks our freedom to invest fully and joyfully in new opportunities. Ungrieved grief, encapsulated grief, condemns a person to live in the past, emotionally and mentally. A person's history is still alive in the present. In a real sense history has not become history.

Thoughts and feelings are attached to an absent person, place, or thing. The body is painfully in the present, while the spirit is tied nostalgically to the past. The transition from the past to the present can be made only through the "valley of the shadow of death" when a death has occurred.

The refusal or inability to grieve deeply enough to release the past condemns us to a future of digging up the dead. We become like the dead, continuously burying the dead. If we dare attempt to go somewhere with our life under the influence of encapsulated grief, we are like the driver who tries to see where he is going by looking in the rearview mirror.

Jeannie's dreams were picturesque symbolic descriptions of the grief process after the death of her mother. In the early weeks she dreamed about being with her mother, only to have her mother disappear before the end of the dream. Then her dreams shifted to hospital scenes and anxious attempts to help save her mother from some unseen danger. After this stage she began to dream about being in large groups of people that made her feel uncomfortable with their seriousness and concern for her.

Her dreams suddenly ceased for several weeks. Then she had a vivid dream of her mother sitting up in a casket and saying to her, "Please let me go to my resting place."

Jeannie awakened with her pillow wet from crying in her sleep. She had only one comment about the dream: "I guess I will have to release her and let her be dead as she actually is."

Our history is very important to us. The longer we live, the more we have. When we complete the stages or work of grief and successfully maneuver the transition, we acquire strength for facing the future. The biggest danger to our future is the incomplete closure of the past. In a paradoxical sense, our history as history is unavailable to us until we finish the chapters that are dead. A major task of the counselor is to help counselees complete those chapters. Then the counselees have freedom and creativity to write new chapters.

Important questions about grief include the following:

Do you find yourself talking about the past as if something were unfinished?
Do you find yourself compelled to return in fact or fantasy to the past?
Do you hold on to hostile or hurt feelings that caused the loss?
Do you hold on to hostile or hurt feelings that resulted from the loss?
Are you so full of the past experiences that you are losing the joy and creativity of the present?

We knew of a man who moved from one state to another and in the process left behind a beautiful, thriving, unusually large and healthy vegetable garden upon which he had lavished a great deal of time and energy. As it happened, he moved to another state almost as good for gardening, but because he never let go of his old garden, he had no enthusiasm for the new one, which he planted and cared for haphazardly. He talked for months about how much nicer his old garden was, but he did not realize he was grieving.

Later he told us how embarrassed he was when he realized he was grieving over tomato plants! Further, he felt silly and embarrassed to tell his family or friends what he was grieving about. He illustrates what so many of us experience in losing what might be significant to us, be it a cat, a car, a garden, a tree, a job, an office, the seashore, a good fishing place—we feel embarrassed to actually name the loss and let it be publicly known that we are grieving over it. Often we try to convince ourselves not to grieve anything so "silly." But we need to grieve what is lost, or risk losing the future!

The grief experience can pull down both the griever and the fragile support system that provides the only means of hope. The grief-stricken person is often told not to cry, not to get too upset! But this advice is more for the benefit of the emotional state of the support person than the griever! Some persons in grief are told the "little lies" of good intention such as: "She is better off now," or "You will get over this very soon," or "Everything will be all right," or "Try to forget about it," or "Stiff upper lip," or "He or she wouldn't want you to cry."

Hospital personnel may give medication to the grieving family as they dispensed medication to the dying relative to lessen the pain. Careful assessment should be made of a person's grief, however, before medication is given. Only persons with known medical risk to high stress should be given medication, and then only to maintain the person's equilibrium. Indiscriminate medication can prolong or encapsulate the grief.

Grief has its own built-in stages to allow for gradual release and relief. The griever needs permission and assistance to pass through the painful steps of grief. In a sense, grief is analogous to natural childbirth. In our time the movement toward natural childbirth came from a revolt against too much or too little help, both of which can hinder the baby and the mother. What is most helpful is the presence of supportive persons who care and who know what to do and when to do it. Only in recent years have we begun to return birthing to the normal life experience it was meant to be. Special help is given only in the emergencies of abnormal births. At the other end of life (death and grieving) are normal processes where informed, caring persons who know what to do or not to do also are needed.

Relating the history of the relationship is one important help for a person in grief. This may be done all at once or in stages according to the available time and energy of the griever. The support person helps the grief sufferer tell the story in a way that facilitates catharsis, which is the flushing out of the grief.

Mrs. Peabody was called to the hospital after an accident involving her husband. She feared that he had the accident while driving under the influence of alcohol and her fears were confirmed at the hospital. She waited long hours with her three teenagers until the surgeon and the chaplain informed them that her husband died during surgery. The chaplain remained in the room with them, listening to the recent history of a husband-father who also was an alcoholic. Mixed emotions of love and anger were freely expressed along with the tears.

The chaplain asked Mrs. Peabody to tell him how she and her husband first met and what they liked about each other. He asked how long they dated, about their engagement, the wedding, their first house, the jobs they had and places they lived. He carefully walked the family through their history, often stopping for waves of tears as they recalled both happy and sad times. He brought them through the painful part of the recent history and to the point of the fatal accident. He was then able to say to them, "Now your husband, your father, is dead. It seems you have a new chapter in your family history." The chaplain helped them review their background before talking with them about important decisions that had to be made for the funeral and the future.

The chaplain was trained in crisis intervention and grief work. Much of what he had learned in order to help facilitate grief can be learned by caring persons. He used what are called the "rearview mirror" approaches to grief work. It is like taking a good look in the mirror when a crisis occurs to see what is behind before trying to look out of the windshield into the future. Naturally, the windshield is more important than the rearview mirror; both, however, are necessary for safe driving.

Listed here are some steps that can be taken to help a grieving person review the history of a person, place, or thing irretrievably lost.

1. Be genuinely interested in the story. Find ways to assist the telling so that facts and feelings about important events are fully expressed.
2. Remain nonjudgmental. A person experiencing grief feels enough guilt and judgment. Listen to their opinion about the story of the deceased and the past relationship.
3. Find the appropriate time and setting for telling the story. Some people are embarrassed or afraid to be honest in front of persons listening to the history.
4. Be prepared for different versions of the history during various stages of grief. A deceased relative who was seen in an idealized

light soon after the death may be viewed differently weeks later.
5. Give encouragement for the expression of feelings. The griever may need to know it is permissible to cry in your presence. Provide tissue or handkerchief as a signal that crying is acceptable.
6. Where the grief has been encapsulated, encourage the person to express the feelings and thoughts through writing a letter (not to be mailed) to the deceased. A visit to the cemetery may uncap the encapsulated grief.
7. Ask the griever to show you a series of pictures or photographs of the deceased. Visualization from seeing the picture may facilitate the grief process even years after the loss.

We need to know what we are doing with grief work and why we are doing it as we help persons allow their history to become history. This is called helping the "almost" dead bury the dead so that they can live again through and beyond their grief. Then and only then are they free to look through the windshield and face the future with confidence.

BLESSED ARE THEY WHO MOURN

The paradox of grief is that although it feels like a curse while we are going through it, we are blessed after having experienced it. Either we are made stronger through the mourning process, or we are weakened by avoiding it. We are released from the deceased through the pain of grief, or we are condemned to bear the weight of the loss for the rest of our lives. No one likes to grieve; however, no one is healed from a significant loss without the purging release of the grief experience.

As Shakespeare wrote: "There is a tide in the affairs of men. . . . omitted, all the voyage of their life is bound in shallows and in miseries." In the context of this work, the "tide" is the experience of pain that comes from the cathartic release of emotion that floods over the grieving person.

Jesus said, "Blessed are they who mourn." This paradoxical statement needs to be seen in light of the consequences of refusing to grieve when an important loss has occurred. The blessing is the result of finished grief. The loss has finally been accepted. The person is whole again and able to establish healthy relationships with others. The individual is a blessing to be around because the heart is actively present in the now, instead of looking with nostalgia to the past.

There are many reasons why people become sidetracked in their grief, and are thereby unable to successfully complete the normal process of mourning over a loss.

Some of these reasons are:

Common Emotional Experiences

- Lack of information about the healthy aspects of grief
- Cultural prohibitions
- Myths about death and dying
- Overintellectualization about the facts and details surrounding the loss
- Lack of time
- Fear of feelings
- Insufficient support
- Embarrassment over loss of usual composure

Persons afraid of strong emotions, as well as those who have the common tendency to label emotions as good or bad, may perceive grief as a threat. There is no mourning without the expression of emotions. The blessing that comes from mourning is the freedom that comes after the emotions are safely and fully expressed. How these emotions are expressed will depend upon individual personality dynamics and the cultural context.

We will now look at the *normal* process of grief, with an example of a griever who kept a careful diary of his experiences at the time of his father's death. He has given us permission to use this material so we can reflect on his stages of grief and compare this with the dynamics of encapsulated grief.

Jim learned that his father was diagnosed as having inoperable cancer. The full impact of this information did not hit him until he made a special trip to see his father. As he left the family home, he was able to drive no more than a block before a flood of tears blinded his eyes, forcing him to pull over to the side of the street.

Jim was in anticipatory grief. The system of denial surrounding him crumbled as he remembered how his father said good-bye. Jim knew he would never again see him alive, and he began preparing himself for his father's death. Two months later his brother called to say their father would die very soon. Jim wrote about his initial reactions:

> *I couldn't believe what my brother was saying. I felt a numbness come over me. I knew my brother would not have called me if Dad was not in serious condition, but I couldn't comprehend the fact that Dad would soon be dead. I felt confused. The fact could not register in my mind. I was dazed. As I made preparation to leave, I avoided the issue. There were no tears, only numbness.*

In the words above Jim describes the most common reaction to a painful loss, whether anticipated or not. Researchers on grief report that shock, numbness, and denial are the first stage of grief in sudden and unexpected loss experiences. The mind and emotions become temporarily numbed to the pain of the loss. The most commonly heard expression is, "Oh, no!" Everything in us says no to the reality of loss.

In encapsulated grief, the mind accepts the fact of the loss, but the emotions are another story. Emotions do not approve the reality and wage war on the mind, refusing to acknowledge the facts. Thus, the person becomes sandwiched in between reality and what used to be. This conflict is fierce and quite painful.

Jim wrote in his diary while flying back home:

> *I love my dad. But I honestly wish he'd hurry up and die. I cannot miss too much work. Let's just get it over with. I know that I sound like a creep, but why should I lie about it?*

A few minutes later he wrote:

> *If my dad is going to die, he'd better wait until I get home. Oh, I don't care. Let's get it over with. I hate to see him—and me—suffer. Why does it have to be this way?*

Jim's emotional reactions were anger mixed with fear. He was afraid of facing the situation involving death. He dreaded going home to face his feelings about his father and honestly portrays his feelings about this death in his diary. In encapsulated grief, the ambivalence is not allowed to surface to conscious awareness. The lost person or place is seen as being totally good or totally bad. Mixed feelings remain hidden or become split between good persons and bad persons. Jim's fear and anger were also expressed toward God when he wrote:

> *I hate you, God! . . . I do not want to be mad at God. I am upset with my dad for dying. God, I dread going home.*

As happens so often when a person we love dies, we are forced to reexamine our relationship with God. Jim's mixed feelings about his father spilled over toward God. Thus, the loss of a significant other [person] may be reflected in the loss of faith in God. The grieving person may in anger blame God for the death or in guilt blame self for not rescuing the dying person.

A common characteristic of persons in unresolved grief is that they have not faced the blame (anger) and the guilt. Someone did someone wrong and they will not be forgiven. This can be projected onto others or

Common Emotional Experiences

incorporated into oneself. Forgiveness is lacking. Resentment prevails. Jim continued his story:

> When I arrived at the airport my brother-in-law met me and immediately informed me that Dad had died. I became angry. Why did he tell me so suddenly? I was mad and relieved at the same time. My heart felt ripped apart. I walked a few steps. My brother-in-law kept talking, but I could hardly hear his words. I asked if I could sit down. I cried body-wrenching sobs. It hurt all over.

This immediate release of emotions through crying that involves every muscle in the body is a healthy reaction to the awareness of the reality of the loss. The sooner and the deeper the grief-stricken person can do this the better will be the recovery. In our grief work, we often facilitate the release of pent-up tears that should have been expressed when the loss first occurred. As one client said, "I feel like I have been walking around with a bucket of tears inside!"

Withdrawal or isolation are common reactions in grief. Jim wrote:

> When I arrived home, I realized immediately that my family was definitely in a different stage of grief than myself. They were not crying but were very calm about it all. Immediately this repulsed me and I sought asylum in a bedroom. Then I cried. Waves of tears came. I tried to hold them back, but they kept coming.

Jim is describing the normal reaction to acceptance of death. The waves of grief offer the best, though the most painful, hope for healing. The griever's health depends upon the release of the emotions. Encapsulated grievers have been cheated from experiencing body-cleansing grief after a loss. Instead, they are condemned to a lifetime of nearly imperceptible grief that keeps the tears locked inside.

Jim's next stage could easily be predicted by persons familiar with the process of grief. He reported:

> I had difficulty and confusion as I walked around the house. I listened to hear my father cough or talk. I expected to see him any minute. My memories played tricks on me. The denial of his death could no longer stand unchallenged in the face of the emptiness of the house. My mind did not give up the fantasy, that he was not really dead, without a struggle.

Jim was aware his mind was playing tricks on him. He stood between life as it had been and the reality of life without the familiar presence of his father. The encapsulated griever often gets trapped in mind games. The loss is accepted factually, but the fantasy games of "if only" or "not really" still prevail. The dead one has only died partially. The living one is only partially alive.

Jim went to the funeral home to view the body of his father. He was still in a form of denial when he saw his father. He wrote:

> *I looked at the flowers and the clothes he was wearing. I thought about the socks that would keep his feet warm. I touched his face. Then the loss hit me in my gut. I knew I had to let him go. I cried and cried and cried. I envied the women who could cry more easily than the men. Maybe that is why they live longer. Most of the men were unable to openly express their grief.*

Jim came to the moment of acceptance of the death when he encountered the lifeless body of his father. With his tears he released his father to the company of the dead. In contrast, the encapsulated griever has not taken the decisive step of releasing the deceased. The lost person is no longer alive, but neither is he or she buried. The encapsulated griever sees all the detailed facts, but fails to experience the personal significance of the loss, just as at first Jim was thinking about the socks.

Jim is on his way through the normal grief process. He still has much grieving to do, though on a different level. He continues:

> *After the funeral, I was depressed and so lonely. I realized more and more that I have actually lost my father. He was such a meaningful part of my life. Why did he have to die? I will miss him. It helped me to cry when I saw the flowers and read each card; I realized how much their sympathy meant to me.*

Depression and loneliness after a major loss are normal reactions for a period of three to twelve months. A short-term depression serves the purpose of conserving energies and allowing the process of healing to reach into various levels of the personality. It is the long-term depression after major loss that we call encapsulated grief. The grief has not been released. The person is stuck in the grief process. Time does heal the brokenhearted, except for the encapsulated griever. For the encapsulated griever, time only prolongs the suffering. A person remains trapped in bondage to grief until release comes from an outside source.

Jim returned to his reflection eighteen months after the death of his father:

> *The most intense period of grieving was basically the six months immediately following my father's death. This was a time when the tears*

> of mourning came easily and usually very unexpectedly. There were several times that I broke down and wept almost uncontrollably months after Dad's death. Comments, memories, or certain mannerisms of people would remind me of Dad and trigger a strong emotional release. During this time of mourning I experienced a tremendous sense of loss, unlike any other I had ever experienced.
>
> I think the initial shock of Dad's death protected me from experiencing all this at once. But as the sense of shock wore off over the days and weeks, the reality of Dad's death became more apparent. It was as if God designed my mind to break the news to me gently. In many ways, the sense of shock is like romantic love. It's blinding and anesthetizing. I believe this enabled me to handle the loss a little bit at a time as I was able.

Jim's suffering during the normal stages of grief was mostly psychological. However, there were physiological effects as well. He writes:

> I felt drained and tired most of the time. I believe this was a result of the increased emotional and mental energy needed to cope with the intensity of the grief experience. My blood pressure went from a normal 125/80 to a consistent 150/110. I've heard that elevated blood pressure is a natural anesthesia. Yet I wondered about the effect it would have on my body.

Jim had reason to be concerned about physical changes in his body. Many studies have documented the high rate of hospital admissions after the death of a close family member. Suicide and deaths from other causes increase during this time. Not enough evidence has been collected to establish the precise correlation of destructive results from normal versus encapsulated grief, but the evidence seems to point in the direction of vast adverse effects, which occur over a much longer period of time for the encapsulated griever. Normal grief gradually restores us to life. Encapsulated grief may gradually lead us to death.

Jim's reflection of his grief experience eighteen months after the death of his father gives us further insight into the spiritual dimension of grief:

> The acute period of grief was accompanied by intense faith struggles. My anger toward God eventually resulted in my questioning the existence of God. When Dad died, God died also. More correctly stated, my concept of God had to change if there was to be a God in my life. Dad's death destroyed my concept of the miracle-working, always intervening God. It took me months to develop a concept of God that saw Him as caring and present, not always handing out "miracles," a God who allowed death. I have a new understanding of God's

> *grace. I didn't have to like Him or even believe in Him for Him to love me. I discovered that He loved me even when I was angry with Him. He believed in me even when I did not believe in Him.*

Jim's faith struggles are common to normal grief. He was honest and open with his feelings toward God. In encapsulated grief, the sufferer still holds a grudge against God for robbing him of the life that once existed. On the other hand, the person in grief may try to appease God for all the hateful thoughts that came out during the intense suffering. Many devout religious persons live in intense fear of a vengeful God who will get back at them for their anger. Some may become religious to overcome their negative ambivalence toward the deceased. Death frees them from bondage to the deceased, but they take on a new bondage called guilt. They are glad the dead person is dead but they feel guilty for feeling that way.

Jim finished his reflection about the positive effects of the grief experience:

> *My grief experience has been a catalyst for personal growth in almost every area of my life. I feel much more aware of my own feelings and I am definitely more sympathetic to others who suffer great losses. I feel like my personality and outlook have gone through positive changes since my dad's death. The grief process is not completely over. Christmas was very hard and quite sad. I still miss Dad and think of him often. The loss was real. The healing has come with hope. Yet, I am still growing through the experience and receiving the help of others who care. But even now I feel better about myself and my future.*

The major difference between healthy and encapsulated grief is that the first produces growth through suffering. The second fails to complete the grief, thereby preventing growth and the healing processes. With unfinished grief the blessing from mourning is yet to be received because the grief continues in the hidden recesses of the griever's life. The bondage of ungrieved grief is the curse of living with the dead.

The case of Jim helps us see the normal stages of grief. Through Jim's experience we can see the blessings from mourning that await those who fully grieve their losses.

CHILDREN AND THEIR GRIEF

Before they reach the teenage years, children probably suffer more losses than others because they have very little control of their world. They must move geographically when their family moves; they cannot stop their parents from divorcing. Their pets die or run away. They can be separated from their friends by the school teacher or principal or by the friends' families moving away. Their losses are both large and small, but to a small child, all losses are big.

The biggest loss to small children is the death of a parent, brother, or sister. The first thing to bear in mind about helping children with this kind of loss is that often, long before or even shortly before the death of a loved one, the child may have wished them dead. Because children have only a relatively simple and unsophisticated sense of cause and effect, they very often assume that their wish was the cause of the death; often, when this is the case, they are terrified to tell anyone else about it.

Sometimes children remember the loved one having said such things as, "You will be the death of me yet," or "You are killing me with your whining," or "You'll drive us to our grave with your complaining." It is important, with *all* children who have lost a loved one, that a caring adult in their life speak with them several times *at length* about what has happened and what the child is feeling and thinking. This gives a chance to make sure that if the child is feeling responsible, there be an opportunity to set things straight.

In this same vein, children need reassurance about any other of the many guilts and regrets they might be experiencing about the loved one's time with them on earth. Regrets about not being a better boy or girl, not being more helpful, not visiting the loved one more or taking better care of the loved one during illness, perhaps forgetting a birthday are just a few of the concerns a child might be struggling with.

Children, especially younger children, may have misconceptions about what death means. Each of these misconceptions needs to be talked through in a reassuring manner. Some of the more common misconceptions include the idea that dead people are only sleeping and will be buried alive. Perhaps they will wake up underground and starve to death or suffocate, or maybe they will be left all alone, forever locked in the coffin. Another is that they are not dead, and that the mortician will kill them.

Children often believe that their loved ones will get lonely for them in heaven. Sometimes they wonder if there will be anything to eat in heaven, or if there will be a Christmas tree and birthday parties, or if there will be friends. Often children think God "did this" to the loved one, and might get the child next. They may also wonder whether the loved one can still hear them.

The younger the child, the more important it is to translate freely and answer questions concretely. For example, we believe the child who asks if Grandpa will have a rocking chair and pipe in heaven could be told yes, because to say no would mean to the child that Grandpa will be unhappy in heaven. If you are unwilling to answer this concretely, you can simply assure the child that Grandpa will have what he needs to be happy in heaven. Although there are those who would disagree, in our opinion, for very young children it is acceptable to speak of pets that have died as having gone to "animal heaven." Surely the Lord does not mind small children believing that their animals live on in happiness? And how do we know for certain that this is not the case since it is not mentioned in Scripture?

Death of a Child's Parent

When a child's parent dies, imagine how confused and hurt the child can be. This mother or father was the very center of the child's life. What will happen now? To add to the problem, others can be so caught up in their grief that the child is not even noticed. The grief of children is often treated as secondary or incidental to that of grieving adults. You often hear such statements as "They will get over it," or "They don't understand," or "They don't know what happened," or "They don't know he or she is dead," or "They have each other." Even worse, sometimes children are simply viewed as another problem caused by the death: "What will we do with them?"

At the wake and funeral, the grieving child or children are often at a loss. Some of their questions and concerns, which often do not get asked out loud, are:

"Am I to blame?"
"What will happen next?"
"Could I die?"
"Who will love me now?"
"Poor Mommy."
"Don't get in the way."
"Somebody hold me, help me, notice me."
"Why are they saying Daddy is so happy but everybody is crying?"

What the grieving child needs is *support* and *love* from the surviving adults. In such a context, one of the tasks for the loving adults is to explain to the grieving child what has and has not happened in the death of the loved one, and what happens at a funeral. Then the child needs to be helped to decide whether to go to the funeral (most will go) and to be comforted at the funeral and graveside services. The child also needs to be held that night and many nights, while he or she cries and remembers the lost loved one with the inevitable tears, questions, and pain. *Support* means held, hugged, talked to, listened to, helped to rage, cry, ask questions, feel bad, be depressed—for as long as several years!

Helping children grieve also means to cry with them, to share emotional reactions with them, and to let them know that adults, too, are sad, depressed, hurt, and bewildered.

Children also need to know of our faith in life after death, assuming we do so believe. They need to learn of our hope; they need to know that we grieve, but not as those who have no hope. Those who believe in life after death must also realize that both believers and nonbelievers grieve, for it is human to grieve at loss. The difference is that believers grieve a loss to themselves, knowing that the lost one lives on in eternity.

Other Losses and Griefs

Children, like adults, are suffering losses all the time. Life brings change. Children lose friends, teachers, their school, their homeroom teacher, pets, homes, bedrooms, toys. Children suffer many losses and mostly because of events which they can neither control, understand, or prevent. These events can become opportunities for helping children learn to grieve and heal from loss. When these losses *can* be prevented, it would be good for us to do so.

For example, if the next promotion means a move, the needs of the children should be considered in the making of the decision. If a move is to be made, be sure to work with the children in helping them prepare for the losses that the move will bring.

Children are children. Their attachments and loves, often poorly articulated and frequently half-hidden, can seem "childish" to adults. Remember they *are* children. As adults we may think how could a child love a stuffed animal enough to cry when it falls apart? How can a child be so attached to a pet as to be depressed and grieve when it is sick, or hurt, or dies?

We knew a teenage girl whose cat was killed. The loss was like losing a close friend and yet she couldn't explain her grief to people for fear of ridicule. She was surprised to learn that such love and such grief did not mean she was sick or crazy. She had invested a good part of herself in this cat. When the cat died, a good part of herself was torn away. A therapist suggested to her that she bring in pictures of her cat to their next session. She brought a full album of pictures, many of which were taken with her own camera. A whole hour was spent in relating the joys and heartaches of loving and losing a pet. Amazingly, too, as she wept over the death of her cat, her depression lifted.

Children, just as much as adults, invest themselves in what they love. Their losses are devastating, but the scale of their world is often too small for adults to notice. For example, the loss of a little friend may seem insignificant to the adults of the family, when they notice that their child has many, many friends who all seem to be alike. A child may be crying herself to sleep while the parents are discussing in another room "how well" she is doing!

Take the grief of children seriously, all of it!

HOW TO GRIEVE

As adults, we may need to complete encapsulated grief. From time to time we will certainly need to grieve new losses; for as life continues and we age we will lose more and more. To grow is to let go.

A way to get going with uncompleted grief is to get *all* the way back into the past and focus on what was lost. If the loss be a loved person, get a picture of the person or go back in time and space until in memory the person is present: *We are together, I am with them in some favorite place or activity, the scene is firmly fixed in my mind's eye. I can hear the voice and the sounds in the background.*

If the loss be a job or some object, get it firmly into focus. If the loss be a way of life or some favorite activity, "relive" a day, an hour, a golden moment, get into the feelings and sensations; imagine it is happening all over again.

After the loss is firmly in focus, let the feelings flow along with whatever sounds, words, speeches, yelling, kicking, screaming, sobbing, and shaking come to you. To do this even for thirty minutes, six or seven days in a row, would be enough to bring the entire grief wound into play and allow us to either commit more deeply to the work of healing or to realize that it is over and we must go forward with our lives. Like the clergyman who watched the grieving widow clutching desperately to her husband's casket as it was ready to be lowered into the ground, we may discover that the time has come. He noticed that the widow was preventing her husband from being buried; she was not about to let go, and she was screaming at the top of her voice, "I can't be without him!" So the minister looked up and gave the funeral attendants instructions to lower her away with her husband and bury them both! She instantly let go! And so can we. The most frequently heard comment after all the grieving has been completed is, "What a relief!" "I feel *so much* better!"

Present Grief

The first thing we need to remember about grieving present losses is that grief is a process: the deeper the loss, the deeper the wound, and the longer to heal. In the case of a loved one, the healing process takes six months to a year or even two years. That does not mean, of course, months and years of nonstop crying and anger.

What we "have to do" is experience the bundle of emotions that we have generally understood to be unpleasant and undesirable: anger, rage, tears, guilt, fear, insecurity, isolation. We must realize that no emotions are bad or wrong. Actually, all are useful and necessary for a fully functioning human being. We get into trouble when we suppress awareness of some and attempt to overuse more pleasant ones.

Not Only in Death

As adults we suffer a great many losses other than death. Perhaps the most frequent loss besides the death of a loved one is a divorce. Here the loved one is definitely lost, except that in addition to the loss there is the blow of rejection which comes from being abandoned by a loved one who is still alive and who, often enough, chooses another lover. Divorce is traumatic for the same reasons that death of a loved one is traumatic. Part of self was invested in the loved one, and now is ripped out with the leaving of the loved one, and the wound bleeds with all the grief hurt. In addition, our self-confidence suffers a serious beating—and we generally assume we must be ugly inside and out.

What is lost in divorce is not only a loved one, but a way of life, a total relationship, a marriage with the friends and relatives attached. There is lost a central relationship of life. Usually with such a loss goes a drop in self-confidence, self-esteem (no one else likes me and neither do I), accompanied by a sense of failure. We also get very angry, very hurt, very depressed, very isolated, very afraid, and very insecure. Letting history become history takes a methodic, organized effort. The effort needs to be scheduled. The tears, the questions, the crying, the standing in front of a mirror and finding good points, the praying; all this needs to be done.

In addition to the loss of divorce are other major kinds of loss, such as destruction of a home, loss of a job, bankruptcy (loss of credit and self-esteem). These sorts of losses, just like death and divorce, represent serious upheaval and personal devastation. They are to be dealt with by grieving over a period of time, until they become integrated into our history, and we become free of the rancor, depression, and constant looking into the past.

"Happy Griefs"

We need also to realize that many many of our adult happy events bear grieving, too—something which is not generally done in our culture. The marriage of a son or daughter, for example, is supposed to be a happy occurrence, and we are supposed to beam as the proud parents! The wedding is to be so joyful, and everyone is to smile and be excited, when in fact our hearts are breaking. We realize they can never be ours again and the place won't be the same without them—the room will be so sad and empty, and we will miss them so terribly. It may seem disloyal to say any of that and grieve, so what do people do at weddings? Some get angry and fight before the wedding and get depressed and withdrawn after the wedding—and they do not express their grief because in our culture the tears are supposed to be hidden in the joy.

So, too, with promotions, which often mean moving away from friends, neighborhood, established routines. We are expected to be all smiles. We saw this in the case of a man who was retiring. He was treated as though this meant only good news: He should smile and be happy. Now he is going to stay home in the mornings instead of coming into work. The retiree received the praise in the speeches and the gift from the company, and he heard how lucky he is now that he is free, and so forth. He could not share his grief, could not say how sorrowful the occasion really was for him, could not cry and beat on the wall and rage and bewail the loss, for the occasion demanded that it not be experienced or perceived as a loss, but as a *gain*! Those who notice the retiree expressing any sadness whatsoever, especially crying, tell him or her not to be sad. So often the retiree *believes* there is nothing to grieve, wonders about the depression, actually suspects something is wrong because he or she does not "feel better" about the whole retirement, and becomes even more afraid to openly express or to even grieve secretly. The grief is covered over, just as at weddings, and a person is considered crazy to insist that there *is* loss, that there *is* grief on the underside of the good news. And there is!

Small Things

Sometimes our losses are not large, but small. These too must be noticed. Sometimes we lose smaller and seemingly "silly" or "trivial" attachments, such as gardens and plants, dishes, and pets. It is important *not to assume* that such losses in our children's lives are trivial. For ourselves, we must not assume that because a loss of ours is trivial, it should be ignored. *All* griefs are waiting to be healed, so all loss needs to be grieved, even if it is the loss of something as seemingly insignificant as a change of offices or the loss of a tennis partner.

In Conclusion

To grieve is to heal.

Blessed are they who mourn . . . not because grieving is fun, and not because sorrow really isn't sorrow—but blessed are they who mourn at a loss as compared with those who will not grieve their losses. Those who are willing to mourn shall be healed of their losses.

To be healed of grief is to become whole and strong enough again to go on living fully with the memory of the lost loved one or thing, but without all the grieving emotions of that loss once the grief is completed and the loss has become history. To mourn is to cheat death of any more than what death has already claimed; it is to let the dead be dead but allow the living to live fully and free from the shadow of death—to not die before our time. It is to accept our history as history, and live until we die, whole and complete, healed of our losses and open to new love and new life.

Grief comes in three basic forms: anticipatory, present, and encapsulated (unfinished and blocked) from the past. Grief needs to be considered in all stages of life. Grief can be over things, events, processes, as well as over living things such as pets or plants. Most of all, grief is over the loss of loved ones. In every case, grief is a loss, a wound. Healing is needed. Time can heal only clean wounds, and grief wounds can only be cleansed with tears.

13
Depression
O. Quentin Hyder, M.D.

WHAT IS NORMAL DEPRESSION?

Normal depression is the experience of grief, or the process of mourning, which are feelings of sadness and emptiness that follow the loss of any significant loved object or person.

Grief is universal, and therefore normal, because everyone experiences a sense of loss many times during a lifetime. It is the natural emotional response to a loss of any kind. It is an experience of deprivation producing psychological, emotional, physical, social, and even spiritual effects. Whenever any valued or pleasurable part of one's personal life is lost, there is grief or mourning.

The commonly recognized signs of grief are: (1) crying, which has the beneficial effect of expressing deep feelings, and thereby releasing tension; (2) depressed mood, leading to temporary withdrawal from others; (3) agitation or restlessness, resulting in insomnia, possibly with nightmares; and (4) reduced daytime functioning efficiency. Other temporary effects include loss of appetite, episodes of anxiety, feelings of guilt or anger, irritability, reduced sexual interest, and a generalized loss of enthusiasm or energy for getting things done.

Anniversary reactions also occur, often long after initial recovery, with a recurrence of the signs and symptoms of grief on such occasions as Christmas, Thanksgiving, New Year's Eve, birthdays, wedding anniversaries, and of course the date of death of the loved one.

Normal grief involves emotional pain, sorrow, low depressed mood, and sometimes feelings of loneliness, anger, or anxiety. Often physical symptoms and even deterioration in interpersonal relationships can result. Its duration may vary from a few weeks to many months depending on the quality of the relationships both in the past with the deceased, and in the future with new friends.

Grief is not only normal and natural. It is also necessary, indeed essential and healthy. It is important to go through a temporary period of mourning after a loss to prevent a more serious reactive depression later. If grief is not appropriately and adequately expressed in the days and weeks following a loss, the bereaved one is more likely to experience the full depth of abnormal or excessive depression up to several months later.

The open expression of grief should therefore be neither stifled by the bereaved nor discouraged by well-meaning sympathetic friends. When grief is not fully experienced, it could be either the result of denial or avoidance, or that there was not a close relationship with the deceased in the first place. This latter could lead to guilt feelings, or delayed but protracted depression, which could occur much later.

Although usually the greatest sense of loss a person experiences is the death of a loved one, grief can also be felt with a wide variety of other kinds of losses or disappointments. Common causes for grief feelings are such life experiences as divorce, retirement, property damage, personal injury, declining health, mugging or burglary, amputation of any body part, or the loss of any object of intrinsic or sentimental value.

Other less tangible losses include: a child leaving home for college, moving one's home away from a familiar neighborhood, death of a family pet, defeat in any important game, sporting event, or election, or such subjective experiences as a loss of a good sense of self-esteem, or the development of doubts in the area of philosophical or religious beliefs.

The process of grief, though a universal human experience, has only recently been scientifically studied. The word *thanatology* means the study of the process of dying and of coping with bereavement. The preeminent work in this new field is the 1969 publication of the outstanding book *On Death and Dying* by the previously unknown psychiatrist Dr. Elisabeth Kübler-Ross.

Almost in parallel with Dr. Kübler-Ross's five stages of dying, there seem to be five fairly well-recognized phases of grief or mourning.

1. *Shock,* with a sense of numbness, disbelief, and even denial.
2. *Emotional release* with crying, and an appropriate normal phase of reactive depressed mood.
3. *Yearning* for the recovery of the lost object or person with a sense of empty loneliness (that transitional period).
4. *Acceptance* of reality with the gradual anxious realization of the inevitability of a need for changes and readjustments.

5. *Reorganizing* of life-style, behavior, and interpersonal relationships leading to eventual overcoming of the grief, with any accompanying residual guilt or anger, and the beginning of a new life.

"Grief work" was a term first used by Freud. It means the task of mourning, which is hard work—slow, painful, and long. It involves untangling oneself from the ties that bound one to the deceased, readjusting to life without him or her, and the forming of new relationships.

It requires breaking through the initial denial or disbelief; accepting the reality that the past and the deceased are dead; rethinking, reflecting, and reexamining the past repeatedly; and reliving past memories, pleasant and unpleasant, again and again, until the past can finally be buried and understood in the beauty and blessing that it had been.

Grieving persons do not need pat answers or sticky-sweet platitudes. They need friends, willing, with patience, understanding, and realistic reassurance to listen to them express their feelings. They need to be given every opportunity to pour out their appropriate feelings to close friends and relatives.

Encourage, but do not pressure, the bereaved one to verbalize every thought and feeling that seems to need to be expressed. Help the widow to talk through her immediate problems, and, where appropriate, discuss with her necessary important decisions that need to be made. Discourage any irrational conclusions and provide practical help whenever possible. Actions speak louder than words.

Out of the process of mourning a new more mature person emerges with new attitudes, new values, new priorities, and new appreciations of life itself. Such changes lead to the personal growth that can make all the suffering worthwhile. This refinishing process is truly a gift or blessing in disguise to anyone who fully grieves.

WHAT IS ABNORMAL DEPRESSION?

Later you will read about depressions of *biochemical* or *neurotic* origin that are not related to loss. In this section we are concerned with *reactive* depression, which is in essence an excessive grief experience following a severe loss of a loved object or person. When does grief go beyond being a normal mourning reaction and become abnormal or pathological depression?

The main evidences of abnormality in the grief experience are undue *delay, intensity,* or *duration. Delay* in grieving may result from a protracted period of unrealistic denial in which the bereaved one fails to mourn appropriately through an inability or unwillingness to accept the objective facts of his loss. This can lead eventually to a severe reactive depression many months later when the passage of time eventually forces the mourner to face reality.

Increased intensity of grief to an abnormal degree may be evidenced by some of the following symptoms: an attitude of helplessness or hopelessness; self-condemnation, excessive false guilt feelings; extreme withdrawal from others; impulsive or antisocial behavior; drug taking or excessive alcohol consumption; development of hypochondriac aches and pains; and threats, veiled or specific, of suicide.

In addition, abnormal grief may be evidenced by the mourner's verbalizing feelings of very low self-worth, unwarranted hostility toward others, preoccupation with the deceased, veneration of objects previously owned by him, hyperactivity, and resistance to accepting advice, comfort, or offers of practical help.

Excessive duration is the third evidence of abnormality in the grief process. Although in our culture a year of mourning is often considered to be appropriate, it could be quite normal for it to be shorter or longer. It could be shorter if there had not been a very close relationship between the deceased and the bereaved, if the relationship was based on ambivalent feelings, of if the bereaved enters quickly into a substituting relationship with someone else. An abnormally short mourning period can lead to profound guilt feelings later, or to a delayed reactive depression.

Mourning for more than a year could be normal if the deceased was a child, especially an only child, or a spouse with whom the bereaved had happily spent the bulk of his or her life span, and there was little prospect of remarriage. Anniversary reactions, feelings of grief on birthdays, wedding days, holidays, and so forth, are of course commonly experienced and normal. Failure to adjust to a new life-style without the deceased within a year or two should be regarded as pathological, and the bereaved in need of counseling or even medical treatment.

WHAT KINDS OF PEOPLE GET DEPRESSED?

Depression or melancholia has been well-recognized and documented since the dawn of human history. Whereas the post-World War II period was often called the "age of anxiety," we are living today in what is frequently called the "age of melancholy." Nathan Kline, M.D., pioneer psychiatrist in the treatment of mood disorders, believed that "more human suffering has resulted from depression than from any other single disease affecting mankind."

Depression in this country is our number-one health problem. As a psychiatrist I see more patients suffering from some form of depression than all other emotional problems put together. Over 50 percent of all

Americans suffer from some form of clinical depression at some point in their lives. At any given time it is estimated that over 20 million of our citizens (almost 10 per cent) are currently depressed for one reason or another.

Depression seems to affect women slightly more than men, and the wealthy more than the poor. Money does *not* buy happiness. Whereas it may occur during any stressful period in life, it is most commonly seen during the late-teenage years, and menopausal or mid-life crisis years, or after retirement.

I myself was depressed for almost a year in my early thirties. It was in retrospect definitely the most protracted painful period I have suffered. Although I thought of suicide, my personal faith prevented it. One blessing that has come out of that experience, however, is that I am now able truthfully to look my depressed patients in the eye and say, "I know how you feel."

It seems, therefore, that *all* kinds of people are prone to depression; indeed probably everyone experiences some sadness and low mood at some point in life. However there are certain factors that could predispose or make an individual more vulnerable to it.

It seems, from thoroughly taken family histories of depressed patients, that childhood influences can become a learned pattern of behavior. Children can learn to identify with chronically depressed parents and acquire a depressive life-style as a way to avoid stress. As they grow, children and adolescents often develop personalities similar to their parents, and learn to cope with stressful situations by this neurotic depressive avoidance.

Pent-up anger turned inwards, stifled from outward expression, can lead directly to depression. Suppression of the healthy verbalization of anger can breed depression in young children.

Depression can also be used to manipulate one's spouse, parents, or children. Individuals, therefore, who grew up in families in which they could get their own way by sulking or withdrawal will more likely be vulnerable to neurotic depression as adults. Young adults with a low sense of self-esteem can also often use depression as a form of self-punishment.

Further on you will read of many different types and causes of depression, from which it will become evident that any kind of person can become depressed at any stage of life from infancy to old age.

WHAT FEELINGS ACCOMPANY DEPRESSION?

In every medical illness it is necessary to make a diagnosis before instituting treatment. Diagnosis is based on the symptoms complained of and the signs observed. In depression symptoms consist of abnormal feelings, thoughts, behavior, and relationships. These overlap considerably, and sharp categories are hard to define.

An *affect* is defined as a subjective feeling-state or emotion, and *depression* is defined as an affective feeling-tone of sadness. "Feeling blue" is a common way of describing the gloomy, painful, low mood of depression. It involves a sense of sorrow, unhappiness, and even misery, very often at its worst on waking in the morning. Some people have poetically described it as a heaviness of spirit, of being cast down, downhearted, disconsolate, oppressed, moody, or melancholic. It is certainly a sense of discouragement, despondency, distress, and even despair.

Although low mood is the predominant emotion experienced in depression, there are several others that are often felt. Hard to describe, but readily understood by anyone who has suffered them, are such feelings as a sense of isolation, loneliness, emptiness, hopelessness, and even helplessness. The depressed person tends to turn his attention away from the world outside, and inward toward himself. He often feels like crying, experiencing a sense of self-pity, rejection, of being alone and unloved, and craving for love from others.

Depression is also frequently accompanied by feelings of anxiety or apprehension, sometimes a sense of dread, often also some repressed anger, resentment, hostility, or easy irritability.

Physical feelings can include a wide variety of real or imagined vague aches and pains, like those of a hypochondriac.

Finally, the feelings of the sexual drive are usually greatly diminished. Libido is significantly reduced both in desire and ability to perform.

The depressed person is DOWN in every area of life, and in every sense of the word. Down, but not out. There is hope. There is help. There is healing.

WHAT THOUGHTS ACCOMPANY DEPRESSION?

Feelings are associated with thoughts, and depressive thoughts accompany depressive feelings. Thinking in depression is slowed down and reduced, but what there is of it is self-deprecating and full of gloom.

The predominant thought in depression is the conscious awareness of how miserable one feels. Morbid self-preoccupation with one's own problems and a negative self-concept with a low sense of self-esteem constantly fill the mind. There is guilt about the past and pessimistic worry about the future, especially in the areas of family relationships, job, or financial security.

The depressed person is full of remorse and shame over relatively trivial matters. He dwells on a persistent sense of failure, lacks self-confidence, and makes frequent self-deprecatory remarks. He is overly self-reproaching and self-critical, and says he is worthless, inadequate, inferior, and useless. There is introspective brooding on the futility and meaninglessness of life, often made worse by a perplexed confusion of contradictory thoughts.

In the depressive there is frequently the conviction that life is not worth living. There is a desire to give up, to quit, a longing to die, and yet a fear of dying. Often he has a masochistic preoccupation with thoughts of death, doom, and self-destruction. The loss of hope that things will improve leads eventually to thoughts of suicide.

In psychotic depression contact with reality is totally lost, with delusions, hallucinations, and a bizarre swarm of unrealistic fantasies.

In the religious area one of two opposites tend to occur. The depressed person might pull away from his former beliefs about God and reduce or discontinue his private and public worship. Alternatively he might become excessively preoccupied with prayer and Bible study, sometimes spending hours a day verbalizing his miseries to God.

Thinking disorders in depression are especially amenable to treatment by medications and psychotherapy.

WHAT ARE THE SUBJECTIVE SYMPTOMS OF DEPRESSION?

In addition to thoughts and feelings there are other internal evidences of depression, both personal and social.

Probably the most painful subjective symptom is *anhedonia,* or an inability to enjoy life. The depressed person has little sense of humor and rarely laughs. He lacks the ability to be amused or entertained. He has no enthusiasm for anything and has lost interest in activities that formerly gave him pleasure. Life becomes dull and uninteresting. His concentration is poor, he has a shortened attention span, and his memory is defective for recent events. He is apathetic, indecisive, and lacks motivation.

Associated with anhedonia are various physical symptoms such as tiredness and fatigue, with loss of energy. Such lethargy leads to inertia and social withdrawal. He pulls back from involvement with other people because it is too much effort to relate normally to them.

Insomnia is another serious problem for the depressive. He either cannot go to sleep at night, wakes too early in the morning, or wakes up in the middle of the night and can't go back to sleep again.

Appetite also is often affected in depression in either of two opposite ways. One can either lose one's appetite, a condition known as anorexia, or turn to gluttony as a means of drowning one's sorrows in the pleasures of eating. Alcohol or drug abuse, of course, are also well-known to be very self-destructive symptoms of, and attempts to avoid, depression.

Other frequent physical symptoms experienced in depression are constipation, dry mouth, and painful, irregular, or decreased menses. A wide variety of other real or imagined symptoms can occur from time to time. The most frequent of these are rapid heart beat, chest pains, overbreathing, sweating, and such gastrointestinal problems as indigestion, nausea, stomach cramps, and diarrhea.

However, remember that there is hope. Depression can be treated, and, even without treatment, tends eventually to go away.

WHAT ARE THE OBJECTIVE SIGNS OF DEPRESSION?

Signs are evidences of illness that another person can observe. In depression the most pronounced sign is called psychomotor retardation, which is a gross and obvious slowing down or reduction of both thought processes and physical activity.

Whereas sometimes the depressed person who is also anxious might show some restlessness and agitation, more often he is the opposite, that is, restrained, inhibited, slow of verbal response, and restricted in bodily movements. He may sometimes sit for long periods, quiet and still, with his head drooped. He might have a recognizable depressive affect, that is with a furrowed forehead and a mournful facial expression with the corners of his mouth turned down. He may sigh, sob, or spontaneously burst into tears for no immediate reason.

Other objective evidences of depression are a lack of hygiene and personal grooming. The depressed person is often untidy, unwashed, slovenly, disheveled, and generally unkempt. Men often do not shave. Women fail to use makeup or to keep their hair combed. There is often a halting speech, a limp handshake, and a dejected attitude and manner.

It is painfully difficult to have an ongoing conversation with someone seriously depressed. He tends to be unresponsive and uncommunicative. There is a loss of spontaneity or initiative in interpersonal relationships, which might become clinging and dependent on supportive close friends or relatives.

Since all activity levels are reduced, the depressive has a serious work-related problem. He feels it is desperately hard to get up and get going in the morning. If he makes it to work, he is liable to be seriously underproductive, lacking in interest and energy, and withdrawn in his relationships with co-workers and authority figures.

Finally, because of his appetite changes he is liable to be thin and emaciated because of anorexia, or obese because of overeating.

The kinds of depression that cause all these objective signs are invariably those caused by a biochemical imbalance, and are especially responsive to medications and somatic therapies.

WHAT ARE THE TYPES OF DEPRESSION?

Depression can be thought of as a *reaction,* a *symptom,* or a *disease.* As such its three major categories are called *reactive, neurotic,* or *endogenous.*

1. *Reactive depression* is a result of, or a reaction to, a loss or other disappointment in the world outside. It is essentially an exaggerated or protracted experience of grief. There are four fairly well-recognized forms of reactive depression, two very common, and two relatively rare.
    a) The most common reactive depression is usually called *depressive adjustment reaction* and is a temporary disorder of variable intensity or duration. It is seen in people with no apparent preexisting mental disorder who are responding to an overwhelming external stress. Time heals this condition as the stressful event fades into the past. Most sufferers usually do not need medical treatment but can be helped by a caring sympathetic ear, and practical support from others.
    b) *Secondary depression* is seen in people whose primary problem is some other physical or emotional disorder. Any illness or injury, especially if it disrupts one's daily routine, or separates one from friends or loved ones can cause this. Very common also is depression secondary to anxiety. I see many patients who complain of depression but underlying it is a severe chronic anxiety. If this is correctly diagnosed, treatment and relief of the primary anxiety will lead to the depression going away by itself.
    c) *Post partum depression* comes on in a small number of women between three weeks and three months after delivery of their first child. Fear and feelings of inadequacy are frequent aspects of this threat of motherhood. The symptoms almost always disappear as the new mother adjusts to her unfamiliar role and gains self-confidence.

Very rarely, however, this depression can become a dangerous psychosis in those genetically predisposed to it, and these women should be under the care of a physician for a few weeks, at least until improvement is in evidence. Although this condition is usually thought of as a reactive

Common Emotional Experiences

depression, there are often also some neurotic (and rarely, psychotic) elements to it.

  d) *Anaclitic depression* is seen in an infant in the event of the sudden loss of its mother. It is characterized by withdrawal, loss of interest in its environment, apprehension, reduction in appetite, insomnia, and a flat facial expression. Lengthy deprivation can lead to death, rare in our culture. More often recovery occurs rapidly with the return of the mother, or gradually with the development of a new relationship with a mother substitute. Anaclitic depression may also occur in the elderly after the loss of a spouse.
2. *Neurotic depression* is essentially a symptom of the development of a life-style, of a way of coping with stress. It is a withdrawal or avoidance of facing up to and dealing with the responsibilities of the hard realities of life. It is not a reaction to a loss or disappointment on the one hand, nor a chemical imbalance on the other hand. It is not a psychosis, which is loss of reality contact. On the contrary the patient is all too well aware of the pain of reality, and his depression is a symptom of an attempt to escape from it.
  a) *Depressive neurosis* is manifested by both biological and social incapacities. The patient is biologically affected by such symptoms as anorexia, insomnia, anhedonia, loss of libido, and potentially any of the evidences cited earlier. Socially he is affected in his work efficiency, deteriorated interpersonal relationships, and a generalized withdrawal from other people.

  Neurotic depression usually lasts, untreated, for several months, (unlike reactive depression which lasts only a few weeks, or endogenous depression, which untreated can last for many months or years). The depressive manifestations of this neurotic syndrome may be either relatively persistent or separated by periods of normal moods lasting a few days to a few weeks at a time.

  Neurotic depressives usually respond to a combination of psychotherapy and a brief course of antidepressant medications.
  b) *Cyclothymic disorder* is a personality or character abnormality in which lifelong patterns of up-and-down moods are evident. It is classified here as a neurosis because it is not a reaction to an exterior stress, nor is it serious enough to be of psychotic proportions.

It resembles a manic-depressive disorder but is not as severe. Throughout life the individual experiences alternating high and low moods which may either be separated by normal moods lasting a few months, or swing directly from one to the other. During the low swings any of the symptoms of depression may be experienced to a minor degree, and, similarly, minor degrees of elation may be felt during the highs.

Since this is essentially a disorder of the inborn personality, medications are of little value other than for short-term control of mood at the peaks of the swings. Lithium has been tried with some success in preventing extremes of mood. Psychotherapy cannot change the personality but can help understanding of the condition and thereby indirectly can potentially lead to improvement in behavior and relationships.

3. *Endogenous depressions.* These depressions are the most serious and are caused by a chemical imbalance in the brain. There are four major conditions in this category: involutional melancholia, psychotic depression reaction, manic-depressive illness, and schizoaffective disorder.
   a) *Involutional melancholia,* though rarely seen in middle-aged men (part of the so-called mid-life crisis syndrome), is most commonly seen in menopausal women. There is usually no obvious precipitating cause, and the woman almost never has a past history of depression.

The most prominent symptom is that of depression, but this is often accompanied by evidences of psychotic thinking (such as paranoid delusions, hallucinations, and incoherence). Other frequent symptoms include severe guilt feelings, anhedonia, anxiety, anorexia, agitation, insomnia, feeling of unworthiness, false hypochondriac fears of disease, and a black, overwhelming cloud of conviction that she deserves punishment for some real or imagined sins.

A combination of electric shock treatment with antidepressant medications is especially effective in this condition.

   b) Psychotic depressive reaction, most commonly seen in middle-aged or older men, is a very severe form of depression with many of the signs and symptoms described previously. In addition, however, there are manifested additional symptoms of the psychotic process, namely, delusions (false beliefs), hallucinations (false sensory impressions, like "hearing voices" or "seeing things"), and incoherence in conversation.

Distorted thinking, often in relation to his own bodily functions are frequently present together with guilt, anxiety, and thoughts of suicide.

Common Emotional Experiences

Hospitalization is invariably needed to prevent this from being carried out. Shock treatment is often necessary.

c) *Manic-depressive illness.* In this condition recurrent depressive episodes of varying degrees of intensity or duration are alternated with high moods in which the patient behaves with a manic euphoria. There are essentially three types: bipolar, unipolar depressed, and unipolar manic. They are called affective disorders.

   (1) The bipolar manic-depressive illness, often called the circular type, is manifested by alternating periods of deep depression and mania. Either or both can be so severe as to be psychotic. The period of alternation can be as little as a few days or as long as several months. One might follow the other directly or be separated by a period of normal mood and functioning.

   (2) The unipolar depressed type is sometimes called "recurrent depression." Mood swings alternate as in the bipolar type, but unhappily for the patient he never enjoys the manic or euphoric phase. Between depressive episodes he experiences normal but not high moods. Symptoms during the depressed phase are much as previously described with the occasional addition of the reality-loss symptoms of a psychotic depression with its attendant dangers of suicidal ideation (thoughts).

   (3) *The manic type* of unipolar affective disorder can occur without alternating depressions but this is rare. In mania, or hypomania (less extreme), the patient experiences, and subjectively usually much enjoys, a feeling of high mood with euphoria and elation. He feels elevated and expansive, but he is also impatient and easily irritated.

He manifests a marked increase in his activity level at work, socially, or sexually. There is physical restlessness, rapid speech, and racing thoughts with quickly changing inconsequential ideas. He tends to dominate conversations with uninterruptible talkativeness, and has inflated self-esteem with grandiose delusions, easy distractibility, and decreased need for sleep.

In addition the manic is liable to become involved in doing things that have a high risk for painful consequences such as uninhibited, inappropriate or excessive sexual activities, buying sprees, and poor financial judgment generally leading to foolish business investments. He may also pursue such self-destructive actions as provocative belligerent threats to other people, reckless jaywalking or dangerous driving.

This condition tends to run in families because of a hereditary predisposition. Patients with this condition, however, need not remain childless. Lithium carbonate therapy is very effective in both the treatment and prevention of manic-depressive illness.

d) *Schizoaffective disorder.* This condition is rare and is essentially a form of schizophrenia with superimposed high or low mood swings as well. Unlike the affective disorders (depression, mania, etc.) which are primarily the result of abnormal moods or feelings, schizophrenia is primarily a disorder of thinking or thought processes, manifested mainly by loss of contact with reality, or psychosis.

When a person's primary condition is schizophrenic, but he has additional manic or depressive episodes, he is described as schizoaffective. The best treatment is antipsychotic medications, though lithium can also be used to control the secondary mood swings.

WHAT ARE THE CAUSES OF DEPRESSION?

Just as there are three major types of depression there are three categories of causes. Reactive depression is caused by a loss or disappointment; neurotic depression is caused by an emotional or psychological maladjustment—endogenous depression is caused by a biochemical imbalance affecting the brain. Depression is not "catching" like the flu.

Another way of seeing the causes of depression is to understand that: (1) Reactive depression results from the precipitating pressure of a situational problem; (2) Neurotic depression is caused by early environmental factors such as unresolved unconscious conflicts of childhood; (3) Endogenous depression is a hereditary medical condition genetically induced.

Causes of Reactive Depression.

There are at least five different kinds of loss:

a) *Real loss* is the actual real-life loss of something precious or valuable such as loss of job, money, health, freedom, an opportunity, a contest, or a prized object. It could also be the loss of persons through death, divorce, prolonged separation, or marital family estrangement leading to loneliness and isolation.
b) *Autonomous loss* is caused by a sense of helplessness or loss of control when something adverse happens vocationally, socially or personally about which one can do nothing. Depression secondary to physical illness is one such example. So also is the inexorable process of aging.

c) *Abstract loss* is more intangible and causes depression through such losses as that of self-respect, power, prestige, status, control of others, or the assurance that one is loved by others. Any lowered feelings of a sense of self-worth or self-esteem can cause depression.
d) *Imagined loss* is caused by delusional thinking in which one becomes suspicious of others with unrealistic (but not psychotic) paranoid feelings of rejection by others. Loneliness or lack of close relationships can lead to all kinds of fantasied losses leading to reactive depression.
e) *Threatened loss* is a real but only potential loss, as experienced for example by a woman who feels a lump in her breast. She becomes depressed before seeing her doctor, through fear of malignancy. Before and after surgery, depression results from fear of eventual fatality, or the possible effect of a mastectomy on her husband's desire for her.

Help for reactive depression through counseling would aim at encouragement toward changing the changeable, acceptance of the unchangeable, and the development of a personal philosophy or theology.

Causes of Neurotic Depression

Neurotic depression is essentially a learned personality defect in which the patient unconsciously uses his symptoms as a means of avoiding stress or responsibilities. It is learned usually from one's parents. (Neurotic parents breed neurotic children.) It represents a life-style of coping or escaping from anything that causes anxiety. It is an attempt at the easy way out, but unhappily it proves to be a way out that merely leads to a different kind of pain. Anxiety is either replaced, or superimposed on, by depression.

Rejecting or status-seeking parents who set unrealistically high goals or standards for their children prepare them for inevitable failure. Discrepancy between expectations and achievements leads to a surrender of effort, and protective depressive withdrawal. Real or false guilt associated with a lack of success in earlier life can set one up for a neurotic depressive episode later in one's middle years.

Negative thinking, seeing only the dark side of life, can also lead to intense hopeless depression. Thinking negatively about one's own inadequacy, the overwhelming wicked world around, and hopelessness for the future leads to neurotic withdrawal and despair.

Anger turned inward also leads to neurotic depression. Any hurt or disappointment can lead to anger. Initially this leads to a desire for revenge, but since this is not acceptable behavior in our culture, it is repressed inward. The recent widow is angry at her deceased husband for leaving her with young children. She cannot express her anger and cannot take any revenge. Her inner hurt and resentment are turned inward and she becomes depressed.

Genetically, much research remains to be done in the area of an inherited tendency to depression. Women are more prone than men to developing neurotic depression, but this could be cultural rather than genetic. Statistically, research reveals that close relatives (parents, siblings, and children) of depressed individuals are more likely to become depressed than the general population. Recent studies indicate that a gene on the X-chromosome may be responsible for the transmission of a manic-depressive predisposition from parent to child, and possibly that of neurotic depression also.

"Bad genes" however are usually overemphasized by people who tend to blame their parents for their problems, when they should be more appropriately accepting responsibility themselves for coping with stress in their lives. Whereas bad genes cannot certainly be blamed for neurotic depression, it is much more likely that they could be responsible for the various endogenous varieties. Some relief of neurotic depression can at times be achieved through psychotherapy. Medications can provide temporary relief from the acute symptoms to the extent that they are the result of a secondary biochemical disruption.

Causes of Endogenous Depression

A variety of chemical-imbalance problems can cause endogenous (internally caused) depression.

Hypothyroidism, or reduced levels of thyroid hormone production, has been known for over one hundred years to cause internal depression. More recently hypoglycemia, or low blood sugar, has been recognized as leading to low mood in some people. Diabetes mellitus can cause depression, and a tumor of the pancreas leading to too much insulin production, the opposite effect, can cause it too. Other hormones from the pituitary or adrenal glands can get out of whack and lead to endocrine imbalance with depressive effects. Electrolyte disturbances in the blood (sodium, potassium, and other elements getting out of balance) are now known to cause recurrent and manic-depressive illness. Viral and other infections, physical fatigue, toxicity, and insomnia also can lead to internal depression at least temporarily. (Premenstrual syndrome, agitation and depression preceding the monthly menses, is discussed later.)

However, the basic cause of most endogenous depression is an imbalance in the biogenic amines. Let me explain what I mean.

Nerve cells in the brain do not actually touch each other like two electrical wires twisted together. Instead they communicate via a minute sac called a synapse. In this sac is a fluid containing millions of molecules of hormones and electrolytes, which are called nerve transmitters because they transmit messages from one cell to the next.

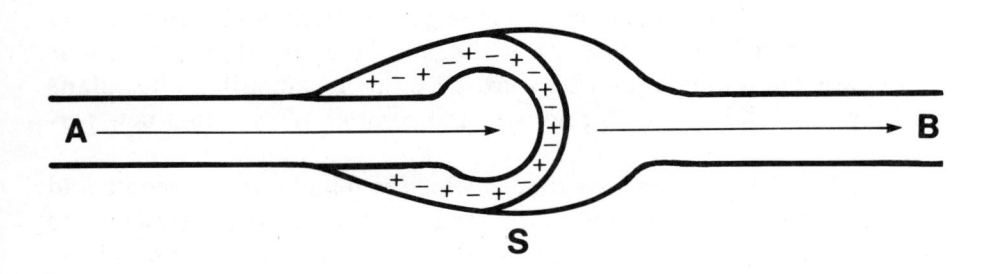

In the diagram, an impulse traveling down nerve cell A ends at the synapse S. There the impulse charges various neurotransmitters, which leap across the gap and stimulate nerve cell B. If enough of them do this, then an impulse is initiated in B which then carries it to the next synapse and so on. Of course all this takes place in a microsecond of time.

After delivering their stimulus, these little messengers return to A to be charged up again for the next time. If not enough messengers stimulate B, or if they do not go back to A for recharging, then B will not carry on the impulse. If this happens in the arms or legs, there develops a loss of their strength or reduction in their major function of motion. If this happens in the brain, you get depression.

The commonest neurotransmitters are called biogenic amines, and the ones presently thought to be the most influential in various psychiatric disorders are norepinephrine (adrenaline), serotonin, and dopamine. The first two are probably involved in depression and anxiety; the latter in schizophrenia. Breakdown products (metabolites) of norepinephrine and serotonin are found to be abnormally low in people who are depressed.

Understanding the biogenic amine theory of endogenous depression is essential to comprehending the use of antidepressant medications.

WHAT ARE THE RESULTS OF DEPRESSION?

We have described most of the subjective and objective effects of depression of any type and from any cause. However there are two other results of depression that, in conclusion, need to be understood. One is potentially good. One is invariably bad.

The potentially good result of depression is that its onset can be protective of the patient. Depression can be a warning of the physical or emotional illness that can lead to a defensive withdrawal. Depression results in a removal of the victim from a stressful environment. His loss of interest and energy enable him to conserve his strength in a debilitating employment, social, or personal situation, or in the case of physical illness or disease. He is able to pull back from his involvement in all his affairs and take a fresh look at his priorities and commitments with a new perspective.

A period of depression buys time in which to rebuild one's strength and rethink one's motivation and plans for the future. It also enables us to forgive and forget the past and start afresh with all our personal objectives and interpersonal relationships. It is better to withdraw from stress by means of a temporary depression than to use such self-destructive means as drugs or alcohol, impulsive or violent behavior, gambling or sexual acting out of frustrations.

The ultimate in self-destructive behavior, suicide, is of course the bad potential result of depression. There is no more thorough a way of escaping an unbearable life situation than to end it. Suicide is especially prevalent in teenagers (second only to accidents as the leading cause of death). It is also higher among middle-aged single (especially divorced) people living alone, and in elderly widows.

More women than men attempt suicide, but more men are successful because they tend to use more lethal means such as shooting, jumping, hanging, or crashing an automobile.

Women usually use an overdose of pills, most often hoping they will be found and rescued. Their suicide "attempt" is of course a cry for help, and demands serious attention initially through hospital treatment of the medical damage. This should be followed by counseling or psychotherapy aimed at exploring the dynamics and motivation behind the act, and the development of new healthy attitudes toward life and living.

The underlying depression needs a temporary course of an antidepressant medication, and follow-up supportive dialogue to help reestablish a normal mood and renewed hope.

MEDICATIONS

Antidepressant medications have only been discovered and developed in the last two or three decades. Prior to that the only available mood

Common Emotional Experiences

elevators were the amphetamines (Dexedrine, for example), and illegal drugs like marijuana, cocaine, or heroin. All these tend to become addictive, with a consequent need for ever-increasing doses to produce the desired effect.

"Down" drugs such as sleep medications, some tranquilizers, and alcohol can also reduce the feelings of depression temporarily, but again are self-destructive in the long run because of the danger of addiction. Caffeine in tea, coffee, cocoa, and cola drinks is stimulating and also addictive.

Look again at the diagram on page 345. We learned there that a deficiency in those little messengers (neurotransmitters) in the little sacs (synapses) between nerve cells (neurons) in the brain causes depression. We do not know what casues deficiencies in these various biogenic amines but we do know now that several recently produced antidepressant medications can act in the synapses to prevent or reduce the loss of the amines, and thereby can elevate a depressed mood back to normal.

The mode of action of antidepressant medications is theorized to be as follows:

The biogenicamine neurotransmitters most certainly known to be involved in mood abnormalities such as depression are norepinephrine (a form of adrenaline) and serotonin.

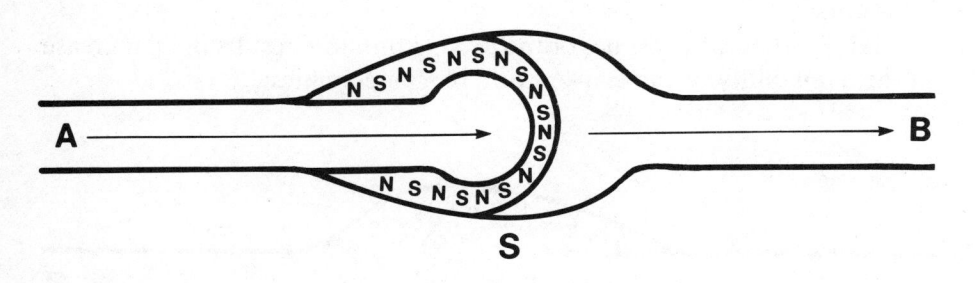

Normal Synapse

Here is a schematic diagram of a synapse between two nerve cells in the limbic system of the brain of a normal person who is not depressed.

(1) The neurotransmitters serotonin and norepinephrine (represented by S and N) are stimulated by an impulse from nerve A. (2) They move across the synaptic gap to stimulate nerve cell B, which then conducts the impulse as shown by the arrow. (3) Their work done, the

neurotransmitters then go back to nerve cell A. This process is known as reuptake. (4) Some may be "recharged" and made ready for the next impulse (microseconds later), but others are metabolized (eaten up) by an enzyme in A called monoamine oxidase, and are thereafter ineffective.

In depression there are not enough little messengers in the synapse in the brain's limbic system or hypothalamus. Compared with the first diagram the synapses look schematically like this:

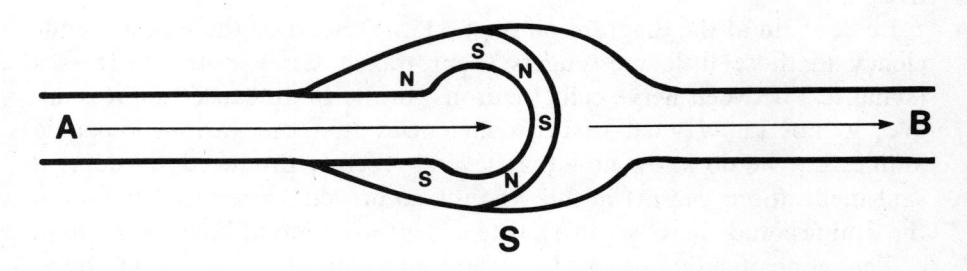

Depressed Synapse

Antidepressant medications are essentially of two varieties: (1) Those that act to prevent reuptake of the neurotransmitters by cell A. These are the tricylic antidepressants. (2) Those that prevent enzymatic breakdown of neurotransmitters by cell A so that they survive to return recharged for the next round of impulses. These are called monoamine oxidase (MAO) inhibitors.

Taking either the tricyclics or the MAO inhibitors results in an increase in the availability of the transmitting biogenic amines:

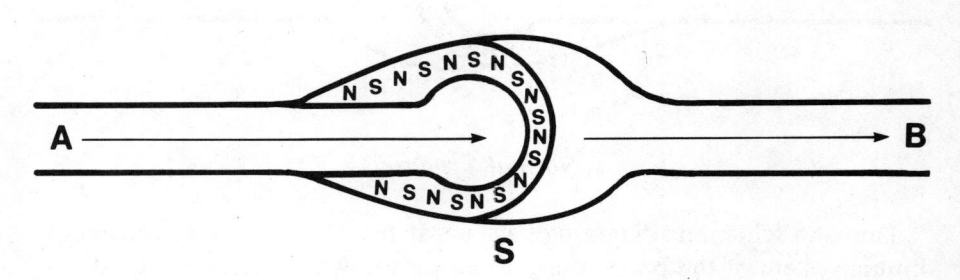

Depressed Synapse with Medications

The most commonly used tricylic antidepressants (which act by decreasing the reuptake of N and S by the presynaptic neuron (nerve cell A) and hence increasing their availability) are as follows:

Common Emotional Experiences

Brand Name	Generic Name	Average Daily Dose
Adapin	doxepin	25–300 mg
Asendin	amozapine	100–300 mg
Aventyl	nortriptyline	30–100 mg
Elavil	amitriptyline	25–300 mg
Endep	amitriptyline	25–300 mg
Ludiomil	maprotiline	75–300 mg
Norpramin	desipramine	25–200 mg
Pertofrane	desipramine	25–200 mg
Sinequan	doxepin	25–300 mg
Tofranil	imipramine	30–300 mg
Vivactil	protriptyline	15–60 mg

The tricyclics are relatively safe. They can be used in rapidly increasing doses if small starting doses are ineffective after a few days. (Even huge overdoses rarely bring about successful suicide attempts.) Their commonest side effects are dry mouth, constipation, and a feeling of sleepiness during the day. They do not work within minutes like an aspirin tablet, but build up a therapeutically effective level in the blood over a period of two to four weeks. Persons under treatment should therefore be patient, stick with the medications, not expect instant miracles, and continue to take them even though no immediate effect is felt. Often sedative effect is "used up" during the sleeping hours leaving their antidepressant effect working throughout the following day. Given time, they are effective in elevating depressed mood in 95 percent of people suffering from internal chemical (endogenous) depression, and also for the brief acute temporary episodes of very low mood seen sometimes in reactive or neurotic depression as well.

However, rarely, a patient does not respond with tricyclics, and needs an MAO inhibitor. These work by preventing (or at least decreasing) the metabolizing (destruction) of the reuptaken biogenic amines in neuron A. They prevent (or inhibit) the destructive effect of A's monoamine oxidase enzyme. There are three MAO inhibitors in common use today:

Brand Name	Generic Name	Average Daily Dose
Marplan	isocarboxazid	10–30 mg
Nardil	phenelzine	15–75 mg
Parnate	tranylcypromine	10–30 mg

Unlike the tricyclics, however, MAO inhibitors can be dangerous without special precautions. They can cause hypertension (high blood pressure) if anyone using them *also* takes in any tyramine. Tyramine is found especially in aged cheeses such as Cheddar and Stilton, and in red wine. It is also found in beer, broad beans, figs, yogurt, chicken liver, chocolate, coffee, licorice, game, pickled products, raisins, sherry, salted fish, sauerkraut, soy sauce, or yeast products. (Cream and cottage cheeses are okay.) If the depressed patient taking MAO inhibitors avoids these foods he will do well. These medications are *very* effective antidepressants.

Finally, it is *strongly* urged of any person who is depressed for any reason not to self-medicate with alcohol or any street drug. Though temporarily effective in helping to avoid facing reality, they are all, unequivocally, in the long run extremely self-destructive.

SOMATIC THERAPIES

The word "somatic" comes from the ancient Greek word *soma,* which means body. Somatic therapies are medical treatments that are applied to the physical body, as distinct from the mind, but attempt to influence the mind.

In less-civilized times psychiatric, including deeply depressed, patients were "treated" with straitjackets, solitary confinement, iced-water dunking, whipping, and forced ingestion of poisons. Many depressed, psychotic old women, thought to be witches, were burned alive in the belief that thereby their souls would be purged and prepared for entering heaven. In the fifteenth century their executioners really believed that they were doing them the favor of rescuing them from eternal hell by putting them to a fiery death at the stake.

In our present century there have been insulin coma therapy and sleep therapy, in which depressed patients were knocked out with drugs for extended periods. Upon recovery some indeed woke up less depressed, and remained so. Others predictably showed only temporary improvement and soon relapsed. These practices are rarely used today.

Psychosurgery was first introduced in 1936 as an experimental attempt to control psychotic behavior (including depression unresponsive to any other therapy). (1) *Prefrontal lobotomy,* done until the mid to late 1950s, was effective at least in controlling the bizarre behavior of acute schizophrenics, including those psychotically depressed. Unfortunately, however, it altered the patient's personality, leaving him without ambition, initiative, or humor. It has now been all but discontinued. (2) A patient who is suffering from the otherwise uncontrollable irritable and aggressive symptoms of temporal-lobe epilepsy can benefit from a very limited and specific surgical procedure into the brain to sever some neuronal connections there. There is confidence that pretty soon specific medications will obviate the need for this type of surgical intervention.

A form of somatic treatment still in use today in selected situations is ECT (electroconvulsive therapy) first tried in 1938.

Today ECT is not dangerous or painful. It is simply like being put to sleep by an anaesthesiologist before an operation.

Once the patient is asleep the doctor applies electrodes to the sides of the patient's head behind the ears or on the temples, and gives him a fifth-of-a-second shock of about eighty volts. Within seconds a generalized epilepticlike seizure convulses muscles throughout the body. It lasts ten to thirty seconds. Soon after, the patient begins to wake up; and within an hour he is usually fully alert with no memory of the treatment.

Five to eight such treatments, a couple of days apart, are usually sufficient to have a dramatic effect in elevating depressed mood. ECT is especially useful in the treatment of severe protracted depression that has failed to respond to high doses of medication. It is also used as a "treatment of choice" (first option) in such conditions as psychotic depressive reaction, the acute depressive phase of manic-depressive psychosis, involutional melancholia, and in acute depressions of any cause in which the risk of suicide is so great that medications would be too slow to rescue the patient from his self-destructive intent. ECT is too risky in someone with a brain tumor or a serious heart disease.

The main complaint following ECT is slight memory loss, especially for recent events, but in fact since depression itself can affect memory, some patients actually regain memory once their depression is lifted. A relatively recent refinement involving shocking only the nondominant hemisphere of the brain (for example, the right half of a right-handed person and vice versa) causes less memory loss.

The theory of ECT is that the procedure increases the local availability of norepinephrine in the brain, thereby elevating mood. Once the course of ECT is finished the patient should be maintained for at least a year or more on tricyclics or MAO inhibitors. Failure to do so would probably necessitate more ECT several months later.

The increased success of antidepressant medications has significantly reduced the use of ECT in recent years; but it remains a final resort to help those who have failed to improve by other means, or who are seriously suicidal.

SALTS, HORMONES, NUTRITION, AND VITAMINS

A lot of attention has been paid recently to the influence of a person's dietary intake on his or her physical and/or emotional well-being. Much has yet to be explored in this area and new facts are continually being discovered.

Salts are not drugs, but the products of the simple chemical combination of an acid with an alkali. Lithium carbonate is an outstanding salt now in wide use in psychiatry.

In 1949 John Cade, an outstanding physician in Australia, first tested lithium on manic patients and discovered it to be far more effective than tranquilizers in controlling high mood swings. Since then lithium has come to be used worldwide both for the treatment of mania and also prophylactically in the prevention of up and down mood swings. It is unquestionably the treatment of choice in any person whose history gives a clear indication of either unipolar or bipolar affective disorder (*see* p. 341).

After over thirty years of use, it is still not clear as to how or why lithium works. What is known is that lithium has the effect of restoring a proper balance in the distribution of sodium and potassium in the cells and synapses of the central nervous system. When these get out of whack they can lead to an increase in available norepinephrine, which can lead to a manic, euphoric mood state. By restabilizing sodium and potassium levels mood is restored to normal. Lithium does this.

For a reason not understood it seems also that if lithium is taken regularly by someone with a history of up and down moods, it can prevent, or significantly reduce, the frequency, duration, and severity of them. Lithium should be considered a preventative for anyone with a definite affective disorder even though he currently has no symptoms.

To prevent any possibility of toxicity (too much lithium building up in the system) federal regulations require monthly blood tests for serum lithium levels. Some patients in this country have now been taking lithium for almost twenty years with no problems.

Lithium is not only effective in manic-depressive illness. It is also good for use in combination with minor or major tranquilizers in the treatment of cyclothymic personality disorder or in schizoaffective schizophrenia.

Hormones are complex chemicals in the body produced by the endocrine glands. Unlike glands with ducts leading somewhere (like the gall bladder, salivary or sweat glands) most of these have no ducts but secrete their products directly into the blood. They used to be called ductless glands. The well-known ones are: the pituitary, in the middle of the head; the thyroid, the parathyroids, and the thymus, all in the front of the neck; the pancreas, behind the stomach; the adrenals, above each kidney; the ovaries, under the brim of the female pelvis; and the testes of the male scrotum. (The pancreas, ovaries, and testes also have ducts—for digestive enzymes, eggs, and sperm respectively—but their hormones [insulin, estrogens, and testosterone] go directly into the blood. They are both ducted and endocrine.)

The conductor of this endocrine orchestra is the pituitary gland, which itself is controlled by the hypothalamus in the brain. Both are only the size of a pea but they control virtually every major function of the body,

Common Emotional Experiences

including its emotional reactions. For example there is a complicated interaction between the hypothalamus and the biogenic amines that effect neuronal transmission, and therefore affect mood. The stress hormone cortisol is elevated in depression, whereas thyroid hormone (energy) and sex hormones (libido) are reduced. It has been known for a long time that thyroid-hormone supplement can energize and elevate mood. Most endocrine imbalances can be treated and restored to normal. Natural or synthetic hormones are readily available to replace deficiencies and in most cases excesses can be reduced. Such hormonal treatment, however, is not the expertise of a psychiatrist, but of an endocrinologist, who can be recommended by your family physician.

A special hormone-related depression is that associated with the monthly menstrual cycle. Some women develop anxiety and/or depression, either during or immediately before their menses. Premenstrual syndrome (PMS) is now a well-documented condition of depression, agitation, and easy irritability, which improves with progesterone treatment. Your gynecologist can deal with most menses-related emotional disorders because he or she can best determine if the problem is related to psychological, cultural, situational, or hormonal factors.

Much has been written recently about the influence of diet or nutrition on physical and emotional well-being. The whole science of the cause and effect of dietary intake on psychological functioning is right now exploding upon the awareness of physicians and other health-care professionals.

As of this writing the main problem is the lack of documented proof from controlled double-blind (neither the patients nor the physicians know who are in which group) studies. Almost all that I have read about the value of nutritional factors in health has been from assertive, almost dogmatic, enthusiastic proponents of diet, vitamins, and minerals. I have spoken to many. They are united in their zeal—but unhappily divided in their specific recommendations. None that I know can show results of reproducible, scientifically monitored, or controlled experiments. If they could produce such proof, they would not need to be so zealous. All the world would believe them and follow their practices. Such is not yet the case, much as I wish that it were.

There are, however, a few basic principles of diet that can be documented as being beneficial for physical health, and therefore indirectly for emotional health, including the avoidance or relief of depression. In summary they are these:

In our North American culture, most people eat too much animal fat, white refined sugar, and flour products, and usually too little high-fiber foods. For both physical and emotional health we ought to replace beef, lamb, and pork with fish and chicken, and eat only moderate amounts of eggs and dairy products. We should consume fewer sugar-containing foods such as cakes, cookies, pastries, candies, ice cream, sweet soda drinks, and of course alcohol. By contrast, we should generally eat a higher percentage of whole-grain breads and cereals, more legumes and other green vegetables, and plenty of fresh citrus and noncitrus fruits. Those who exercise regularly can also benefit from pasta and baked potatoes.

Nutritional deprivations of course can cause a variety of physical and psychological disorders. Anorexia nervosa, related usually to female adolescent schizophrenia, can lead to secondary infection and death. Malnourishment certainly can lead to depressed mood and reduced drive. Eating mainly junk foods (fats and sugar-filled) can cause one to be overweight but malnourished (*see* also p. 94).

Vitamin deficiencies in the diet can lead to physical diseases that have emotional, including depressive, overtones. Supplements of vitamins known to be deficient will directly improve mood abnormalities. In particular, B_6 and B_{12} have occasionally apparently produced beneficial effects. Vitamin C is claimed to protect from the common cold.

Megavitamin therapy, massive doses of gross excesses of the United States Recommended Daily Allowances, has produced, predictably, some success and some failures. I strongly encourage the enthusiastic proponents of those therapies to continue their studies, specifically in the direction of producing *objective* and documented proof that their theories work in controlled double-blind studies (*see* also p. 111).

HOSPITALIZATION

Many believe that to be hospitalized for a psychiatric reason is the second-worst possible fate, next only to imprisonment for a crime. The stigma of such a situation is widespread in our culture and society. I believe it should not be so, because, as a physician, I see most psychiatric disorders as just as much a medical problem as a broken leg, acute appendicitis, or pneumonia.

Certainly in the cases of serious depression, acute anxiety, schizophrenia and bipolar affective disorder, biochemical imbalances in the central nervous system account for almost all of the symptoms experienced, and medical treatment can most effectively be administered for the seriously ill in a hospital setting.

When someone is severely depressed with many of the feelings, thoughts, symptoms, and signs described earlier, he or she almost always needs medical treatment. If he receives none, he will probably recover gradually over a period of twelve months or more provided he doesn't commmit suicide first. If he takes antidepressant medications and receives weekly psychotherapy on an outpatient basis, he will probably recover in three to six months. If he submits to hospital treatment, he will most likely start feeling better in a week, be discharged in a month, and be back to work in five or six weeks.

The best form of treatment depends on the type and severity of the depression. *Mild* depression not affecting work efficiency or social relationships can usually be treated with psychotherapy without medications, thereby avoiding the dry mouth and sedative side-effects most of them produce. *Moderate* depression in which work, social life, and sleeping are adversely affected are better treated with a combination of outpatient psychotherapy and medication provided there is no psychotic or suicidal thinking.

Hospitalization is generally the treatment of choice if the person is so depressed that he is unable to go to work, or is seriously ineffective at work, is totally socially withdrawn, is psychotic or on the brink of psychosis, or if he has thought of suicide. If someone is so depressed as to need intensive treatment, it is usually better to obtain it on an inpatient basis. The period of suffering will be shorter, and full recovery with return to a normal life will be sooner. Although most depressions lift eventually, the duration of pain and the level of incapacitation will in the long run be less with hospitalization.

The advantages of hospitalization are:

1. Intensive individual, group, and other forms of therapy are available daily from physicians, nurses, and other members of the staff.
2. Changes and dosage adjustments in medications can be made much more rapidly than on an outpatient basis.
3. If electroconvulsive therapy is needed, it is safer when given in a hospital.
4. The patient is removed from his stressful environment into a safe retreat with a friendly supportive and helpful atmosphere.
5. He will meet other depressed patients who are recovering successfully and who will be a source of encouragement to him.
6. He will be closely observed at all times by nurses and other staff to prevent suicide attempts, and, as he recovers, he will be enabled to gain insights into the causes and cures of his condition.
7. Since it is generally covered by insurance, hospitalization in the long run is usually less expensive to the individual than prolonged outpatient therapy. Also he is usually able to return to full employment sooner.

The disadvantages of hospitalization are:

1. Among people of lower socioeconomic life-style especially, psychiatric hospitalization is a stigma. The poor usually end up in city or

state hospitals with overcrowded conditions. The more well-to-do tend to go to more comfortable, even opulent, institutions. Since members of higher socioeconomic groups tend to have more education, they are usually better able to understand the problems and assign less stigma to them.
2. A history of being in a hospital for a psychiatric disorder can affect getting a new job, promotion on the job, or even sometimes obtaining a driver's license.
3. Some very dependent people begin to enjoy the security, care, and even the comfort of a hospital, and desiring to continue to stay in such a place, feign the symptoms of depression (easy to do) when a psychiatrist or other staff member is around.
4. Without major medical insurance, or welfare payments, hospitalization is very costly, running in excess of two hundred dollars per day in 1984. Even with adequate insurance it is unethical, even illegal, for either patient or doctor to arrange for inpatient stay any longer than is absolutely necessary.
5. After discharge from the hospital, although a patient is usually feeling fine—even happy and enthusiastic—his friends and family remember him as he was before he went in. They may be understandably aloof and hesitant to ask questions about what has happened since they last met. Although it isn't intended to be, a sensitive patient might interpret their reserve personally as a rejection.

ECONOMIC SECURITY

It follows logically after a discussion of hospitalization to discuss the effects of economic security, or lack of it, on depression and its treatment.

Lack of funds over a long period of time can be seriously depressive, especially when a person gets to the point where he cannot see how expected income can possibly meet anticipated expenses. Parkinson's "Second Law" states that expenditure rises to meet income; so the rich are just as vulnerable as the poor in this regard.

There are many nontechnical books on the subjects of living within a sensible budget and managing money. It is outside the scope of this writing to digress to such matters, but a few comments are made here in the general area of economic methods that can lead to avoidance or elevation of depressed mood.

The Bible says that the love of money is the root of all evil. This may seem a somewhat exaggerated statement to some, but it does seem to be true that worshipping the god of money often brings misery in the long run. There is a big difference between wanting money to buy pleasures, which almost never satisfy, and wanting money to get out of debt, which is a moral duty, and depressing if not quickly accomplished.

To avoid financial depression one needs (1) to earn money honestly, (2) to spend it on needs rather than luxuries, (3) to invest it carefully, and (4) to give it away joyfully to others in need.

Money can lead to depression if one develops distorted values about its worth. Materialism, or the excessive desire for the "good things" in life, never satisfies. If you own a Chevy, extra money might lead you to desire a Mercedes; if you have a Mercedes you might desire a Rolls Royce. If you own a twenty-foot yacht, you might covet a thirty-foot one.

Even if you get what you want, you'll soon get over the novelty of it. Also, your friends and relatives will not think more highly of you for your Rolls or a large yacht. They will merely think, "So he's made it," with not a little envy or jealousy! Friendship can actually be lost through the accumulation of possessions. Pride that sometimes comes with wealth can lead to alienation from loved ones.

Covetousness, greed, and the desire to get rich quickly in this country came as a shock to Aleksandr Solzhenitsyn when he saw our "fantastic greed for profit and for gain which goes far beyond all reason, all limitations, good conscience." Our economic system, taken to this excess, leads to national inflation, unemployment, high interest rates, and, on a more personal level, to unmanageable debts and family discord.

In the middle and lower income groups, avoiding certain specifics will help prevent the development of depression. Impulse buying, carelessness in budgeting, uninformed speculations, gambling, cosigning for a risky venture, being tempted by a sale to purchase things not really needed, and buying on credit can all lead to financial problems and hence depression.

Depression associated with money problems can be compounded by worry and anxiety over inability to pay bills, family and marital discord caused by disagreements over financial priorities, and loss of friends due to nonrepayment of loans, with attendant embarrassment. When those whose fulfillment comes from the accumulation of possessions are disappointed, unhappiness and emotional emptiness can be devastating.

Here are a few guidelines for the prevention and treatment of financially induced depression.

1. Create a monthly budget. Write down all sources of income in one column and all expenses in another. Balance the totals.

2. If you agree with the Judeo-Christian ethic, assign 10 percent of your gross income to charitable contributions, especially to the poor and to your place of worship.
3. Be sure to allow for taxes and other compulsory items.
4. Of the remaining amount of spending money—"workable income"—domestic economists often recommend the 10–70–20 plan. Put 10 percent to savings, 70 percent to living expenses, and 20 percent to pay off debts. When all debts are paid, that twenty percent should be divided among contributions, savings, and essential expenses.
5. For peace of mind be sure that you have adequate insurance; life, major medical, property, disability income, and liability.

EXERCISE

Someone once said, "I've never met a depressed jogger!" There may be some exaggeration in such a statement but the principle is certainly true.

In addition to watching one's diet it is necessary to take adequate exercise to keep the body in great shape; and keeping the body in great shape is a major contributing factor in avoiding depression and other neurotic illnesses.

A famous high school in England, dating back to the thirteenth century, has as its motto the Latin statement, *Mens Sana in Corpore Sano*. "A healthy mind in a healthy body."

Quoting the ancient Greeks, then President-elect John F. Kennedy, in the December 26, 1960, issue of *Sports Illustrated* wrote, "Physical fitness is not only one of the most important keys to a healthy body, it is the basis of dynamic and creative intellectual activity. Intelligence and skill can only function at the peak of their capacity when the body is healthy and strong; hardy spirits and tough minds usually inhabit sound bodies."

One of the reasons exercise contributes to preventing depression, or elevating depressed mood, is that the expending of physical energy results directly in an increase in adrenaline (norepinephrine). This increased production, from the adrenal glands, goes via the blood not only to the muscles involved in the exercise but also to the brain. Hence the expression "runner's high," which is a feeling of euphoria that is frequently experienced subjectively after exercising for several minutes.

Another major contributing factor that physical fitness makes in the treatment or prevention of depression is the great feeling of achievement that most people experience during and after exercise. Also the satisfaction and sense of good self-esteem one obtains from having a physically fit body more than outweighs the time and effort expended to achieve it.

Depression tends to occcur less often in people who are in excellent physical shape, especially if that condition is the result of regular exercise. Consider yourself. Where are you at right now in terms of physical well-being?

Let's do a quick self-evaluation. How are you feeling today? Tired, yawning, sleepy in the afternoon, drowsy after a heavy meal, listless, fatigued, depressed in mood? Are you anxious, irritable, impatient, uptight, hostile, worried, fearful? Any indigestion? Too much or too little appetite? Nausea, constipation, or diarrhea? Poor interpersonal relationships? Problems with authority or fulfilling responsibilities? Sleep poorly at night? Are you more than ten pounds overweight? Flight of stairs, short run for a bus make you breathless? Mowing the lawn, raking the leaves, shoveling the snow lead to collapse? Losing interest in your job, work around the house, the kids, social, or church activities? Less interested in sex (granted your age) than you used to be? Or less able to perform? Too tired? Too tired!

The medical signs and symptoms of inactivity are scary. A body that isn't used, quickly deteriorates. Astronauts have to do vigorous exercises out in space to compensate for the ease of living in a weightless environment. If the extent of your exercise consists of walking from your car to your television set, you will eventually fall apart: Your lungs will become less effective in the task of oxygen and carbon-dioxide exchange; your heart will grow less efficient; you will lose muscle tone; your bones will become more brittle due to loss of calcium; your blood vessels will become less pliable; and your body will become weaker, especially in the matter of the blood's ability to resist infection. You will then become much more vulnerable to colds and other upper-respiratory infections. If you suffer any injury to bone or muscle, you will take longer to heal. Worst of all, your mind will become affected, as evidenced by yawning and a drowsy feeling all day, slowed thought processes, a frequent sense of being "too tired" to do even minor tasks, and eventually by failing memory and declining ability to think logically and rationally.

By contrast, consider these rewards of physical fitness: increased zest for living, generally; increased available energy for all daily tasks; ability to work efficiently, without fatigue; increased sexual libido, both desire and ability; significantly improved performance and health of all organs, especially the heart, lungs, and blood vessels; greater speed of healing of all bone and soft tissues in case of illness or injury; greater resistance to infections; better tolerance of emotional stress; much-improved sleep at night, and ability to rest and relax properly, when necessary, during the day; reduced fat deposits and, therefore, better control of body weight; decreased pulse rate and blood pressure (signs of cardiovascular health);

decreased reaction time (quick reflexes); fewer gastrointestinal symptoms, such as indigestion or constipation; less chance of emotional depression or anxiety, general feeling of well-being, leading to attitudes of optimism, increased productivity, improved interpersonal relationships; and, considerable sharpening in thought processes, due to the total dependence of the cerebral cortex (conscious mind part of the brain) on efficient heart-lung functioning.

A healthy body is fun to have, but to be unhealthy is miserable. A healthy body is delightful, comfortable, and pleasant to look at; while an unhealthy or fat body is ugly, or even grotesque.

Some pain and discomfort, either in physical or emotional form, can happen to anyone; but much that we suffer we have brought upon ourselves by our own neglect.

Think about this: If, right now, starting this week, you begin a slowly progressive, nonpainful diet and exercise program, here's what would happen: You'd start to feel better; you'd function better; you'd relate to others better; you'd not only enjoy a renewed zest for life, but you'd also retain or return to good or even excellent health; and incidentally, you'd probably live longer.

Whatever you choose as your health-giving, weight-controlling exercise, it must be: (1) something you can learn to enjoy sufficiently to be willing to do it thoroughly and regularly (a minimum of three times weekly); (2) something that produces sufficient caloric expenditure first to reduce and then to control your body weight; and (3) something that results in sufficient oxygen consumption to produce a training effect that promotes fitness in the essential organs—the heart, blood vessels, and lungs.

All these requirements could be fulfilled very adequately by simple brisk walking, preferably progressing to jogging short distances, and ultimately to running to a good pace for longer distances. Walking and running have the added advantages of being easy to do, are usually the most convenient, the least expensive, the least demanding of equipment and facilities, and by far the most efficient in terms of calories and oxygen used in the time available.

Becoming physically fit has tranformed my life: I feel healthy every day, and this has led to immeasurable improvement in my functioning in all areas.

Many of the patients I see daily in my psychiatric practice would never have needed to come if they had been in excellent physical condition. Obviously not all, but I am certain that many of the men and women who go to their family physicians or pastors, and through them to a psychiatrist or marital counselor, complain of a multitude of minor problems that

Common Emotional Experiences

often might not have arisen if all members of the family had been diet and weight conscious and had been in a more regular exercise or conditioning program. (*See* chapters on *Flab,* p. 16, and *Fitness,* p. 62.)

I have, furthermore, found that the pursuit of a good nutritional and activity routine by patients seeing me for a wide variety of minor neurotic problems has led to many quite dramatic improvements without the use of medications or protracted in-depth psychotherapy. In many instances, a depressive mood has been elevated, moderate anxiety attacks partially alleviated, poor self-image problems improved by an increased sense of identity and ego strength, and marital and family conflicts reduced or eliminated through the development of new, shared activities and better communication arising out of great feelings of physical well-being.

Double-blind studies have proved the value of exercise in treating depression. Studies in the southern states and in California with two large groups of depressed patients, one on antidepressant medications, the other simply on a jogging program, have shown conclusively that the exercising group came out of their depression more quickly and remained well while continuing their regular physical activity.

This sounds as if it were some kind of magic, or at least too good to be true. Of course, not all emotional or interpersonal-relationship problems can be cured by simply dieting and jogging! Obviously, also, merely getting the body into first-class shape doesn't automatically cure problems. The underlying causes of many neuroses and personality problems still need to be discovered, understood, and either accepted or changed where possible. However, this much is certainly true: A life-style that has respect for bodily well-being, by careful attention both to what is put into the system and also to the physical effort put out by it, leads to a significant reduction of aggravating symptoms, both subjectively and with respect to relating to others. This is a good biological example of the cause-and-effect principle.

PSYCHOTHERAPY AND COUNSELING

I do not like the word *psychotherapy* because it leads too many people to believe that there is something either scientific or magical about the process. Penicillin unquestionably cures bacterial infections because it kills the bacteria. Psychotherapy cannot "cure" depression or any other mental or emotional illness. It can, however, help the patient to feel better, and therefore to suffer less, and to make some decisions and changes that can improve his situation.

I much prefer the word *counseling* to psychotherapy because most people understand that counseling is essentially advice from a professional based on his or her training and experience. To use the word *counseling* removes any delusion that the client or patient might have that the process is either "scientific" (logical cause-and-effect sequence), or "magical" (that the process is somehow beyond reason). Counseling puts the emphasis squarely on the dynamic of an interpersonal relationship (between counselor and counselee) without the fantasy or confusion of some imagined outside influence.

In practice, of course, counseling is a lot more than giving counsel or advice. The process also consists of listening with concern and attention to the unburdening description of the multitude of thoughts and feelings the sufferer is experiencing. The act of ventilating (talking out) these thoughts and feelings is most of the therapeutic value of the encounter. Only a little is derived from advice, reassurance, or verbal contribution of any sort from the professional.

Actually the most important contribution that a psychotherapist or counselor makes is in the creation of a caring relationship in which the depressed person can gradually feel free to express everything that has been troubling him. This would include such major related factors as guilt or anger about the past, anxiety about the present, and a sense of hopelessness about the future. Indeed virtually every feeling or thought described earlier could benefit by being talked through by the sufferer in the presence of someone whom he trusts and believes cares.

There are many different types of psychotherapy, from Freudian psychoanalysis to Glasser's Reality Therapy, Transactional Analysis (I'm OK, You're OK) to Behavior or Conditioning Therapy, and from Cognitive Therapy to Rational Emotive Therapy. All of these are well-described not only in professional literature but also in popular magazines. There is no need (or space) to elaborate on them all here except to say that the very fact that there are so many different approaches to the "talk treatment" of depression is evidence in itself that no perfect solution has yet been found, or that in the present state of knowledge is likely to be found in the foreseeable future.

In fact most competent professionals do not always use one theory, or practice, with all patients. People are different, their depressions are different, and the best therapeutic approaches to them are also different. There are, however, a few basic objectives that need to be constantly in the mind of the therapist or counselor seeking to help someone to come up out of a depression.

When I see a depressed person for the first time I spend almost the entire session listening to what he wants to say and encourage him with leading questions to go ahead and say it. At the end I will leave him with the hopeful comment that his depression is not only temporary but also that it is amenable to significant relief in the relatively near future. Hope *must* be rekindled in the heart and mind of a depressed person. The resigned "what is the use?" attitude must be replaced by one of optimistic expectation that the future will be happier than the past.

Reaching out with reassurance and hope combined with listening patiently to often repetitive complaints are both essential parts of the therapeutic process. Certain specific issues also must be dealt with. If the patient does not raise them himself the counselor must do so because they have to be worked through. These issues include such problems as anger, which needs to be verbalized instead of turned inward; guilt, which could be either true or false; low self-esteem, negative thinking, and the sense of helplessness.

In cases of grief or reactive depression the patient must be encouraged to talk out his or her feelings and thoughts about the lost loved object or person. The grief work of the mourning period should be brought out into conscious awareness, preferably by verbalized expression.

Endogenous depression is primarily treated by medications or somatic therapies, but the patient can also benefit from the supportive understanding caring relationship of a therapist who can regularly talk with him, listen to him, and let him talk through the feelings and thoughts that accompany the recovery period.

Neurotic depression is the most difficult to deal with in the counseling situation. The whole life-style, family history and relationships, and early methods of coping with stress need to be exposed and talked through thoroughly. Reality Therapy, with emphasis on the need to deal with situations and relationships in a responsible manner, is especially useful.

Most people do not "snap out" of depression. The road to recovery is long and often painfully slow. Both the counselor and the sufferer must be patient. Recovery takes place eventually, sooner rather than later if treatment is sought and received. A major responsibility of the therapist is of course to listen for suicidal ideation. Even veiled allusions to self-destruction should alert him to the probable need for immediate hospitalization.

Finally remember that physical and mental activities can contribute significantly to elevating depressed mood. Patients should be encouraged to become involved in activities that bring them into contact with other people. Relating to others will help to take the mind off themselves.

SOCIAL ACTIVITIES

Loneliness is a major contributing factor to persisting depression. No man is an island. There is really no such person as a happy hermit. Loneliness is painful: Everyone needs friends for emotional health.

How do you make and keep friends? Through shared activities and interests.

I have scores of friends at a wide variety of levels of intimacy. We have at least one interest or activity in common, which keeps us both in touch and friendly. I have friends who participate in the same sports that I do. I have friends whom I've met through cultural or social events. Others have become friends through my academic or professional interests. Some friendships have developed through church or religious activities. Several of my wife's relatives have become good friends of mine through our family ties. By far my closest friend is my wife herself.

Friendships are made and kept through talking about things of common interest and doing things that are mutually enjoyed.

Something that is very important also is to be friends with oneself, to have a good sense of self-worth: to enjoy some times alone with a good book, creating a recipe, doing needlepoint, or some other hobby, mowing the lawn, or going out for a jog. An intelligent person is never bored. Boredom can lead to depression, and depression will lead to less and less involvement in activities with others. It is a vicious circle.

It is very hard to summon up the energy to be outgoing and gregarious when feeling depressed, but the depressed person must be encouraged, even cajoled, into becoming involved in relationships with others. It is hard, but it is not impossible; and as with so many things in life that are really worthwhile the hardest step is the first. Once the depressed person has taken the plunge and become involved in whatever activity he has chosen, he will find that persisting in it will become progressively easier.

Becoming interested in the cares and concerns of others, and giving of one's energies in sharing time with others helps to take the mind off oneself. Especially helpful to a depressed person is making a commitment to doing something for someone needing help, or simply giving of oneself by listening to and sympathizing with someone who is suffering. There is nothing like appreciating and attempting to alleviate other people's pain to divert thoughts from one's own depression.

The more you give, the more you get. Giving of oneself in caring service to others, will gain relief from a low mood and self-pity. It must not be overdone, however. Nonstop or frantic activity can lead to anxiety or a sense of lack of accomplishment. There should be time to be alone to savor the happy recent memories. These will help take the mind off the causes of depression.

Depressed people should be encouraged to get away from their familiar environment every day for at least a few hours. Those who are not employed could benefit enormously from making a commitment to some regular, preferably daily, volunteer work in a church, hospital, school, li-

Common Emotional Experiences

brary, Red Cross, senior citizens groups, or any other local community institution or project. Those who are employed should strive to arrange at least one thoroughly enjoyable activity every week to which they can look forward.

Even on a daily basis a depressed person should at the very minimum arrange for just one little special pleasure. How about having lunch with a friend, going to visit a shut-in or a loved one, seeing a movie or a favorite TV show, attending a concert, art exhibition, or other cultural activity, accepting a party invitation, or inviting a friend to dinner. Simply going for a walk with your dog in the park, or, if you are not a city dweller, just bursting out into a country walk in the invigorating pollution-free fresh air can help you feel better.

I cannot know your personal circumstance, but think for yourself, if you are depressed, of things you can do, people you can meet and relate to, that will help to get your mind off yourself. A depressed person invariably feels better if he or she dresses "special," with clothes, hairdo and makeup not usually used, or serves a meal with the best china and silver.

Could you take a part-time or evening course at a local school, attend lectures or other events? Could you join some service group that welcomes local newcomers; organizes blood donors, fund-raising events for charity, or a political election campaign? Would you offer to babysit for a young couple, or go shop for an elderly couple? Discover your hidden talents. What you find out about your abilities might *really* elevate your depressed mood!

The gist of this message, I am sure, is quite clear: The more the depressed person avoids his familiar routine and environment the better able he will be to focus his mental and emotional activities on the cares and concerns of others. He will also thereby be more likely to find interesting and/or pleasurable pursuits of his own, which will help to take his thoughts and feelings off himself and thereby significantly reduce the pain of his depressed mood.

To give is better than to receive: But if you *do* give of yourself, depressed or not, you *will* receive more than you dreamed possible.

RELIGIOUS ACTIVITIES

I once saw in a children's coloring book a diagram of a man in a clerical garb under which was the caption: "This is a priest. Color him gray"!

To many people gray represents dull. Young children taken with adults to church are bored to the point of embarrassing agitation. To an adult, however, religion can be either all-absorbing, possibly affecting one's daily life, or the very opposite, an empty ritual practiced by people who nonetheless seem somehow dependent on it.

Depressed people also are affected by structured religion in one of two different ways. Religion either inspires them and elevates their mood, or they become even more depressed by being with others who appear joyful when they are not. Religion also can have one of two opposite effects on other factors often associated with depression.

An example is guilt. Religion can either cause one to become even more guilty because of the higher moral standards self-imposed by religious people, or by the finer sense of right and wrong they tend to have. Or, religion can help depressed guilty people to develop a sense of having been forgiven, which can significantly reduce the burden. (Anger and anxiety, both often associated with depression, can also be much reduced through one's religious belief system.)

Institutional religion, for all its faults (and pastors, priests and rabbis readily admit to several of these) nevertheless does offer some benefits that can help someone who is depressed.

First is the Judeo-Christian doctrine of the love of God. To those who believe, this truth can shine through the black clouds of depression with the message of hope for the future. The concepts of God as sovereign and of His care for us as individuals have sustained multitudes through the ages in times of adversity, danger, and depression. The knowlege that "thou art with me" when we pass through "the valley of the shadow of death" is warm comfort to the negative thinking of the depressive, and is to many a means of elevating low mood.

Second, churches and synagogues can provide a supportive fellowship of sympathetic and helpful friends. It is a great source of comfort to anyone suffering from depression to know that there are others who are concerned about them, praying for them, visiting them, and providing practical support and help to whatever extent is possible.

Third, adherents to traditional church doctrines and values can often obtain much uplift from such institutions as the eucharist (taking bread and wine), the confession (talking with one's religious leader about one's problems and sins), and participation in corporate acts of worship, which include the singing of hymns, the reading of Scripture, and prayers of thanksgiving, praise, and intercession. The joyful spirit of other worshipers can be catching.

Finally, the individual who is depressed can obtain much relief from his own reading of the Old and New Testaments and other religious writings. Private prayer also is a valuable source of healing. Talking to God in prayer can be a lot better than talking to another person if one is a believer.

PERSONAL FAITH

While this is not primarily a religious book, the consideration of treating and relieving depression would not be complete without some mention of the therapeutic value of personal faith.

Over and above the contributions of formal religion discussed previously, there is a certain respect in which an individual's direct relationship with God can provide uplift and joy.

This spiritual resource is, unhappily, generally not available to the unbeliever or sceptic. There is certainly no reluctance on God's part to be a source of comfort, but it is rather that the unbelief itself prevents the appropriation of the help that God can give.

By contrast the man or woman of faith is able to believe that God cares and is not only able but willing to bring healing and relief.

There are many verses of Scripture in both the Old and New Testaments that can bring hope and optimism to the hearts and minds of those who are depressed. If through private prayer the believer can appropriate these to himself and apply them to his particular situation they can be of inestimable help in uplifting low mood.

Personal faith is itself a gift from God that is offered to all, but effective only to those who receive it. Once received, faith leads to a direct individual relationship with God, in the case of Christians, through the accepting of Jesus Christ as one's personal Savior and Lord. Thereafter the influence of God's Holy Spirit enables the humble seeker to find inspiration and hope in the divinely inspired words of Scripture.

God apparently never intended that this life would be invariably happy, but He *does* promise to go with men and women of faith throughout all their sufferings and to bring them eventually into His eternal presence.

Perhaps no one suffered as much as the old patriarch Job; yet in his darkest hour he was able by faith to say to his friends, "Though he slay me, yet will I trust in him. . . . He also shall be my salvation. . . . For I know that my redeemer liveth . . ." (Job 13:15, 16; 19:25). At the end of the book we read, "And the Lord turned the captivity of Job, when he prayed for his friends. . . . So the Lord blessed the latter end of Job more than his beginning. . ." (Job 42:10, 12).

There are countless verses in the Psalms that can provide hope and joy to believers who can claim God's promises for themselves. The same Spirit who inspired the writers can inspire those who read them three millennia later. David sang, ". . . for the Lord hath heard the voice of my weeping" (Psalms 6:8) and "God is our refuge and strength, a very present help in trouble. Therefore will not we fear . . ." (Psalms 46:1, 2).

David also testified, "He hath delivered me out of all trouble . . ." (Psalms 54:7) and the psalmist promised, "He will regard the prayer of the destitute, and not despise their prayer" (Psalms 102:17).

To the faithful, God promises: "When thou passest through the waters, I will be with thee; and through the rivers, they shall not overflow thee: when thou walkest through the fire, thou shalt not be burned. . . . For I am the Lord thy God. . . . thy Saviour. . . . Fear not: for I am with thee . . ." (Isaiah 43:2, 3, 5).

Jesus said: "Let not your heart be troubled: ye believe in God, believe also in me . . . and I will pray the Father, and he shall give you another Comforter, that he may abide with you for ever. Peace I leave with you, my peace I give unto you. . . . These things have I spoken unto you, that my joy might remain in you, and that your joy might be full" (John 14:1, 16, 27; 15:11). In the Sermon on the Mount He also said, "Rejoice, and be exceedingly glad: for great is your reward in heaven . . . (Matthew 5:12).

Paul wrote to the believers in Rome: "And we know that all things work together for good to them that love God, to them who are the called according to his purpose." His conclusion began with the prayer, "Now the God of hope fill you with all joy and peace in believing, that ye may abound in hope, through the power of the Holy Ghost" (Romans 8:28; 15:13).

In conclusion here is a stanza of a poem by an unknown Christian author who had found at least a partial answer to his depression in his personal experience and encounter with his Creator and Redeemer:

> How thou canst love me as I am
> And be the God thou art
> Is darkness to my intellect
> But sunshine to my heart.

Read that again. The concept could not only elevate depressed mood; it could change your whole life, and even affect your eternal destiny.

14
Anxiety
O. Quentin Hyder, M.D.

Closely rivaling depression in prevalence in modern industrial society is the painful neurotic condition commonly called anxiety. Anxiety is an affective (feeling) state characterized by apprehension, uncertainty, and helplessness, *not* relative to any real external danger, which distinguishes it from fear. Anxiety neurosis afflicts 5 to 10 percent of the general population in the United States. It is especially common in young adults and affects women about twice as commonly as men. By definition neurotic means not psychotic, which is a loss of contact with reality. The psychotic lives in a world of fantasy as a means of avoiding the pain of his or her environment.

By contrast the neurotic suffers the pain of his world, with which he is fully in contact, through such common subjective feelings as generalized anxiety and depression. Less commonly he may experience such symptoms as panic attacks, phobias, obsessive thoughts, compulsive rituals, hysteria, vague physical aches and pains, and hypochondriac complaints. These are all neurotic, not psychotic, conditions. He is not mentally ill, but emotionally disturbed. Anxiety is not a disorder of thinking but of feeling.

Is anxiety normal?

Yes, some degree of anxiety is essential for survival. Without some ability to respond protectively to the alarm signal of anxiety, the human race would never have survived. Some anxiety enables us to study hard for an examination, work well to avoid being fired from a job, or keep alert properly when driving a car.

What is abnormal anxiety?

The point at which anxiety becomes abnormal is when a person's functioning capacity is seriously disrupted by an excessively anxious response to any stress or threat. If, for example, a person's anxious feelings are severe enough to impair clear thinking, decision making, or appropriate actions in any given situation, then the anxiety has reached pathological or abnormal levels. Even though such experiences are excessive or abnormal, they are nevertheless quite common events in daily life.

We have all experienced temporary acute anxiety: a slip while climbing a ladder or walking on ice, hearing the harsh squeal of brakes of an oncoming car, misplacement of a wallet, pocketbook or keys with fear of permanent loss, hearing any piece of news or information that might jeopardize our job or sense of security, or the fear of some symptom or finding by a doctor that might indicate a serious illness in ourselves or our loved ones.

If these remain temporary, they can be regarded as just part of the wear and tear or stress of life. But if they become protracted to the point of disturbing our inner peace, interpersonal relationships, or ability to cope with responsibilities, then they are abnormal and might necessitate medical treatment.

What kinds of people get anxious?

Any and everyone experiences anxiety from time to time throughout life. People are different, however, in their ability to cope. Some highly sensitive or vulnerable people, often described as having a neurotic personality, seem to go through life in a constant state of anxiety. It is almost as if they are not happy unless they have something to worry about. As defeated Christians, they seem to lack faith, with the philosophical attitude: "Why pray when you can worry?"

Others by contrast seem to have remarkable equanimity. Nothing phases them. Some simply don't care what happens, others deny to themselves the reality of consequences. A more positive Christian attitude is one of trust in a sovereign God, with faith that He is protectively and mercifully watching over and controlling every detail of one's daily life in accordance with His perfect eternal plan.

What are the subjective symptoms of anxiety?

Anxiety is an inner feeling tone describable as apprehension, uneasiness, concern, worry, dread, impending danger, doom, damage or destruction, and a pervasive sense of helplessness. The sufferer often decribes himself as tense, nervous, or uptight. There is a generalized

Common Emotional Experiences

awareness of tension both in the chest and in the muscles of the neck and back.

Chronic anxiety can last for days or even months with a vague sense of uncertainty about the future with accompanying insomnia, chronic fatigue, headaches, and a variety of multiple, vague aches and pains.

Acute anxiety, sometimes described as a panic attack, is a highly painful episode lasting from a few minutes to an hour or two. There is a subjective terror for no evident reason, with a haunting dread of some imminent catastrophe, which can totally prevent rational thinking or logical actions. Nausea, diarrhea, dizziness, feelings of pins and needles, or numbness around the mouth, or at the tips of fingers and toes, and muscular weakness may accompany the acute phase, with a distressing feeling of unreality or loss of contact with people or objects in the immediate environment.

What are the objective signs of anxiety?

Visible to others, or detectable on physical examination, are the manifest signs of anxiety produced by stimulation of the sympathetic nervous system. The most frequent and easily elicited are dilated pupils, perspiration, increased heart rate (rapid pulse), raised blood pressure, palpitations, tremors, obvious agitation, and loss of ability to converse logically. Respiration rate may also be greatly increased because of a sense of "air hunger" leading to what is called the hyperventilation syndrome.

Although these signs are most obviously detected during an acute anxiety or panic attack, they are also present to a lesser degree during chronic anxiety. Indeed it is the long-term effect of these chronic factors on the heart that can lead to permanent hypertension (high blood pressure) which causes strokes, or to excessive stimulation of the heart rate which can lead to a heart attack. These chronic effects can also affect the digestive system, leading to such conditions as indigestion, gastritis, stomach ulcers, and colitis. These can often lead to poor digestion and eventual weight loss.

What are the types of anxiety?

As in the case of depression, anxiety can be thought of as a reaction, a symptom, or a disease, and as such it can be categorized as reactive, neurotic, or endogenous.

Reactive anxiety is a usually normal response to any threatening situation. Any real or imagined event in a person's life that could portend something unpleasant in the immediate future can lead to either an acute panic attack or the development of chronic anxiety. The passage of time with either the removal of the potential threat, or the coping with the actual threat, leads eventually to the disappearance of the symptoms and signs.

Neurotic anxiety is a symptom of a developed life-style in which the anxiety response is an attempt to cope with stress. As with neurotic depression this form of anxiety can represent a withdrawal or avoidance of facing up to and dealing with the responsibilities of real life. This is commonly called generalized chronic anxiety to distinguish it from the following more specific types of neurotic anxiety which are:

1. *Obsessive compulsive disorder,* which is characterized by the presence of recurrent ideas and fantasies, and repetitive impulses or ritualistic actions.
2. *Hysterical conversion reaction,* in which there is a dissociation or separation between internal mental contents (such as memories ideas, feelings and perceptions) and conscious awareness. This can lead to such phenomena as sleepwalking, amnesia, multiple personality, and temporary paralysis of a limb, or blindness.
3. *Somatization disorder,* in which are experienced multiple vague aches, pains, or dysfunctions in or of any part of the body with no diagnosable or even demonstrable physical cause.
4. *Hypochondriacal neurosis* in which there is a morbid preoccupation with bodily functions and a fear that one is suffering from some serious disease. This particularly affects menopausal women, though "mid-life crisis" men can also be affected.

Endogenous Anxiety. Again, as in the case of endogenous depression, this form of anxiety is the most serious and is caused by a chemical imbalance in the brain.

The two main types are *acute anxiety attacks,* just described, and *phobic disorders.* These disorders are characterized by the presence of irrational and exaggerated fears of objects or situations not inherently dangerous or the appropriate sources of anxiety. By far the commonest are:

Claustrophobia, or fear of being trapped in an enclosed space such as elevators, tunnels, and airplanes (though fear of flying is often more related to fear of heights [acrophobia], or accidents).

Agoraphobia, which is a fear of open, public places, or situations where there are crowds. The sufferer's activities are seriously restricted even to the point of being unable to leave the security of his or her home. There are a great number of other phobias, many with very fancy Greek names such as pyrophobia (fire), nyctophobia (night or darkness), and xenophobia (foreigners). Other common phobias include fears of dirt, germs, strangers, animals, and water (hydrophobia).

What are the causes of anxiety?

The subjective feeling of anxiety is essentially caused by abnormal biochemical reactions in the fluid contained in the minute synaptic gaps between nerve cells in the brain. (*See* the diagram and explanation of the causes of depression. p. 348.)

As in depression, anxiety is caused by an imbalance between the various hormones and electrolytes contained in the fluid in the cerebral synapses. Arousal of frightening inner impulses and emotions sets in motion complicated discharges of these substances at these synaptic junctions. This is known as the fight-or-flight reaction. It is a very fundamental physiological mechanism, which enables the animal, including man, to deal with or escape from any potentially threatening or dangerous situation. It is mediated by the sympathetic component of the autonomic nervous system originating in the hypothalamus, a very primitive part of the mid-brain, and as such is not subject to the voluntary control of the cerebral hemispheres. In other words, it is automatic. You cannot prevent it.

Now, whereas the immediate cause of the actual feelings of anxiety are biochemical, the causes of those biochemical upsets are enormously varied. As stated earlier, virtually any theatening situation or experience can fire off the biochemical response. Much has been written in the psychoanalytic literature about the psychological causes of anxiety, both reactive and neurotic.

For example, the classical psychoanalytic explanation of anxiety by Freud was that it is the product of internal conflicts between the primitive urges of the id, and the socially controlling influences of the superego, which the mediating will, ego, or real self is unable to reconcile. The basic drives of aggression and sexuality, pulling against the conscience, causes acute tension within when no compromise is reached. Anxiety feelings therefore are a warning from the ego to the individual that appropriate actions (flight or fight) are immediately needed to deal with the stressful situation.

Karen Horney taught that anxiety is the result of personal and collective insecurity. Harry Stack Sullivan emphasized that anxiety was caused by disturbances in our interpersonal relationships, especially if they involve rejection or disapproval by others that lead to loneliness or loss of self-esteem. Erich Fromm considered anxiety to be the result of meaninglessness in our lives. In his existentialist thinking Rollo May said that it is essentially the inevitable result of apprehension of the future. It is brought about by a perception of either real or imagined changes to either one's physical safety or sense of security in any area.

More-modern therapies have also attempted to give explanations. Behavior or Conditioning Therapy, Transactional Analysis (I'm OK, You're OK), Rational Emotive Therapy, and so forth, have all made their contributions. Reality Therapy (William Glasser), perhaps the closest secular equivalent to biblical counseling, sees anxiety as a result of a failure to meet one's needs by responsible behavior guided by the demands of facing reality and having respect for the needs of others.

What are the results of anxiety?

As touched upon earlier, acute anxiety can result in a paralysis of function with a variety of cardiovascular and respiratory symptoms and signs. Chronic anxiety can lead to ulcers, high blood pressure, and heart attacks, and withdrawal from normal activities and relationships.

Any anxiety therefore, acute or chronic, which extends beyond the limits of acceptable normal life's experience probably needs medical treatment, which will now be considered.

Treatment of anxiety

A review of the section on the treatment of depression will find many parallels in the treatment of anxiety and need not therefore be repeated. For example, the arguments for and against hospitalization would be essentially the same for admission for anxiety as for depression. The discussions on the importance of economic security, involvement in social and religious activities, and the great value of regular vigorous physical exercise apply equally to anxiety as depression. For instance the high adrenaline levels of the anxious person can often be very effectively reduced by the high metabolic burning process involved in aerobic energy expenditure. In other words go for a jog or a brisk walk and you'll feel a lot less uptight!

Some differences prevail however. There is no equivalent to electroshock therapy in the treatment of anxiety. ECT would only make anxiety worse. Nor are lithium or hormone treatments effective in anxiety as they are in mood-swing disorders. Nutrition and vitamin enthusiasts of course would have their recommendations for treating anxiety—usually at great expense and with no guarantees. In spite of my lack of personal or professional experience with these, however, I can nevertheless support a trial run with the dietary approach. At the very least it is unlikely to do any harm, and if you luck into the correct combinations of food for your particular problem, you might be greatly helped.

Three areas remain worthy of some comments on the special needs in the treatment of anxiety: psychotherapy or counseling, medications, and the healing blessings of a strong, personal faith.

Psychotherapy or counseling in the treatment of anxiety can only be aimed at eliminating the causes of the basic chemical imbalance. If external precipitating factors can be lessened, both chronic anxiety and acute episodes can be significantly reduced.

Common Emotional Experiences

Insight therapy attempts to uncover unconscious conflicts. This can lead to increased self-understanding and toleration of internal drives. *Supportive therapy* can reduce symptoms through reassurance and the development of a sympathetic, understanding nonjudgmental relationship between the sufferer and his therapist or counselor. *Relaxation techniques* such as meditation can exert some voluntary control over psychological and muscular tension.

Most often effective in treating anxiety is for the therapist to help the patient identify the causes of his or her apprehension. Attempts should then be made to do all possible to change the stressful environment to make it less intolerable. In situations in which the precipitating stress is unavoidable the counselee must be helped to confront them directly, admitting his anxiety, and to move ahead in spite of them. *Courage consists not of an absence of fear, but of the capacity to conquer in spite of it.*

Medications. Please look back to the section on the treatment of depression through the chemical approach, especially the section describing the changes in the neurotransmitters in the synapses resulting from the introduction of antidepressant medications (pp. 348–49).

In anxiety the problem, much oversimplified of course, is that there is too much adrenaline or norepinephrine in the synapses. This results in an overactivity in transmitting nervous impulses from one nerve cell to another. This overactivity in the arms and legs leads to restlessness and agitation; in the chest muscles and diaphragm to overbreathing; in the heart to increased pulse rate and blood pressure; and in the brain to anxiety.

Anxiolytic (antianxiety) agents, commonly called the minor tranquilizers, work by reducing the norepinephrine levels in the synapse, and thereby reducing the signs and symptoms of anxiety. (Major tranquilizers also calm anxiety but are of a different chemical class from the anxiolytics and are used mainly in the treatement or prevention of the psychoses—schizophrenia, and so forth.)

The most commonly prescribed anxiolytics are:

Brand Name	Generic Name	Average Daily Dose
Atarax	hydroxyline	50–400 mg
Ativan	lorazepam	1–6 mg
Equanil	meprobamate	1200–2400 mg
Librium	chlordiazepoxide	10–100 mg
Miltown	meprobamate	1200–2400 mg
Serax	oxazepam	30–120 mg
Tranxene	chlorazepate	15–60 mg
Tybatran	tybamate	750–3000 mg
Valium	diazepam	2–40 mg
Vistaril	hydroxyline	50–400 mg
Xanax	alprazolam	1–6 mg

These drugs are relatively safe. Even very large doses taken all at once are very rarely effective in suicide attempts. Also side-effects, such as sedation and hangover, are mild in therapeutically effective doses.

Finally, remember that minor tranquilizers are only intended to be used temporarily. Reduction of the symptoms of anxiety in the early phase of treatment enables the patient to think more clearly and articulate his thoughts more logically. He can thus more rapidly benefit from the psychotherapy or counseling he receives. When this has led to a reduction in anxiety-producing stressors in his life the medications can be discontinued.

Personal Faith. As in coping with depression the spiritual dimension can be very valuable in helping the believing Christian to become less fearful and anxious. There are many verses in the Psalms and elsewhere in the Old Testament where we are encouraged to fear not, and to trust in the Lord. Jesus also said "Peace I leave with you, my peace I give unto you.... Let not your heart be troubled, neither let it be afraid" (John 14:27).

Paul exhorted us to rejoice, to show a considerate gracious attitude toward others, to be anxious for nothing, to pray and give thanks, to let one's requests be made known to God and to think about things that are true, honest, just, pure, lovely and good. If we do these things he promised that "the peace of God which passeth all understanding, shall keep your hearts and minds through Christ Jesus" (*see* Philippians 4:4–8).

15
Nervous Breakdown
O. Quentin Hyder, M.D.

We have considered in this section the interrelated experiences of grief, depression, and anxiety, all of which, if not adequately treated, can lead to what is commonly called a "nervous breakdown." However this term is also used to describe not only a neurotic, but a psychotic, mental collapse as well. This collapse can be either so mild and chronic as to be almost indistinguishable from a personality disorder, or so acute and even violent as to necessitate drug treatment and hospitalization.

The word *neurotic* is used to describe an abnormality of feeling such as anxiety or depression, whereas *psychotic* describes an abnormality of thinking, a thought disorder. The mental illness most often associated with this condition is called schizophrenia. Pastors, counselors, and concerned relatives of victims of this illness need to know enough about its symptoms to be able to distinguish it from the simple neurotic conditions. This is because, in addition to counseling, schizophrenics almost always need medical treatment at some point during the progression of the disease.

Schizophrenia classically develops in late-adolescent or early-adult life, except for the paranoid type, which tends to delay onset until middle age. In the early 1950s almost half of all hospital beds in this country were occupied by schizophrenics. Now, more than thirty years later, that figure is down to about a quarter thanks to the widespread use of drugs. These have enabled at least half of all treated schizophrenics not only to leave the hospital but also to live acceptably productive lives including even full-time employment, and marriage, and parenting.

Schizophrenia has a higher prevalence among the lower socioeconomic classes (whereas the higher classes tend to be more neurotic), probably because of the greater stresses of social disorganization and because mentally ill people tend to drift gradually down the social scale.

Schizophrenia is caused by a complex interaction between inherited and environmental factors. Almost all victims give a family history of someone in a parallel or senior generation having had some form of mental or emotional disorder. A genetic predisposition, therefore, is almost certainly a necessity for schizophrenia to occur at all, but the actual precipitating causes are almost always evident in the form of faulty patterns of upbringing, disturbed relationships, or stressful life experiences.

The immediate physiological cause of the thinking disorder and the emotional upsets in schizophrenia is a biochemical imbalance in the brain. Dopamine and salts in the synapses in the central nervous system get out of whack for a reason not clearly understood. This imbalance affects the transmission of nervous impulses from one nerve cell to another and this causes the aberrations in thoughts and feelings experienced by schizophrenics.

Although no simple personality type is recognizable as predisposing to the onset of schizophrenia, most victims show such traits as sensitivity, shyness, unsociability, lack of emotion, paranoid attitudes, poor interpersonal relationships, and social isolation.

The term "borderline" is used to describe someone who is not fully schizophrenic but who manifests several personality characteristics suggestive of it. These people are defined as schizoid personalities. A few of these develop schizophrenia later in life, often in the form of a brief psychotic breakdown usually caused by some temporary acute stress. Most, however, remain borderline in their functioning without breaking down, especially if they are taking small doses of preventive antipsychotic medications.

The schizoid personality is introverted, withdrawn, solitary, reticent, emotionally cold, and distant. He or she is usually fearful of closeness or intimacy with others and is most often absorbed with his own thoughts and feelings. He is given to daydreaming and prefers theoretical speculations to practical actions. If he begins to deteriorate in the direction of psychosis, a sharp counselor or close relative will be able to recognize such warning signs as the display of oddities of thinking, paranoid ideation, perceptual abnormalities, loss of good interpersonal communication skills, and inappropriate behavior.

The key to diagnosing schizophrenia is the evidence of a loss of contact with reality, a condition in which the patient's thoughts and feelings are apparently not in touch with, or appropriately relating to, the real world around him. The onset is almost always preceded by a period of several weeks or months of increasing withdrawal and disorganization of the previous level of functioning. In the early stages of this deterioration the patient might be uneasily aware that his psychological integrity is becoming impaired.

Evidence of a thought or thinking disorder is found in the loss of clear, goal-directed or consequential speech, which can become quite diffuse and vague. Sudden, incomprehensive changes of subject and obvious flaws in reasoning may occur. He may experience sudden thought blocks, or develop paranoid delusional beliefs that somehow his mind is being controlled by others.

Emotional (affective) changes such as blunting (dullness) or inappropriateness of overt feelings are usually easily observed. Any extreme of mood disturbance from elation, through anxiety, to depression may occur. Perceptual disorders such as visual or auditory hallucinations occur in severe cases. Paranoid delusions are also common, especially those involving thoughts of persecution, personal grandeur, or ideas of a sexual or religious nature.

One of the most serious manifestations of schizophrenia, especially of the paranoid type, is the danger of a resort to physical violence. Self-mutilation or suicide may occur during an acute psychotic breakdown. Violence to innocent people, seen erroneously as a source of the patient's suffering, is especially common. Unhappily this most often involves either someone close, such as a wife or husband, lover, parent, child, or teacher, or a popular idol or prominent political leader. In his tormented thinking the schizophrenic is seeking recognition, but at the same time often expects and even welcomes death as both a punishment and an escape from his suffering.

The prognosis of schizophrenia is not as hopeless today as it used to be. About one-third of all patients recover completely, and most of the rest can show significant improvement in symptoms if they cooperate with medical treatment. Whereas there is no known guaranteed cure of the illness, sufferers can eventually live reasonably stable and fulfilling lives within the limits of their disability. With effective medications even a full-blown psychosis can commonly be controlled within four to six weeks with residual defects of varying severity possibly persisting for a few further weeks. Relapse, however, is an ever-present threat, but this can frequently be prevented by persisting with maintenance (low) doses of medications.

Treatment of schizophrenia consists primarily of medications known as neuroleptics or major tranquilizers. These are very effective in restoring the biochemical balance in the neuronal synapses back to normal. Specifically they act by blocking the dopamine receptors in the brain.

Clinically their effect is to reduce significantly such major disruptive symptoms as paranoid delusions and visual or auditory hallucinations. They also markedly calm the associated anxiety and indirectly also elevate secondary depressed moods. In summary they restore contact with reality.

After a complete recovery from an acute psychotic episode, drug treatment usually need not be continued more than six months with gradually decreasing doses. Long-term chronic schizophrenics and those with a definite borderline personality, however, are more safely maintained indefinitely on doses one-quarter to one-third of the acute level.

Here are the dozen most commonly used neuroleptics:

Brand Name	Generic Name	Usual Daily Dose
Haldol	haloperidol	1–50 mg
Loxitane	loxapine	20–250 mg
Mellaril	thioridazine	50–800 mg
Moban	molindone	20–200 mg
Navane	thiothixene	6–60 mg
Permitil	fluphenazine	1–20 mg
Prolixin	fluphenazine	1–20 mg
Serentil	mesoridazine	25–400 mg
Stelazine	trifluoperazine	2–60 mg
Taractan	chlorprothixine	30–600 mg
Thorazine	chlorpromazine	30–1000 mg
Trilafon	perphenazine	4–64 mg

Treatment, however, consists of more than just taking pills. Hospitalization is sometimes necessary, even involuntarily, to protect the patient from his own self-destructive impulses, or to provide day-to-day supportive care when his capacity to meet his own needs fails. In or out of the hospital a very important adjunct to treatment is the development of a good therapeutic relationship with a skilled counselor. The patient while recovering also needs social support and rehabilitation. This can sometimes best be provided in a day-care center or a halfway house, a residential haven, for several months after hospitalization, before returning to home and work.

Psychotherapy with schizophrenics is virtually useless during the acute psychotic phase, but once reality contact has been reestablished, working with the patient and his family helps to alleviate distress and problems of work and personal relationships. Restoring patterns of readjustment and uncovering and working out an understanding of the stresses that precipitated the acute event are very important in reducing chances of a recurrence. Occupational therapy directed to vocational retraining and gradually increased social involvement are helpful as progress continues. In many areas sheltered workshops are available to give meaningful employment as preparation for return to the competitive working world.

Shock treatment, minor tranquilizers, lithium salts, and hormones are generally not at all effective in the treatment of schizophrenia. The nutritional approach with special diets and vitamin supplements has apparently effected significant improvement in several documented cases. The approach, however, tends to be very expensive and quite hit or miss—a trial and error system—worth at least a trial if you can afford it.

Careful control of environmental pressure is an essential therapeutic objective. Overstimulation of a recovering schizophrenic by high expectancies, overly emotional involvement with relatives, or excessive work loads can cause a reexacerbation of symptoms or protective withdrawal. On the other hand understimulation such as by overprotective parents tends to reinforce passivity, dependency, and habitual helplessness. Individual psychotherapy combined with medications and an appropriately stimulating family helps the healing process to foster direct reality-oriented communication between the patient and his world.

Part V

Physiological Needs

Three healthy normal physiological needs not previously considered in this book are mentioned briefly here for completeness.

In the stressful lives characteristic of most people in our modern industrialized societies there is the need for adequate rest and relaxation. Recommendations are made for reducing stress and refreshing the body and mind with changed activities in periods of time alternating with those committed to work and similar stressful responsibilities.

A few thoughts are added about the need for adequate sleep, and some suggestions as to how to overcome insomnia are given.

Sexual activity, or rather the subjectively assumed need for it, is seen as a developed habit. Those who have avoided developing the habit are apparently in many cases able to live full and satisfying lives without the pursuit of it. The point is also made that the only biblical provision for meeting this need is within marriage, other forms being usually disappointing at best, or mutually destructive at worst.

16
Relaxation and Sleep
O. Quentin Hyder, M.D.

All of creation is in a constant state of alternating periods of high and low energy output. The entire universe is presently expanding. One theory has it that eventually it will contract and then expand and contract again, and so on, perhaps forever. Many of the cosmic electromagnetic radiations that reach us from outer space are pulsating. The sun alternates periods of more and less heat radiation. The tilt of the earth, relative to its plane of orbit around the sun, gives us our alternating hot and cold seasons.

Biology is no different. Many animals hibernate through the winter and become reactivated in the spring. The earth alternates its day and night cycle, with man and most other living things adjusting activity levels accordingly. Sleep is part of the cycle of life, and in adult humans should occupy about one third of it: But, during waking hours, most people also need periods of alternating relaxation from the stress of daily duties.

Stress is unavoidable for most people, especially those with pressured city-business life-styles, though country folk also experience some different forms of stress. Although some people experience anxiety without stress, the vast bulk of human suffering in the form of nervous tension or apprehension is caused by the various emotional stresses and strains of daily living. Generally speaking, stress is worse in this generation than in most previous ones. The pace of life in this twentieth century is certainly much more stressful for most people than it was a hundred years ago.

Urban living is generally more stressful than suburban or country living. The hostility, rudeness, and selfish behavior in crowds is inevitable

Physiological Needs

in cities. Noise is very stressful. Fire and police sirens, construction and repair squads with compressed-air drills, trucks and motorcycles, buses and subways—all add to the constant stress of city life. The poor have anxiety about how to make ends meet, but the rich are anxious about their investments, business deals, and the state of the market. Performing well on the job and getting on well with the boss or fellow workers can also be very stressful. Unemployment and physical illness are great threats to one's tranquility. Hatred, boredom, frustration, and fatigue are common causes of internal stress.

Stress is the wear and tear of life, but it is not the stress itself but the effects it produces on our bodies and minds that are damaging. Some stresses are good. A game of tennis, a thrilling movie, or an exciting, happy piece of news are stresses which, like anxiety, cause rapid heartbeat, but they are not damaging, in reasonable quantities. Some stress is necessary. We are at our least stressful on first waking in the morning. We have poor physical coordination and some mental confusion, initially, but the stress of having to get up and dressed for the day helps us to pull ourselves together quickly.

We all have to live with stress, which is defined by Dr. Hans Selye of Montreal as the nonspecific response of the body to any demand made upon it. Stress is not in itself harmful to the body or mind, unless it is too severe, lasts too long, recurs too frequently, or is not alternated with periods of adequate relaxation. By contrast, stress which is too severe, protracted, recurrent, and unrelieved leads to definite physiological effects on the body.

The commonest biological defensive reaction to stress is an increased outpouring of adrenaline and other hormones from the adrenal glands. This is known as the biologic stress reaction and leads to a condition now commonly called "the general adaptation syndrome." This is manifested in two distinct groups of symptoms, the immediate and the delayed, the acute and the chronic.

The acute results are such effects as raised blood-sugar level, raised blood pressure, increased pulse and respiration rate, and other signs such as sweating, dilated pupils, and subjective feelings of anxiety. Added together, these results are known as the "fight-or-flight" response. This primitive defensive reaction to protect from danger is essential to life. Without it, man and animals would never have survived.

If, however, the stress or stresses on the organism continue beyond the acute episode, there follows a period of attempted adjustment. The success or failure of the adjustment depends on the severity and continuity of the stressor and the adaptive ability of the one being stressed. Adaptation, however, can lead to many well-recognized secondary diseases, some of them more painful to the sufferer than the original stress. Best known of these are high blood pressure, heart attacks, gastric ulcers, allergic reactions, and such neurotic conditions as anxiety attacks and depressive mood swings.

Remember, however, that stress is not all bad. It can be the spice of life. Life would be terribly boring without frequent moderately stressful events. We need the stimulus of moderate and frequent, but not constant, stress. Work is a form of stress, whether it be in an office, a shop, or in the home. Doctor Selye teaches that hard work is a biological necessity both for personal happiness and for a long, satisfying, and successful life.

The key to the balance, however, and therefore the key to a health-giving life-style, is the well-disciplined, constant alternation of stress with relaxation. We need both. The stress of unemployment is boredom and frustration. The person who has no regular daily work or occupation must find some alternative activity to fulfill his needs for the expenditure of both physical and intellectual energy. If he does not find some such outward expression, his very inactivity can lead to the same stress reactions as the overworked person.

It is hard to define work and play. One definition is that work is what we have to do; play is what we want to do. Happy, indeed, therefore, is the person who thoroughly enjoys his work, and sad by contrast is the person who has no satisfying or enjoyable play or leisure activity. Disliking your work and having no fun in life are both very stressful. They have different causes, but the same results.

The biologic rhythm of stress and relaxation, of work and play, of activity and rest is essential to health. The unemployed must find work or some other satisfying commitment from which he can derive a sense of personal fulfillment. The hard worker needs some regular means of dissipating his pent-up energies, hostilities, anxieties, and frustrations. If he does not meet this need, he will eventually develop some of the signs and symptoms of the general stress syndrome.

How then can we relax? What should we do to develop this balance in our lives? What really is relaxation?

Relaxation is not the same as inactivity. It is not doing nothing. It is doing something different, or creating a change of pace in one's life. An ideal vacation, in my view, is not one spent lying on a beach all day, getting sunburned. It is, rather, going to new places, doing new things, meeting new people, learning new ideas, or even new philosophies. Releasing tension is an essential part of the cycle of life. It is good to stop the pace of life frequently and allow time for thinking, for meditating, for daydreaming, for reading things of interest, for pursuing hobbies, games, and sports, doing relaxation exercises, even for having a little cry occasionally. A great doctor once said, "The sorrow that has no vent in tears will make other organs weep." In other words, it is better to have a good cry than to develop high blood pressure or a stomach ulcer. However you do it, relaxing from the stress of your daily routine is essential and must be done regularly. The biological cycle of alternating activity and rest is an integral part of maintaining bodily health and emotional stability.

Many people have different ideas on what is best for them to achieve relaxation and produce inner tranquility and peace of mind. I personally have successfuly tried three totally different, but all very effective, methods—one spiritual, one physical, and one psychological.

As a Christian, my daily times of personal prayer and devotional Bible study, most effectively enjoyed at the beginning of the day, prepare me for the stresses of my work. I am much better able to handle the intellectual challenges and the emotional pressures of my daily work as a psychiatrist, if I have had my first session of the day alone with God.

Regular strenuous physical exercise I also find essential, not only to bodily health, but also to the preservation of a mind at peace with man and God. Playing squash or running six days every week enables me to work out of my system any bottled-up anger, impatience, frustration, or anxiety.

Psychological relaxation has been practiced in both Eastern and Western cultures for centuries. Meditational techniques of yoga and Zen Buddhism have demonstrated for thousands of years many people's remarkable ability to gain control over the mind and certain other physiological functions which can lead to profound mental and physical relaxation. Transcendental Meditation (TM), popularized in the United States by Maharishi Mahesh Yogi, is an old yogic technique adapted to be acceptable to the Western mind.

Some years ago, for professional reasons, in order more practically to understand the problem of how best to relax, an important part of my teaching psychotherapy to those needing it, I paid my money and went through the initiation ceremony and beginner's training of TM. I was given by my teacher a personal, secret *mantra,* a meaningless sound upon which I was to focus my attention and repeat over and over while meditating. I was somewhat shocked and uncomfortably embarrassed, however, to discover that the initiation was actually some form of Eastern religious ceremony. I also found that I simply could not readjust my daily schedule to devoting two periods of twenty to thirty minutes, morning and evening, to its practice. So I quit.

However, several months later, I read the excellent little paperback, *The Relaxation Response,* by Herbert Benson, a professor of medicine at Harvard. Doctor Benson has painstakingly examined many meditation methods, and states that the same result as TM can be achieved, without any religious overtones, by fulfilling four basic conditions. If these conditions are met for ten to twenty minutes daily, great relaxation is experienced and more energy and acuteness apparently become available for any physical or mental activity which follows.

Doctor Benson's four conditions are:

1. A quiet environment.
2. A comfortable position (in an armchair is probably the best).
3. A passive attitude (of "let it happen" and "don't be bothered by distracting thoughts").
4. A mental device. This could be any sound or word, which should be repeated over and over again. The word *one* is a sufficiently adequate sound to focus upon to achieve good relaxation. An alternative could be any object upon which to fix one's gaze. Either of these merely help the mind to shift away from logical, externally oriented thought to conscious awareness of the ever-deepening relaxation of all the muscles of the body.

I do not practice this meditation regularly, but I have found that something similar to Dr. Benson's technique is very helpful occasionally. If, for example, I get a headache, become very worried about something, lose my concentration at work, or if I'm becoming very anxious about having too many things to do all at once, I find that a brief period of meditation is very calming. I find I only need about five to seven minutes of this type of nonreligious meditation to achieve a beautiful sense of relaxation in both body and mind, after which I can get on with dealing with my responsibilities.

Two words of caution: first, for Christians. There is for some the question of what might happen if they allow their minds to drift away from conscious control. Some have voiced fears that they would be exposing themselves to demonic intrusion if they were not at all times in contact with the external reality of their immediate environment. This has never been a problem for me. I know that, for me, my mind is in control at all times, and I have never experienced any demonic influence. I also know both by faith and by experience that He that is within me, God's Holy Spirit, is far too powerful to permit any evil influence to enter my mind and soul for as long as I remain faithful to Him.

Second, as a psychiatrist, I have serious reservations about recommending the relaxation-response technique to anyone who is mentally or emotionally unstable. Those with a very low self-image or poor reality contact might not be able to experience the benefits without some confusion. So, if you have any serious psychological or spiritual problems, bet-

Physiological Needs

ter not use this technique. If, however, you are healthy, it can be an occasional, useful adjunct to your prayer and exercise practices to maintain peace and calmness within.

What about your sleep? If you get too little, consistently, over many weeks, it may adversely affect you both physically and emotionally. Severe insomnia for extended periods can lead to disorders of thought and perception that are similar to some of the symptoms seen in acute schizophrenia, the most serious of the mental illnesses.

Newborn babies sleep up to sixteen hours every day, but this amount rapidly decreases through infancy. Teenagers and children every day need about nine hours sleep. Young adults need eight hours, middle-aged people seven, and elderly folk six hours every day, though senior citizens can sometimes also benefit from an additional afternoon nap, if they get very tired. As you get older, your basal metabolic rate falls, and you get by with less sleep.

Sleep researchers have discovered that even within an average seven- to eight-hour night there is an approximately ninety-minute sleep cycle. About every one and one half hours throughout the night, a normal person experiences REM sleep, lasting a few minutes. REM stands for Rapid Eye Movements, a trembling of the eyeballs, which can be observed under the sleeper's eyelids. REM sleep is associated with dreaming and occurs four or five times during the night, the later ones, during the lighter sleep of the early morning hours, being slightly longer. This ninety-minute cycle corresponds with the basic biological rest-activity rhythmicity associated with waxing and waning within the central nervous system.

Some common causes of insomnia are:

1. Discomfort due to noise, light, an uncomfortable bed, physical illness, or extremes of external temperature or humidity.
2. Inability to unwind and forget the day's stresses, fears, pressures, apprehensions, or anxiety caused by overwork or worry.
3. Depression of mood in any form which can cause difficulty in getting to sleep, staying asleep, or cause early morning waking.
4. Guilt, denial, and other protective psychological defense mechanisms which either prevent sleep altogether or repress conscious thought into the unconscious mind, which then resurrects them in the form of unpleasant dreams and nightmares.
5. Extended jet travel, especially from West to East, across several time zones.
6. Poor physical fitness associated with not enough exercise, resulting in inadequate general muscular tiredness and need for rest. Tired

mind and muscles guarantee a good night's sleep. Athletes and people in good physical condition usually sleep well and arise refreshed. People in poor shape often sleep fitfully and tend to get drowsy in the afternoon.

Your eight hours minimum sleep should preferably be had during darkness. It is more healthy to be up and about when the sun is up. In other words, let your sleep be from 11:00 P.M. to 7:00 A.M. rather than from 3:00 A.M. to 11:00 A.M.! Habitual late nights are not good for general health. This "day-night reversal" involving lying-in long hours in the morning can lead to decadence, lazy habits, and avoidance of responsibilities. It also is sometimes an early indication of mental illness.

The following prebedtime habits can help to ensure good sleep regularly:

1. Avoid caffeine in any form after 6:00 or 7:00 P.M.
2. Avoid either strenuous exercise or a large meal within two hours of going to bed.
3. Relax in a deep armchair or a hot tub within an hour of sleep.
4. A hot milk drink is an excellent relaxant for both body and mind.
5. Sexually well-adjusted married couples often find that they sleep deeper and longer if they have intercourse immediately before going to sleep.
6. Sleep medications should only be taken as an absolute last resort, especially by anyone under sixty years of age. In any event, take them only if your physician suggests them. If he does, ask him to prescribe a nonbarbiturate which does not cause hangovers or addiction. Do *not* mix sedatives with alcohol.
7. Prayer before retiring can also help achieve a natural deep sleep. Committing worries, fears, and guilt feelings to God, confessing and repenting of sins and accepting forgiveness for them, trusting that He will take care of tomorrow as He has today, and just fully resting in God's loving and protective care, bring a deep peace to both mind and spirit. "I will both lay me down in peace, and sleep: for thou, Lord, only makest me dwell in safety" (Psalms 4:8).

17
Sexuality
O. Quentin Hyder, M.D.

Sex—who needs it? Or, rather, who *thinks* he needs it? Here is at least a partial answer: He or she who "needs" it is he or she who has become accustomed to it. As with so many things in life, actions lead to habits, and habits lead to cravings for more actions.

This is not a book devoted to theology, philosophy, practical Christianity, social morality, or ethics. It is concerned with bodily well-being, and I am simply asking the question as to whether sexual activity is needful for it. The answer you get to the question depends on whom you ask.

The celibate, or sexually unaroused, adult male or female might be able, truthfully, to claim that he or she has been able to remain in good physical condition without any sexual activity. If you ask him or her, however, about the effects of adult celibacy on his or her *emotional* well-being, answers will vary from confession of acute frustration or anxiety at one extreme, to total equanimity, with peaceful acceptance of the deprivation, at the other.

The fact of human experience is that we are different. Many people can go through life with no sexual experiences, even in fantasy; many others seem to be in constant need of both emotional and genital expression and fulfillment. "If you've never had it, you don't miss it" is an old saying, and one that is as true for sexual craving as for any other desire or need.

Sexually, we differ. Some apparently have a much greater craving and need for sexual activity than others. Some, for example, are able to make a lifetime commitment to celibacy. Some are easily able to be faithful to one marital partner. But some others find it almost impossible not to desire a variety of sexual partners. Christians are no different in terms of their varying natures and appetites. They *are* different, of course, in both the motivation and ability they possess to control their natural cravings.

Sadly however most Christians do not develop or fully utilize this potential, and thereby remain undisciplined in mind and body. This so often leads to consuming guilt, anxiety, and depression of mood which cripple the joy in the Christian experience and can destroy emotional health. God does not give easy victory over sexual sins or any other sins. He does, however, give power to help the Christian who is prepared to suffer the pain of the struggle.

The main theme of this book, however, is not the rights and wrongs of sexual morality, but the consideration of the body's health needs. A healthy body, though, is closely integrated with a healthy mind. For this reason, emotional problems such as anxiety, guilt, or frustration caused by sexual problems or attitudes can adversely affect the healthy functioning of the physical body. Let us therefore briefly consider the matter of sexual activity as either a contributor to or a detractor from bodily well-being and general health. I will not, however, totally evade matters of Christian morality. Issues such as guilt and sublimation are relevant to this book and will be mentioned later in this chapter.

Let us first consider married couples. In the first book of the Bible we read, "And God blessed them, and God said unto them, Be fruitful, and multiply . . ." (Genesis 1:28). In the next chapter is written, "Therefore shall a man leave his father and his mother, and shall cleave unto his wife: and they shall be one flesh." The next verse states, "And they were both naked, the man and his wife, and were not ashamed" (Genesis 2:24, 25).

In response to a letter from Corinth, the apostle Paul wrote:

> Nevertheless, to avoid fornication, let every man have his own wife, and let every women have her own husband. Let the husband render unto the wife due benevolence [love]: and likewise also the wife unto the husband. The wife hath not power of her own body, but the husband: and likewise also the husband hath not power of his own body, but the wife. Defraud ye not one the other, except it be with consent [mutual agreement] for a time. . . .
> 1 Corinthians 7:2–5

From these Scriptures, we understand that in God's eyes the purposes of the gift of sex within marriage are threefold:

1. Continuing propagation of the species
2. Mutual satisfaction of sexual needs

3. Reciprocal expression of commitment and love for each other, symbolizing Christ and His bride, the church (Ephesians 5:31-33).

These three principles lead us to understand three instinctual drives: the reproductive, the physiological, and the emotional. As just stated, the last two of these are closely related and are our concern in this book.

Whereas it is possible for most healthy people to remain physically fit without sexual activity, there are, nevertheless, certain respects in which meeting of sexual and emotional needs do contribute to one's total well-being. For example: It has been the discovery of many married couples that having intercourse after going to bed at night enables them to fall asleep more quickly and to sleep more soundly, due to the total relaxation that usually follows orgasm.

By contrast, sexual deprivation or lack of satisfaction, for whatever reason, can lead to emotional disturbances such as anxiety, depression, resentment, frustration, anger, guilt, hostility, frigidity, or impotence. These symptoms are characteristic of many of the shaky or frankly disintegrating Christian marriages I see daily in my practice. Middle-aged male impotence is often caused by the man's body being unfit. It can also be caused through his wife's inability any longer to excite him. Even the prettiest young girl starts to sag and slump as she gets older, and unless she keeps herself in good physical shape, her overweight, bulging stomach and hips will be likely to turn off her huband's desire towards her. His own unfitness also can of course lead to her frigidity. A fit body is an attractive body.

Emotional responses (for example, to sexual rejection) can lead to such physical manifestations as appetite changes leading to significant weight gain or loss, development of gastric ulceration, high blood pressure, colitis with diarrhea, skin disorders, insomnia, and a variety of other psychosomatic manifestations.

Sexual intercourse within marriage, therefore, should be enjoyed as frequently as it is mutually pleasurable, and should be refrained from only, as Paul recommended, "with consent for a time."

Now, for single people: The comments above referring to the emotional and physiological effects of sexual deprivation in marriage are, of course, for the most part, as true for singles, once they become sexually active, as for married people. If not genitally, certainly emotionally, any healthy adult experiences some sexual, or at least affectional, needs. (These are the needs to love and be loved.)

A single person who has experienced sexual enjoyment or fulfillment before marriage may develop a continuing craving for both the sexual and affectional satisfaction such relationships can bring. When these satisfactions cannot be met, for whatever reason, there is the tragic possibility of the development of resentment, bitterness, jealousy, and feelings of rejection and loneliness. These emotions, in turn, can lead to some of the physical problems just indicated, which are definitely harmful to bodily health.

By contrast, single people who have never been sexually active, and therefore have not developed the habit of obtaining sexual satisfaction, whether by intercourse or masturbation, seem better able to go through life without strong cravings for sexual activity. This is rare, however, especially in men.

Although most parents still hope that their daughers are virgins on their wedding days, the fact is that mature but sexually unaroused women are approaching the endangered-species list. The sexual needs of women have long been underrated and, until recent times, underresearched. Most people in our society today realize that it is healthy and normal for a woman to enjoy sex as much as a man. She may no longer be satisfied to take a passive role in the sex act, as were, for example, many women in her grandmother's generation. Women now often participate and enjoy sex equally with men, though they usually need, more than men, the security of a committed relationship.

Furthermore, in one generation, we have experienced the development of sexual permissiveness in Western culture, which was undreamed of a few years ago. We have also witnessed the emergence of the women's liberation movement, the breakdown of the double standard, the change of attitude toward virginity, the easy access of birth-control methods, legalized abortion, and the single-parent family.

In spite of these powerful influences, however, some women still choose, for moral or religious reasons, to remain chaste and to keep themselves for their future husbands. Such a woman will, of course, have emotional needs for love and companionship, and she will be obliged, therefore, to find ways to meet these needs from sources other than from a husband or lover. The same holds true for men, of course, but because of the much easier availability of casual sex for males and their usually much more intense genital cravings, their motivation for chastity, and the strength to achieve it, generally need to be very much more disciplined.

If, for the present, marriage seems not to be your lot, you can still achieve some measure of peace within yourself and in your relationships by the development of attitudes of sublimation. Sublimation consists of diverting the energy of sexual drives and the cravings for affectional needs into alternative satisfying and fulfilling pursuits. Total diversion is of course neither possible nor even needful. Sublimation can, however, reduce or take the edge off the acuteness of the pain of unfulfilled desires

Physiological Needs

in these areas. It is basically a healthy defense mechanism. Repression, by contrast, which is the attempt to forget or deny one's needs, is unhealthy, unrealistic, and can lead to anxiety or depression. In our culture, both men and women can become actively involved in vocational, avocational, religious, social, cultural, or sporting pursuits, which can satisfy many emotional needs. Single people who have successfully achieved such diversion can realistically function happily without a mate, even for a lifetime.

A major personal problem about which there is a real division among Christians is the question as to whether or not masturbation is a sin. I have found very little written in any Christian books which can be of help to unnecessarily guilt-ridden young people agonizing over this matter. Read an excellent book on this called *My Beautiful Feeling* by Walter Trobisch.

I have a close friend who has told me that he never masturbated and very rarely even felt the urge to do so. He is now happily married, considers his sex life to be normal, and has no extramarital activities or fantasies. I know one or two single priests and nuns who have made lifetime commitments to celibacy, and since their unwavering mental attitudes are that all sexual activity is permanently off limits, they say they are not troubled by sexual temptations. Such saints really exist, but they must be extremely rare. I'm not sure if I envy them or feel sorry for them. I *am* sure that for the majority of Christians, complete chastity is not God's calling for their personal lives; marriage, of course, being the only biblical provision for meeting sexual needs.

Masturbation, now known to be almost as common in women as in men, can provide some measure of temporary reduction of internal tension. In the case of women, though their physical well-being may not require it, most who have been sexually aroused need some sexual or at least some affectional fulfillment for their emotional well-being and stability. In our culture, often, emotional needs for love and companionship, though present, tend not to be as much a source of craving for a man as for a woman. On the other hand, a man's genital sexual needs somehow tend to be more acute than that of most women, probably because they are more physiologically bound.

In the adolescent and adult male, from puberty to advanced old age, sperm are constantly being manufactured by the testicles, transported towards the base of the bladder, mixed with fluid secreted by the prostate gland, and stored in two small sacs called seminal vesicles. Some absorption takes place, but this rarely, if ever, keeps pace with production, especially in younger men. Sooner or later, the vesicles become full and their contents need to be discharged. If this does not happen through intercourse or masturbation, it will occur spontaneously, during sleep. This nocturnal emission is often associated with an erotic dream and, without other sexual activity, will normally occur every two or three weeks.

Much more often, however, a male does not experience these emissions, because his sexual cravings tend to lead to intercourse or masturbation long before the vesicles are full. One cannot say dogmatically that the regular ejaculation of seminal fluid is essential to the body's physical well-being. It does seem, however, that attempts to resist the urge to masturbate, for both sexes, can lead to increasing anxiety and inner tension in those used to its regular practice.

Another problem to be faced is that of the guilt which almost always develops in those who have been taught that masturbation is morally wrong or sinful. I can feel and suffer with them. I have lived through this myself. Single to the age of thirty-seven, I know what it is like to live for twenty years as an adult male, struggling with healthy and natural desires for sexual gratification. Far from claiming to be sin free, I have, nevertheless, personally experienced the fiery conflict within of the "ought to" versus the "want to," the spiritual versus the carnal, that Paul described so vividly: "For the good that I would I do not: but the evil which I would not, that I do" (Romans 7:19). Like Paul, I have experienced both defeats and victories.

I have, therefore, two key thoughts to share with any young person now going through what I have been through:

First, there is no question that one's sexual drives can be at least partially diverted into other channels. For me there were three:

1. Intense academic study for many years, developing my professional career. (For the creative rather than scholarly person it could be art, music and so forth.)
2. Extensive physical activities, recreational pursuits, and sporting endeavors several times each week.
3. Religious commitments of preaching or teaching, and the disciplined pursuit of my personal spiritual development, which necessitated hundreds of hours of private prayer and devotional Bible study during my formative years. I permitted myself very few idle moments. An idle mind easily gravitates to sensuous thoughts.

Second, I kept short accounts with God. I never let my unrepented sin remain as a barrier between me and my Lord. Failure to have victory over any temptation or sin was at once confessed so that fellowship could be immediately restored. Nor have I ever allowed the certainty of future sin to become a barrier. It was a matter of living one day at a time, trusting God to provide for all one's needs, whether it was the need for strength to conquer, or the need for forgiveness and encouragement after failure.

There have been times when the temptations of the flesh seemed to be more than one could bear. These are not easy times, nor is there a simple solution to find relief if one chooses to live within the parameters of Christian principles. I have found prayer is invariably a comfort and source of needed power. It helps one through the darkest hours of loneliness and frustration, and it provides light in the darkness. I am always helped, also, by these words of Paul, "There hath no temptation taken you but such as is common to man: but God is faithful, who will not suffer you to be tempted above that ye are able; but will with the temptation also make a way to escape, that ye may be able to bear it" (1 Corinthians 10:13).

We are creatures of habit, and most sex practices in and out of marriage are developed between couples in conformity with habitual actions or needs. The celibate habitually excludes sexually tempting thoughts, and for him practice makes perfect. He who habitually masturbates yields easily whenever the urge hits him, and ceasing this practice becomes harder the more often it has happened. Married couples develop habitual sex practices which are mutually pleasurable or satisfying. These usually become gradually less frequent with age, or if their relationships deteriorate. After the first adulterous experience, it is very easy for extramarital episodes to become a habit. Actions lead to habits, but it is never too late to change or to break a habit.

It seems to me then that for both men and women, whereas regular sexual activity is not absolutely essential for the body's healthy functioning, it does seem to be an important ingredient in the emotional and psychological well-being of those who have become accustomed to it. Conversely, let us not overlook the opposite consideration of the role of physical fitness in sexuality. The healthy and fit person almost always enjoys an increased ability to perform sexually, for which reason it is preferable for husbands and wives to participate jointly in their exercise programs. For the single person, there is no doubt that a strong, fit body is not only more attractive to the opposite sex, but also bestows on the owner much-enhanced self-confidence in all interpersonal relationships with others of either sex.

In conclusion then, it seems that the celibate can do without sexual activity. The profligate apparently cannot, at least, unless and until he decides he wants to change his habit patterns. Paul said: "But if they cannot contain, let them marry; for it is better to marry than to burn" (1 Corinthians 7:9). But if, for any reason, marriage is not possible for the

Christian single adult, since there is not any very effective fire extinguisher to quench the burning, he or she can, at the very least, through both sublimation and prayer, somewhat control the supply of inflammable fuel!

Part VI
The Spiritual Dimension

18
The Spiritual Dimension
O. Quentin Hyder, M.D.

This book has been concerned so far primarily with physical and emotional health. In my view, however, one cannot have "whole health" unless one is also healthy in the spiritual dimension. To me this necessitates a personal relationship with God that means something far more than having a mere intellectual assent that He exists.

The Bible nowhere attempts to prove the existence of God. It assumes it. The scientific principle of cause and effect can logically lead us to the conclusion that since the universe exists there must have been a First Cause which brought it into being. To believe that there is no God, as the true atheist does, requires a far greater act of faith (that it all just happened without a cause) than to believe what the Bible teaches, that God was the creator of the heavens and the earth and that He continues to sustain them today.

Most men and women in our culture who are not Christian believers would tend to call themselves agnostics. They believe that God must exist, but that after starting the ball rolling He is now simply sitting back and watching with either sadistic pleasure or with a bland indifference at how human events are working themselves out. For them, therefore, there is no possibility of communicating with God because either *He* does not care, or they are themselves so wrapped up in the problems of struggling through daily life that *they* do not care.

In contrast with this is the fact that the same Bible that speaks about creation, albeit as a story rather than as scientific treatise, also speaks about the God who *does* care about humankind, and in fact has done a great deal to reveal Himself to us, and to relate to us as individuals. If therefore God has not only created us, but continues to care about us personally, it is only rational and sensible for us to respond by allowing Him to communicate with us. I believe that God's primary method of communicating with us is through the pages of Scripture, which most Christians believe to be divinely inspired.

Whatever one might believe about the Garden of Eden story in Genesis, Chapters 2 and 3, describing the origin of sin and the "fall," it is manifestly evident that humankind is sinful. It does not require much humility on anyone's part to look within and admit that he or she is far from capable of living a perfect, sinless life. Yet the Bible reveals to us a pure, holy, and righteous God into whose presence nothing imperfect can enter without being instantly burned up by the brilliant light of His glory. Furthermore there is nothing you or I can do about it. It is a fact of human experience that we can in no way live the perfect lives that could possibly earn us the privilege of standing before God's glorious throne.

God, however, was not unaware of our predicament. Since there is no way that we by our own efforts could achieve reconciliation with a holy God, He Himself had to step through the veil of separation to make a way for us to go. That is precisely what He did in Jesus Christ, God incarnate in human flesh.

We cannot understand why God chose to effect humankind's redemption in this way, but for a reason we will only be able to understand in eternity this is the way He did it. The history of the sacrifices of animals as recorded in the Old Testament gives us a glimpse through the symbolism of the ancient Israelite temple worship of the principle of atonement. The slaying of an unblemished lamb one day each year by the high priest was accepted by God as a sufficient sacrifice to satisfy the payment of the penalty for all sins committed by the Children of Israel during the preceding year.

An innocent lamb killed annually was sufficient for the sins of the small nation of Israel for one year. But the sins of all humankind, of every nation, and in all times, required nothing less than the human sacrifice of God Himself in human form. No ordinary human could die for the sins of the whole race. It had to be one without blemish, Jesus Christ the righteous. Every sin therefore that you and I have ever committed, or ever will commit, was potentially forgiven on the cross that April day in A.D. 33. God accepted Christ's sacrifice as the full payment of the penalty for all our sins.

I said potentially forgiven because the transaction cannot be complete without our response to it. We need to receive the gift of forgiveness for it to be effective. If I give you a check for one hundred dollars, but you leave it in your pocket and never cash it, it is as if I never gave it to you.

Christ, by His shed blood on the cross, has given us the gift of full forgiveness, which enables us to stand sinless in God's presence. We can now be redeemed, saved from a lost eternity, and enter into everlasting life.

Now, the response on our part which transforms this potential salvation into an actual real experience is simply our willingness to be humble enough to repent of our sins and confess to God our hopeless inability to save ourselves. Salvation costs nothing. We cannot purchase it with good works, nor earn it by attempting to live a godly life. Our confession and repentance is what God has been waiting for. Immediately he or she turns to God, the humble sinner receives the gifts of faith and the ability to acknowledge Jesus as his personal Savior and Lord.

Salvation to eternity in God's presence, however, is only half the blessing God bestows on the repentant sinner. This assurance of future life after death is a source of real comfort and security to the believer, but we have far more than this promise, wonderful though it is. The other half of God's blessing is the experience in *this* life of God's continual presence with us in the here and now. Only those who have experienced some spiritual transformation can fully appreciate the contrast between the former life lived outside Christ, and the new life in Him.

The initial act of repentance with the gift of faith that accompanies it is variously described as seeing the light, being filled with the Spirit, receiving salvation, getting converted, or, as recounted in John, Chapter 3, in Jesus' dialogue with Nicodemus, becoming born again. This spiritual experience leads the repentant sinner into a personal relationship with God through Jesus Christ. The remainder of one's earthly life is never the same again. One is now a child of God, a sheep in the flock whose shepherd is Christ, and, together with all other redeemed souls, part of the worldwide Church, the body of Christ on earth; and, in eternity, the beloved bride of Christ.

The many blessings of the Christian life on earth are the various products of the greatest fundamental attribute of our sovereign God: His love for humankind in general, and for redeemed sinners in particular. These various blessings are freely given to all who believe and who can therefore appropriate them by faith. Together they constitute the spiritual dimension of total health without which a person cannot be truly whole.

The key ingredient that God gives the person who has repented and surrendered his life to His authority is a love for God, and for the Kingdom of God on Earth. This love leads to a growing willingness to draw closer to God as evidenced by a desire to communicate with Him regularly through private prayer and study of the Bible. As he or she matures in his intimate daily walk with God the reborn sinner develops an ever-increasing understanding of God's will for his life as He progressively reveals it. He or she also experiences a parallel, ever-increasing desire to follow that will in obedience, knowing both by faith and by experience that he is at his most fulfilled when he has most completely brought his own will into conformity with that of his Creator and Redeemer.

Naturally following love for God and for submitting to His guidance is a love for the people of God, other believers, who, prior to one's spiritual conversion, had been generally either ignored or even despised. This newfound love for brethren and sisters in the Lord leads to new friendships, new social activities, a new life-style, and a progressive change in one's estimation of priorities. Love for God and love for others together contribute a most healthy influence on the development of wholeness in a person's total being.

Belief that God is sovereign and loves the newly regenerate sinner gives him or her a profound sense of security as he goes through life. God's providence and protective care of His children gives joy and peace within such as was never enjoyed before conversion. He or she can affirm with the apostle Paul: "All things work together for good to them that love God and are the called according to his purpose," and with the old patriarch Job who cried out in faith: "Though he slay me, yet will I trust in him."

The believer is also given the faith to know that God is guiding him daily one step at a time. He also knows that nothing will happen to him without God. All the joys and sufferings, the successes and the failures, the achievements and the disappointments of life are known to God, and He lovingly gives and permits all experiences in order to enable the believer to grow to spiritual maturity and personal holiness.

The greatest evidence of the validity of the Christian experience is seen in the way that believers are able to face death. I once saw an old missionary die in a hospital when I was an intern. His death was a profoundly moving experience to us his physicians, nurses, and immediate family. But to him it was an experience of joy—truly a graduation to Glory. To the last moment he knew he was about to see the Lord he had loved for a lifetime.

I know that I shall not die one second before or after the time that the Lord has ordained for me; but I know that when my time comes He will be waiting for me. When I drop off to sleep at night, my next conscious awareness is glorious sunlight flooding in through the morning window. When my soul and spirit slip quietly out of my physical body as I expire my last breath, the next experience I shall have is seeing the glory of the face of Jesus flooding my whole being.

The spiritual dimension, in the light of eternity, is the one most vital to total health. It not only gives us assurance for the next life, but love, faith, hope, joy, and peace in this. Adding these qualities to a fit body and a sound mind gives us the total health and wholeness with which God so much desires to bless us in this life.

INDEX

INDEX

Acceptance, 200–02
  of loss, 316, 319
Action for Children's Television (ACT), 104
Adaptability, 207–08, 210
Addiction, 259
  See also Alcohol, Drugs, Smoking
Additives, food, 98–102
Adipocytes, 19–20
Adrenaline, 184, 197, 239, 288, 345, 358, 375, 385
  See also Norepinephrine
Aerobic exercise, 17–19, 29–30, 56–58, 75, 230–31, 232–36
  effects of, 17–19, 30, 57, 59–60, 233–34
  types of, 17, 36, 39, 230
  and weight loss, 17–19, 29–30, 50–51, 61
Alcohol, 144, 156–59, 275, 347, 350
Alcohol (Hyder) 156–59
Alcoholism, 156, 158, 195
Allergy, 289–90
Anaclitic depression, 339
Anaerobic exercise, 29, 75–76, 230, 232
Anderson, Dr. Robert, 197
Anger, 334, 343–44
Angina pectoris, 220
Anorexia, 338, 354
Anxiety, 150, 294, 335, 343, 369–76
  causes of, 373–74
  medication for, 375–76
  results of, 374
  signs of, 371
  symptoms of, 370–71
  treatment of, 374–76
  types of, 371–72

Anxiety (Hyder), 369–76
Anxiolytic agents, 375
Appert, Nicolas, 96
Armentrout, David P., Ph.D., 247–69
Arteries, 164–66, 213, 214
Arthritis, 25
Ascorbic acid, 123–24
  See also Vitamin C
Atherosclerosis, 217–18, 227
  See also Coronary artery disease
Atria, 213

Bailey, Covert, 21, 23, 32, 33, 57–58, 61
Bennett, Dr. William, 54–58
Benowicz, Robert J., 111, 133
Benson, Herbert, 387–88
BHT (butylated hydroxytoluene), 100
Biochemical imbalance, 344–45, 373, 379–80
Biogenic amines, 344–46, 347–50
Biotin, 122–23
Bipolar manic-depressive illness, 341
Birdseye, Clarence, 96
Blood
  flow, 213, 215–17, 278
  lipids, 24
  tests, 225–26
Body
  caring for, 285–90
  density, 74–75
  rebuilding for pain relief, 255–56
  as temple of Holy Spirit, 153–54
  See also Fitness
Body fat, 19–20, 21–24, 24–27, 50–51
Boenisch, Edmond, 202

Booze Battle: A Common Sense Approach That Works, The (Maxwell), 195
Borden, Gail, 96
Breathing, 79, 80–81, 292–93
Brenner, Harvey, 192–93
Brody, Jane, 74
Brozek, Dr. Josef, 106
Butterworth, Dr. Charles E., 146–47

Caffeine, 99, 144, 197, 288, 347, 390
Calciferol, 124–25
Calcium, 130
Calisthenics, 230, 231–32
Calories, 20, 28, 40, 43–44, 45
   See also Weight control
Cancer, 140, 160–63, 169, 170
Carbohydrates, 20, 40–41, 285–87
Cardiopulmonary resuscitation (CPR), 221
Cardiovascular system. See Heart
Carotene, 115, 116
Celibacy, 391, 395, 397–98
Chafetz, Morris, M.D., 158
Chastity, 394
Children
   grief of, 322–26
Chlorine, 130
Choate, Robert B., 103
Cholesterol, 223, 225–26, 287
Choline, 123
Christian life, 11–13, 154–55, 157, 392–93, 400–04
   See also Faith, God, Prayer, Spiritual life
Chromium, 130
Cigarettes. See Smoking
Citrus bioflavonoids, 127–28
Civil obedience, 154–55
Cobalamin, 120
Cobalt, 130
Cocaine, 153
Collins, Dr. Gary, 190, 194
Complete Junk Food Book, The (Lasky), 102
Connotations of Movement in Sport and Dance (Metheny), 68
Copper, 130
Coronary angiography, 222
Coronary artery disease, 164–66, 217–19
Coronary thrombosis, 218–19
Counseling
   for anxiety, 374–75
   for depression, 361–63
   need for, 12
   for pain relief, 264, 266
   for stress, 210, 242

Cyanocobalamin, 120
Cyclothymic disorder, 339–40

Dairy products, 43
DDT, 101
Denial
   and grief, 309
   of loss, 317–18, 320
Depression, 25, 47, 59, 150, 209, 330–68
   causes of, 250–51, 259, 342–45, 356–58
   as grief reaction, 303, 320–21, 330–32
   medications for, 346–50
   results of, 345–46
   signs of, 337–38
   symptoms of, 336–37
   types of, 338–42
Depression (Hyder), 330–68
Depressive adjustment reaction, 338
Developing a Personal Heart Strategy (Losoncy), 229–46
Diabetes, 25, 222, 223–24, 344
Diet
   for fitness, 42–45, 133–34, 223, 226–27, 241, 353–54
   for weight loss, 16–17, 40–42, 73–74
   See also Food, Nutrition
Dieter's Dilemma, The (Bennett and Gurin), 54–58
Dinkins, Burrell, S.T.D., 302–29
Divorce, 327
Dopamine receptors, 379–80
Drugs, 150–55
Dudley, Dr. Donald, 199

Electric shock treatment. See Electroconvulsive therapy
Electrocardiogram (EKG), 226
Electroconvulsive therapy (ECT), 340, 341, 350–51
Electrolytes, 344, 352, 373
Emotions, 47
   in depression, 334–35
   development and consequences, 281
   in mourning, 317, 330–31
   and pain, 249–51
   problems of, 12–13
   See also Anger, Anxiety, Depression, Grief, Guilt, Pain, Stress
Emphysema, 166–67
Endocrine glands, 352–53
Endogenous anxiety, 372
Endogenous depression, 340–42, 344–45
Enzymes, 56–58
Ergosterol, 124–25

Index

Executive Health (Goldberg), 196, 197
Exercise
    aerobic, 29–30, 56–58, 75, 230–31, 232–36
    benefits of, 65, 91–92, 208–09, 255–56, 290–92, 358–61, 387, 390
    in heart-attack prevention, 227–28, 229–36
    routines, 32–33, 77–80, 81–84, 84–90, 235, 290–92
    types of, 75–76, 230–31
    and weight loss, 17–19, 29–30, 56–58

Fairness Doctrine, 171, 173
Faith, 321–22, 367–68, 376
Family, 190–91, 200–02, 208
Fat. *See* Body fat
Fats, 40, 44, 287
Feingold, Dr. Benjamin F., 104–05, 106
Feelings, 200, 334–35
    See also Emotions
Fiber, 41, 43
"Fight-or-flight" response, 184, 385–86
Finances
    as cause of depression, 356–58
    guidelines for, 357–58
    role of, in stress, 192–93, 203–05
Fitness, physical 62–93
    benefits, 63–66, 358–61, 389–90
    problems 72–73
    tips, 92–93
    See also Diet, Exercise
Fitness (Murphey), 62–93
Fit or Fat? (Bailey), 21, 32, 57–58
Flab, 16–61
    See also Fitness, Overweight, Weight control
Flab (Krafft), 16–61
Fluorine, 130
Folacin, 120–21
Folic Acid, 120–21
Food
    additives, 98–101
    allergies, 289–90
    as cause of headaches, 277
    contaminants, 101
    convenience, 94–95
    dye, 100
    fortified, 140–42
    groups, 42–43, 135–36, 285–90
    preservation, 95–96, 99–100
    processed, 141–42
    See also Diet, Nutrition
Food and Drug Administration, 98, 112–13, 132, 134, 139
Food, Drug, and Cosmetic Act, 98

Forgiveness, 401–02
Fortified Vitamin and Mineral Insurance Formula, 114
Freud, Sigmund, 175
Friedman, Dr. Meyer, 188–90
Friendship, 364
Friendship Factor, The (McGinnis), 201
Fromm, Erich, 373
Functions of Sleep, The (Hartmann), 196

General adaptation syndrome, 385–86
Glasser, William, 362, 363, 374
Goals, 48–51, 71–72, 207–08
God
    healing by, 13
    help from, 179–80, 267–69, 367–68, 376
    love of, 402–04
    Word of, 154–55, 392–93
    See also Christian life, Faith, Prayer, Spiritual life
Goldberg, Philip, 196, 197
Gout, 25
Greeden, Dr. J. F., 197
Greist, Dr. John, 209
Grief, 302–29, 330–33
    of children, 322–26
    as healing process, 326–29
    helping in, 314–16, 332
    incompleted, 302–06, 307–09, 318, 320
    physiological effects of, 321
    signs of, 330
    stages of, 312, 314, 317–18, 331–32
Grief (Dinkins and Losoncy), 302–29
Guilt, 244, 307–08, 318–19, 396
Gurin, Joel, 54–58

Habits, 264–65
Habituation, 259
Haney, Dr. Michele, 202
Happiness Is a Choice (Minirth and Meier), 200
Hartmann, Dr. Ernest, 196
Hauri, Dr. Peter, 196
Headaches, 270–300
    causes of, 270–72, 290
    log, 300
    migraine, 273–75
    overcoming, 280–85
    survey, 295–99
    types of, 272–77
Headaches (Miller), 270–300
Healing, 13, 328–29
    Christian, 13

Health, 13, 139–40
    See also Body, Fitness, physical
Heart
    diagrams of, 214, 215, 216
    failure, 220
    rate, 30–32, 35
    rhythm, 220–21
    structure of, 213–14
    valves, 214, 221
    working of, 215–17
Heart attack, 211–46
    complications of, 221
    effects of, 220–21
    prevention, 225–28, 229–36
    risk factors for, 221–25
    statistics, 212, 213
    symptoms of, 219–20
    warning signals, 221–25
Heart Attacks (MacNeil and Losoncy), 211–46
Heredity, 341–42, 344
Hernias, 25
Hesperidin, 127–28
Higdon, Hal, 29, 39
High blood pressure. See Hypertension
Holmes, Dr. Thomas, 186–88, 198–99
Hormones, 344, 351–53, 373, 385
Horney, Karen, 373
How to Survive Being Alive (Dudley and Welke), 199
Hyder, O. Quentin, M.D., 9, 11–13, 150–55, 156–59, 178–80, 330–68, 369–76, 377–81, 384–90, 391–98, 400–04
Hypertension, 24, 222, 223
Hypoglycemia, 286–87, 344
Hypothalamus, 348, 352–53, 373
Hypothyroidism, 344

Immunity system, 239
Inositol, 128–29
Insomnia, 294, 389–90
    See also Sleep
Involutional melancholia, 340
Iodine, 130
Iron, 130–31
Isometric exercise, 76, 230, 231–32
Isotonic exercise, 76

Jackson, Dr. Don D., 190
Jacobson, Edmund, M.D., 282
Jane Brody's Nutrition Book (Brody), 74
Jarvick, Dr. M. E., 174
Job stress, 191–92, 202–03
Jogging, 17, 18, 30, 34–36, 39, 232–35

Joy of Feeling Fit, The (Kounovsky), 68
Joy of Running, The (Kostrubala), 39
Junk food, 94–110, 289
Junk Food (Rohrer), 94–110

Kales, Dr. Anthony, 196
Kennedy, John F., 358
Kline, Nathan, M.D., 333
Kopolow, Dr. Louis, 193
Kostrubala, Dr. Thaddeus, 39
Kounovsky, Nicholas, 68
Krafft, Dr. Jim, 16–61
Kram, Kathryn, 107–08
Kübler-Ross, Elisabeth, 312, 331–32
Kuntzleman, Dr. Charles T., 51–53

Laird, Dr. Dean M., 105–06
Lance, Kathryn, 68
Language of Feelings, The (Viscott), 200
Lasky, Michael S., 102
Laurie, Peter, 155
Learn to Relax: Thirteen Ways to Reduce Tension (Walker), 207
Lee, Tom, 47
Lithium carbonate, 340, 342, 351–52
Loneliness, 320–21, 363
Lortie, Dr. Gilles, 105–06
Losoncy, Larry, Ph.D., 229–46, 302–29
Loss
    acceptance of, 316, 319
    as cause of depression, 342–43
    children's, 322–26
    grief over, 309–12, 326–28
    from pain, 251–52
Lungs, 233
    cancer of, 160–63, 169, 170

MacNeil, Daniel, M.D., 211–28
Magnesium, 131
"Magnitude of Life Events and Seriousness of Illness" (Wyler, Masuda, and Holmes), 198–99
Manganese, 131
Manic-depressive illness, 341–42
Marijuana, 144, 150–55, 182
Marijuana (Hyder), 150–55
Mason, Benard, 107
Masturbation, 394, 395–96
Masuda, Minoru, 198–99
Materialism, 357
Maxwell, Ruth, 195
May, Rollo, 373
Mayer, Dr. Jean, 25, 103, 109
McGinnis, Alan, 201–02

Index

McMillen, S. I., M.D., 160–77
Media, 102–04
Medical examination, 225–26, 277–78
Medications
  antidepressant, 346–50
  for anxiety, 375–76
  for headaches, 278
  for pain, 258–60
  for schizophrenia, 379–81
  side effects of, 259, 349, 376
  for sleep, 390
  withdrawal from, 260
Megavitamin therapy, 354
Meier, Dr. Paul, 200
Menaquinones, 126
Metabolism, 29–30, 54–58, 111–13, 136, 288, 389
Metheny, Eleanor, 68
Migraine, 273–75, 278
Miller, Joan, Ph.D., 270–300
Minerals, 42, 129–32, 288–89
Minirth, Dr. Frank, 200
Molybdenum, 131
Money management, 203–05
  See also Finances
Monoamine oxidase, 348–50
Monoamine oxidase (MAO) inhibitors, 348–50, 351
Monosodium glutamate, 100–01
Moods, 335, 339–40
  See also Anxiety, Depression, Nervous Breakdown
Moore, Peter, 154
Mourning, 316–22, 330–32
  See also Grief
Murphey, Cecil B., 62–93
Muscle, 16, 24, 278
Myocardial infarction, 218–19

Narigin, 127–28
Nerve cells. *See* Neurons
Nervous breakdown, 377–81
Nervous Breakdown (Hyder), 377–81
Neuroleptics, 379–80
Neurons, 345, 347–48
Neurosis, 339–40, 369, 372, 377
  See also Anxiety, Depression, Nervous Breakdown
Neurotic anxiety, 372
Neurotic depression, 339–40, 343–44
Neurotransmitters, 345, 347–48
Niacin, 118–19
Niacinamide, 118–19
Nichols, Dr. Lynn M., 60

Nickel, 131
Nicotinamide, 118–19
Nicotine, 144, 173–75, 275
  See also Smoking
Nicotinic acid, 118–19
Norepinephrine, 345, 347–48
  See also Adrenaline
Nutrition, 142–43, 144
  for children, 107–10
  in headache prevention, 285–90
  in treating depression, 353–54
  in treating schizophrenia, 381
  See also Diet, Food

Obesity. *See* Overweight
O'Conner, Barbara, 26
Oral Roberts University, 17–18, 25–26, 37–38, 47
Overcommitment, 206–07
Overeating, 142–43, 196–97, 338
Overweight, 19–20, 24–25, 196–97, 222, 223, 224
  See also Body fat, Weight control
Owen, Dr. George, 107–08
Oxygen, 215, 217, 219

Pacemaker, 215
Pain, 247–69
  effects of, on relationships, 252–53
  emotions concerning, 249–51
  getting help for, 253–55, 262
  medication for, 258–60
  sources of, 247–48
  spiritual help for, 267–69
  treatment units, 266–67
  See also Headaches
Pain (Armentrout), 247–69
Panic attack, 371
Pantothenic acid, 121–22
Para-aminobenzoic acid, 129
Patrick, Dr. Ben, 201
PCBs (polychlorinated biphenyls), 101
Peace, inner, 243–46
Personality
  disorders, 340
  type, 189–90, 224, 274, 378
Phobic disorders, 372
Phosphorus, 131
Phylloquinone, 126
Physical fitness. *See* Fitness, physical
Pituitary gland, 352–53
Pollock, Dr. Michael, 52
Post partum depression, 338–39
Potassium, 131

Pot smoking. *See* Marijuana
Prayer, 387, 390, 397
   in relieving depression, 366
   in relieving stress, 244–46
Premenstrual syndrome (PMS), 353
Protein, 20, 40, 41, 285
Psychosis, 377
Psychotherapy, 361–63, 374–75
Psychotic depressive reaction, 340–41
Pulse rate, 30–32, 35
Pyridoxal, 119
Pyridoxamine, 119
Pyridoxine, 119

Rahe, Dr. Richard, 186–88
Rapid Eye Movement (REM) Sleep, 196, 389
Reactive anxiety, 371–72
Reactive depression, 338–39, 342–43
Reality therapy, 362, 363, 374
Reconciliation, 243–44
Redemption, 401–02
Reed, Barbara, 106–07
Relationships
   with God, 268–69
   as affected by pain, 252–53, 265–66
   and coping with stress, 190–91, 200–02, 208, 238–39
Relaxation, 384–90
   overcoming headache by, 281–84, 292–95
   for relief of pain, 256–57, 292–94
Relaxation and Sleep (Hyder), 384–90
Relaxation Response, The (Benson), 387–88
Religious activities, 365–66
Repentance, 402
Rest in preventing stress, 241–42
   for relief of pain, 256–57
Retinol, 116
Riboflavin, 117–18
Ritalin, 105
Rohrer, Norman, 94–110, 111–48
Rohrer, Virginia, 94–110, 111–48
Rosenman, Dr. Ray, 188–90
Row, Dr. Clarence, 195
Running. *See* Jogging
Rutin, 127–28

Salt, 131, 287
Salvation, 402
Satir, Dr. Virginia, 190
Schauss, Alexander, 106
Schizoaffective disorder, 342
Schizophrenia, 342, 352, 354, 377–81
Schollmeier, Sally, 38

Schuler, R. S., 206
Secondary depression, 338
Sehnert, Keith, 190–91, 203, 209
Selenium, 131
Self-discipline
   and alcohol, 156–57
   and sexuality, 392–98
   and smoking, 177, 178–80
Self-talk, 264–65
Self-worth, 245
Selye, Dr. Hans, 184–85, 385–86
Serotonin, 345, 347–48
Service to others, 243, 364–65
Setpoint theory, 54–58
Sexuality, 391–98
   biblical attitude on, 392–93, 397–98
   affect of depression on, 335
   effect of smoking on, 167
   and physical fitness, 393
   sublimation of, 392–95, 396–98
Sexuality (Hyder), 391–98
Shealy, Dr. C. Norman, 267
Sin, 401–03
   sexual, 395, 396–97
Sinus, 276
Sleep, 196, 241–42, 294–95, 389–90
Smith, Lendon, 108–09
Smoking, 145, 160–181
   as cause of cardiovascular disease, 164–66, 223
   as cause of lung cancer, 160–63
   effect of, on children, 170
   effect of, on nonsmokers, 167–68
   effect of, on sexuality, 167
   quitting, 175–77, 178–80
   and stress, 197
   withdrawal symptoms, 178
Smoking (McMillen and Stern), 160–77
Social activity, 363–65
Social Readjustment Rating Scale, 186–87
Sodium, 31, 131, 287
   ascorbate, 123–24
   benzoate, 99
   nitrate, 99
   nitrite, 99
Somatic therapies, 350–51
Spiritual Dimension, The (Hyder), 400–04
Spiritual life, 11–13, 59, 244–46, 267–69, 367–68, 400–04
   See also Christian life, Faith, God, Prayer
Stern, David E., M.D., 160–77
Stress, 184–210, 224, 236–42, 384–86
   causes of, 185–90, 237
   coping with, 143–44, 199–210, 240–46 386–89

Index

family-related, 190–91, 200–02, 208
financial, 192–93, 203–05
job-related, 191–92, 202–03
results of, 198–99, 239–40, 271, 334, 389
stages of, 184–85
warning signals, 237, 240, 241
wrong methods of coping with, 194–98
Stress (Young), 184–210
Stressmap—Finding Your Pressure Points (Haney and Boenisch), 202
Stress Power (Anderson), 197
Stress/Unstress (Sehnert), 190–91
Sugar, 97–98, 144, 198, 285–86, 353–54
Suicide, 321, 346, 351, 376
Sullivan, Harry Stack, 373
Sulphur, 132
Surgery, 146–48
Switzer, Katherine, 68
Synapse, 345, 347–48, 373, 375, 379–80

Taste, 97–98
Taylor Johnson Temperament Analysis, 47
Teenagers
  drugs use by, 150–51
  suicide of, 346
Temptation, sexual, 396–97
Tension, 292
  as cause of headaches, 271, 272–73
  See also Stress
Thiamin, 117
Thinking
  disorder, 379
  distorted, 340–41
Thoughts
  accompanying depression, 335–36
  power of, 264–65
Time management, 205–07
Tobacco. *See* Smoking
Tocopherol, 125–26
Tranquilizers, 143, 196, 347, 375–76, 379–81
Travel, 145–46
Tricyclic drugs, 348–50, 351
Type A and Type B behavior, 188–90, 224
Type A Behavior and Your Heart (Friedman and Rosenman), 188–90
Tyramine, 349–50

Unipolar depression, 341
United States Department of Agriculture
  dietary guidelines, 136–37
United States Department of Health, Education and Welfare
  dietary guidelines, 136–37

United States Recommended Daily Allowances (USRDAs) 112–13, 354

Valium, 196, 259
Values, 243–45
Vanadium, 132
Veins, 25, 213
Venting, 242
Ventricles, 213
Ventricular fibrillation, 220–21
Viosterol, 124–25
Viscott, Dr. David, 200
Visualization, 293, 294–95
Vitamins, 42, 111–48, 288–89, 354
  definition of, 111–12
  as dietary supplements, 139–40, 143–48
  myths concerning, 133–43
  natural vs. synthetic, 132–33
  RDAs of, 112–13, 354
  role of, 114–15
  Vitamin A, 116, 135
  Vitamin B_1, 117
  Vitamin B_2, 117–18
  Vitamin B_3, 118–19
  Vitamin B_5, 121–22
  Vitamin B_6, 119
  Vitamin B_{12}, 120
  Vitamin B complex, 117–23, 128–29, 135
  Vitamin C, 123–24, 135
  Vitamin D, 124–25
  Vitamin E, 125–26, 135
  Vitamin H, 122
  Vitamin K, 126–27
  Vitamin P, 127–28
Vitamins and You (Benowicz), 111, 133
Vitamins (Rohrer), 111–48
Vows
  role of, in grief, 306–09

Walker, Eugene, 207
Walking, 17, 18, 34, 35, 39, 51–54, 360
Water, 132
Weight control, 16–61
  attitude toward, 45–48
  benefits, 24–27, 47, 224
  and calories, 28, 43–45
  through exercise, 17–19, 29–30, 50–51
  and quick loss, 16–17, 36–37
Welke, Elton, 199
Wellness, 11–13, 58–60
  See also Fitness, Physical
Williams, Dr. Roger J., 113, 114

Withdrawal
   from alcohol, 159
   as grief reaction, 319
   from medication, 260
   from pain, 261–62
   from smoking, 176, 178–79
Wyler, Allen, 198–99

You Can Profit from Stress (Collins), 190, 194
Young, Dr. Angharad, 184–210
Your Active Way to Weight Control (Kuntzleman), 52–53

Zinc, 132